The making of cognitive science

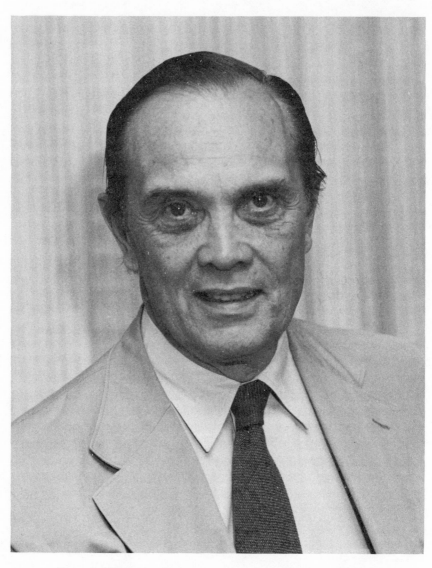

George A. Miller

The making of cognitive science

Essays in honor of George A. Miller

Edited by

WILLIAM HIRST

Department of Psychology, Graduate Faculty of the New School for Social Research

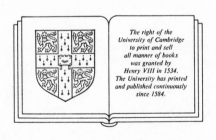

The right of the
University of Cambridge
to print and sell
all manner of books
was granted by
Henry VIII in 1534.
The University has printed
and published continuously
since 1584.

CAMBRIDGE UNIVERSITY PRESS

Cambridge
New York   New Rochelle   Melbourne   Sydney

Published by the Press Syndicate of the University of Cambridge
The Pitt Building, Trumpington Street, Cambridge CB2 1RP
32 East 57th Street, New York, NY 10022, USA
10 Stamford Road, Oakleigh, Melbourne 3166, Australia

© Cambridge University Press 1988

First published 1988

Printed in the United States of America

Library of Congress Cataloging-in-Publication Data
The Making of cognitive science : essays in honor of George A. Miller
/ edited by William Hirst.
p.   cm.
Bibliography: p.
ISBN 0 521 34255 4
1. Cognition.   2. Psycholinguistics.   3. Neuropsychology.
4. Miller, George Armitage, 1920–   . I. Miller, George Armitage,
1920–   .   II. Hirst, William.
BF311.M196   1988
                                                             87-12492

British Cataloging in Publication data applied for.

Contents

Preface   *page* vii
List of contributors   ix

Part I   Mathematical psychology   1
1   George A. Miller and the origins of mathematical psychology
    William J. McGill   3

2   The contribution of information theory to psychology
    Wendell R. Garner   19

3   Writing *Plans . . . Eugene Galanter*   36

4   George Miller's data and the development of methods for
    representing cognitive structures *Roger N. Shepard*   45

5   The magical number seven: information processing then and
    now *George Sperling*   71

6   Cognitive recollections *Ulric Neisser*   81

Part II   The Center for Cognitive Studies   89
7   Founding the Center for Cognitive Studies *Jerome Bruner*   90

8   Life at the Center *Donald A. Norman and Willem J. M. Levelt*   100

Part III   Psycholinguistics   111
9   The psychological reality of grammar: a student's-eye view
    of cognitive science *Thomas G. Bever*   112

10   Psychology and linguistics in the sixties *Eric Wanner*   143

11   Language use and linguistic diversity *Jacques Mehler*   153

12   The immanent form of phonemes *Morris Halle*   167

Part IV   Studying the lexicon   185

13   On opening the dictionary *Philip Johnson-Laird*   186

14   Lexical development – the Rockefeller years *Susan Carey*   197

15   Methodical semanticism considered as a history of progress
in cognitive science *Keith Stenning*   210

Part V   Cognitive neuroscience   229

16   Life with George: the birth of the Cognitive Neuroscience
Institute *Michael S. Gazzaniga*   230

17   Cognitive psychologists become interested in neuroscience
William Hirst   242

Part VI   Cognitive science   257

18   Cognitive science? *Gilbert Harman*   258

Biographical information   269
Publications   271
Name index   279
Subject index   282

Preface

George A. Miller's contribution to the field of psychology is enormous. He is in large part responsible for the dramatic shift away from behaviorism, which dominated the field for over thirty years, to cognitivism, which allowed one to study not just learning but memory, not just speech but language, and not just stimulus and response but the processes that mediate them. His career can be viewed as a series of research programs that not only motivated much empirical and theoretical work but also moved the field of psychology into new territory. The people that he worked with closely – either as colleague or as teacher – became or were the movers of the field of cognitive science.

Several years ago, George wrote about the Symposium on Information Theory held at MIT on September 10–12, 1956:

I went away from the Symposium with a strong conviction more intuitive than rational that human experimental psychology, theoretical linguistics, and computer simulation of cognitive processes were all pieces of a larger whole, and that the future would see progressive elaboration and coordination of their shared concerns. I have been working toward a cognitive science for about twenty years beginning before I knew what to call it. (Miller, 1979, p. 9)

This quote set the tone for the present collection of papers. Rather than being a collection of essays written by former students and colleagues on present research interests, the present book traces the twenty years of work of George and others and, in the process, provides at least a fragmentary history of cognitive science. It is probably no exaggeration that much of what cognitive science is today could be gathered from an intellectual biography of George. He has written several of the seminal papers in the archives of cognitive science, has trained and influenced numerous first-rate scientists, and has been a constant spokesman for expanding the range of "admissible evidence," pushing not just for an experimental psychology of cognition but for sciences of cognition such as cognitive psychology, artificial intelligence, linguistics, neuroscience, and anthropology joined together by common interests. Although George is by no means solely

vii

responsible for the current flourishing of cognitive science, much can be gained by understanding the battles that George fought.

When compiling a list of contributors, no attempt was made to provide a complete survey of a history of cognitive science. Artificial intelligence and anthropology, for instance, are not really represented in the current collection, but both, especially artificial intelligence, have played an integral part in the development of cognitive science. I was interested in inviting people who had worked with George in one capacity or another. Such a selection policy might produce a jaundiced history, but the dual purpose of the present collection made it inevitable.

Each contributor was asked to write a chapter on his or her personal view of the intellectual contribution of George and, more generally, of the theoretical concerns with which George has been associated. They were asked to concentrate on one particular aspect of George's career, or, to put it more generally, one phase in the development of cognitive science. Within these constraints, the chapters were to discuss the intellectual environment of the time of interest and to provide an understanding of what people were thinking about at the time and what was actually done. The chapters were to emphasize not present-day cognitive science but history – history with a personal feel to it.

As might be expected, the resulting chapters approach this mandate in different ways. Some of the chapters are straightforward recollections. Others are more formal historical accounts. Still others take an idea or experimental result of George's and trace how it was subsequently used by the field, thereby providing a history of an idea rather than a history of an intellectual movement.

The book is organized into what I conceive as important segments in George's life, and the contributors are assigned to each part because they figured in George's life at that time. But the different parts of the book also represent different eras in cognitive science, from its nascent form in the formalism of mathematical psychology through the work on language – with the inevitable interchange among psychologists, linguists, and philosophers – to the current age of hopeful maturity.

I want to thank the Sloan Foundation for its generous support, especially Eric Wanner at Sloan, who offered much helpful advice. I also want to thank Mike Gazzaniga for his guidance, David Stark, Michael Long, and Andrew Morral for handling many of the clerical details, Susan Milmoe at Cambridge University Press for her help, and most of all, George, for providing an opportunity. Proceeds from the book will go to fund the George A. Miller Prize for Cognitive Science at Princeton University.

New York, New York   William Hirst

Contributors

Thomas G. Bever
Department of Psychology
University of Rochester

Jerome Bruner
Department of Psychology
Graduate Faculty of the New School
for Social Research

Susan Carey
Department of Psychology
Massachusetts Institute of Technology

Eugene Galanter
Department of Psychology
Columbia University

Wendell R. Garner
Department of Psychology
Yale University

Michael S. Gazzaniga
Department of Neurology
Cornell University Medical College

Morris Halle
Department of Linguistics
Massachusetts Institute of Technology

Gilbert Harman
Department of Philosophy
Princeton University

William Hirst
Department of Psychology
Graduate Faculty of the New School
for Social Research

Philip Johnson-Laird
MRC Applied Psychology Unit,
Cambridge

Willem J. M. Levelt
Max-Plank-Institut
für Psycholinguistik

William J. McGill
Office of the President
Columbia University

Jacques Mehler
Laboratoire de Sciences Cognivites et
Psycholinguistique, CNRS

Ulric Neisser
Department of Psychology
Emory University

Donald A. Norman
Department of Psychology
University of California, San Diego

Roger N. Shepard
Department of Psychology
Stanford University

George Sperling
Department of Psychology
New York University

Keith Stenning
Centre for Cognitive Studies
University of Edinburgh

Eric Wanner
Russell Sage Foundation

PART I Mathematical psychology

In the 1950s and early 1960s, there was a flurry of activity in the field of mathematical psychology, broadly defined. People were searching for metaphors and formalisms with which to describe and explain not only human behavior but human mentation. Psychologists were reading textbooks on group theory and learning about stochastic models such as Markov chains. They were reading about information theory, designed in the context of electronic communication but readily transferred to the psychological world. They were not only attending to but actively participating in the nascent field of artificial intelligence. If cognitive science speaks to interdisciplinary study, then the search for the right formalistic model in the 1950s was cognitive science in the vanguard. Psychologists, computer scientists, mathematicians, statisticians, physicists, electronic engineers, and linguists were all talking to each other.

In the next few chapters, several students and colleagues of George Miller write about this period. The story told here centers mainly on Harvard and Lincoln Laboratories of MIT, but the same tale could be told by others from different parts of the United States. William McGill, as a student of George's, provides background information about the intellectual climate of the time and discusses some of the modeling that was then of interest. Wendell Garner was a fellow graduate student of George's. After graduation, he went to Johns Hopkins as a junior faculty member, while George stayed at Harvard. Consequently, Garner's work in information theory was not done in collaboration with George, but he outlines the issues and captures the tenor of the period.

Eugene Galanter wrote with George and Karl Pribram a book that was to revolutionize psychology: *Plans and Structures of Behavior*. As George wrote in a recent autobiography (Miller, 1987, p. 22), *Plans* "all seems pretty obvious now, but at the time it excited a lot of people. The ideas came from everywhere, but they were integrated in terms of their bearing on Newell and Simon's ideas about cognitive simulation. The centerpiece was to be the TOTE unit – Test whether the goal was realized, Operate to reduce discrepancies between the actual situation and the goal, then Test again, and Exit when the test was satisfied

1

– which was the informational equivalent of the feedback loop that had played such an important role in theories of regulative behavior.'' Galanter's chapter chronicles the writing of this seminal book.

Finally, we hear from three students of George's – Roger Shepard, George Sperling, and Ulric Neisser. Shepard shows how some of George's empirical work played an integral role in the development of a formalized means of extracting the underlying relations in similarity data (multidimensional scaling). This methodology proved central to work in representation, an important issue in contemporary cognitive science. Sperling traces the history of the concept of the magical number seven plus or minus two. George wrote as his presidential address to the Eastern Psychological Association a paper about human capacity limitations. The paper integrated work on information theory and psychophysics and became one of the most cited papers in cognitive psychology.

Neisser is in some sense the lone dissenter in this section. The others uncritically chronicle an active search for appropriate formalisms, whether in the form of stochastic models, information theory, computer simulations, or methodologies such as multidimensional scaling. Neisser, then and now, takes a more skeptical view of the success formalism has had in furthering psychologists' understanding of human nature.

1 George A. Miller and the origins of mathematical psychology

William J. McGill

Mathematical models have played a significant role in psychology from the very beginning. G. S. Fechner (1860) used a model when he attempted to scale sensation by integrating just-noticeable differences. In fact, a good case can be made for dating the earliest quantitative work to the laws of color mixture devised by Sir Isaac Newton (1704). Even the relatively late color theories of Helmholtz (1852) and Grassman (1854) antedate psychology's conventional origins.

When mathematical psychology came along as a new research area a century later, it was greeted at first with understandable skepticism. Traditionalists argued that mathematical reasoning had reached its zenith in psychology at least twenty years earlier when Thurstone published his path breaking study of factor analysis, *Vectors of the Mind* (1935). Granting all of these antecedents, it is nonetheless apparent today that the tentative mathematical explorations of the early 1950s constituted the initial stirrings of cognitive science. Something important and refreshingly new was being invented in the early 1950s. It is evident too that George Miller was a pioneer figure among the inventors.

In the beginning, mathematical psychology was nurtured by the early alarms of the cold war. That shadowy struggle of the late 1940s and 1950s gave powerful impetus in the United States to information technology and systems engineering. Scientists designing computer-based air-defense systems were motivated to model the complexities of human perceptual, communicative, and intellectual processes more realistically than ever before. Cognitive science evolved in part from these early efforts. Only gradually did it win acceptance in its own right. Miller played a critical role in that transformation too.

Shortly before 1950, a group of researchers, most of them young and irreverent, undertook to critique each other's work and to circulate manuscripts well in advance of publication. The papers dealt with a variety of topics connected by little more than sophisticated mathematics. To a casual observer this outburst of energy in information theory, statistical learning theory, choice theory, detection theory, multidimensional scaling, psycholinguistics, and artificial intelligence seemed to come from nowhere. Actually, an enhancement of capacity had been

3

solidifying since the war years, 1941–5. During the cold war era, mathematicians and psychologists found themselves again pressed into service on projects for the military. Each was sensitized by direct contact with the other. The mathematicians became interested in psychological data about which they understood little, while the psychologists were made to feel uncomfortable by confronting their quantitative shortcomings.

Looking back now, it was inevitable that some hitherto unrealized benefit would emerge from these interactions. One immediate benefit was a generation of World War II–era psychology graduate students who worked uncommonly hard to acquire mathematical training at the dawn of the computer age, when such training was bound to be especially valuable. Miller was among the first.

In August 1948, another of those graduate students (the writer) set out from the subway station in Harvard Square, looking for the Harvard Psychology Department. On a blazing summer afternoon, with waves of heat shimmering over the pavements and burning the unshaded sidewalks, I followed a zigzag path through Harvard Yard past Widener Library and Emerson Hall to a gate close by Appleton Chapel. Memorial Hall lay just outside at the intersection of Broadway and Cambridge streets, flanking the fire station.

Memorial Hall is a churchlike Victorian structure never really intended as an academic building. It was erected in 1876 to honor the sacrifices of Harvard's sons during the Civil War. Shortly afterward it became a dining commons for students unable to afford their own kitchen facilities. William James once commented on "Mem" Hall's curiously ambiguous role of "dispens[ing] honor to the dead and food to the living."

Eventually a new generation of Harvard houses provided better dining arrangements, and Memorial Hall lay almost abandoned. The old building spent the 1930s aloof from the hourly tides of students flooding in and out of the Yard, except when a weekend dance might be scheduled in the dining commons or when a lecturer or evening concert brought audiences to Sanders Theatre at its east end. Even the gingerbread trim that once gave the roof an almost jaunty appearance was taken down during World War II in an ill-conceived gesture to a patriotic drive for scrap metal.

Shortly before the war, space shortages developed everywhere at Harvard, anticipating the coming crisis. In 1940, S. S. Stevens was urged by the military services to expand his auditory research laboratory, but there was no place to expand it except in Memorial Hall's decaying basement. The basement offered one of the few places at Harvard where sound pressure levels of 115 dB might be generated without offending the neighbors.

A minor miracle of construction was accomplished. Where once blackened furnaces, dust-coated steam pipes, and rusting kitchen equipment had stood, a shiny new laboratory bloomed. Even by modern standards, the wartime Psychoacoustic Laboratory was outstanding. The federal government underwrote the full cost of construction. The military wanted quick action. Money was no object. The result was one of the best acoustic research centers in the world, built more than a decade before the competition in American universities could catch up.

Not long after the war, the Psychology Department in Emerson Hall gave a convulsive heave and split in two. The reasons were never made entirely clear but seemed to involve ideological disagreement between "soft" and "hard" psychology coupled with personality conflicts among a few key senior faculty. In any event, nearly all of the experimentalists moved their activities across the Yard to the basement of Memorial Hall, adding their numbers to the people already working in the Psychoacoustic Laboratory. Thus the Psychological Laboratories came into being in 1946.

To the left of Mem Hall's main entry on Cambridge Street was a concrete walk leading to a modern glass door beckoning visitors down into the basement. Beside the walk, a neatly lettered sign on a stake driven into the soil announced: "Psychological Laboratories." I stood in the heat, surveying the prospect in August 1948, and thought, how like the condition of psychology: always an afterthought, either in the attic or the basement!

Inside, the air was cool and the prospect far more inviting. The hallway was brightly lit, modern, and spotless. To the left lay the office of Professor Edwin Garrigues Boring, author of the monumental *History of Experimental Psychology* (1929) and advocate of the prescribed eighty-hour work week for graduate students. Around the corner, a long corridor ran past Chairman Edwin B. Newman's office. Across the hall on the right were the psychology library and a shop facility bracketing a large, brightly lit seminar room. The corridor wall outside displayed, in simple black frames, a printed year-by-year record of the department's Ph.Ds dating back to the nineteenth century. It included many of the great names of American psychology.

Farther down the long corridor, past the library and study rooms assigned to graduate students, were offices and laboratories forming the domain of B. F. Skinner. Skinner had arrived a few months earlier from Indiana amid intense intellectual excitement. He had brought with him a group of graduate students and postdoctoral fellows committed to his behavioristic position with a devotion bordering on religious zeal.

Skinner had recently published a utopian novel, *Walden Two* (1948), describing a community governed by Skinnerian principles. Unexpectedly, he became a guru for dozens, sometimes hundreds, of passionate disciples who would willingly shape their lives according to his prescriptions. This peculiarity marked

Skinner's devotees as a cult and thus an object of great interest in a discipline that, although never actually dull, could rarely generate the excitement of theoretical physics.

Skinner's charisma was palpable and instantly communicated. He also had a wonderful flair for publicity. During my time in Memorial Hall, he taught pigeons to play pingpong for *Life* magazine. More precisely, his graduate students trained the pigeons, while Skinner lectured *Life*'s reporters and photographers on operant conditioning.

The opposite end of the basement laboratory, the Sanders Theatre end, belonged to S. Smith Stevens, director of the Psychological Laboratories. It was the site of the wartime Psychoacoustic Laboratory. PAL had conducted vitally important research for the military services, helping to protect the hearing of their personnel from the worst effects of aircraft engine noise. It had also produced crucial papers on methods of voice communication in a high-noise environment, as well as much top-quality basic research on hearing and psychophysical scaling.

Smitty Stevens directed all of this work. He brought in spectacularly gifted graduate students and young faculty, whom he trained in his characteristic rock-hard approach to auditory scaling and psychophysics, as well as the art of good scientific writing. By 1948 these young people were just beginning to make a dent in American psychology. All of the pent-up energy of the Psychoacoustic Laboratory was released with the end of wartime military supervision. The result was a torrent of manuscripts giving the Psychological Laboratories at Harvard a sudden big national reputation.

Polarization along the Skinner–Stevens axis was one of the most tangible realities of Memorial Hall in 1948. Stevens encouraged theorizing. Although notably shy and hesitant in speech, Stevens was brilliant, stubborn, and intellectually aggressive. He hammered away regularly at his psychological theories, often badgering new graduate students unmercifully. An argument with Stevens was like an encounter with a soft-spoken, cold-eyed prosecutor conducting a cross-examination.

Skinner discouraged theorizing, although he was partial to anecdotes applying his principles to human behavior. He observed at the time that his early ideas on the reflex reserve had not held up under careful scrutiny. It seemed to me that the beautifully ordered data Skinner and his students were producing from pigeons via operant methods were nearly perfect candidates for analysis as stochastic processes. Skinner himself seemed undecided, but his coterie stood adamantly opposed on aesthetic and philosophical grounds.

Among serious experimenters, especially those with a keen interest in animal behavior, strong attachment to basic data is sometimes coupled with outright hostility to mathematical models. The early Skinnerians were like that. They dealt in purely descriptive empirical analysis: "knees," "elbows," "bursts," and the like. It was considered objectionable ever to depart from terms directly verifiable in the cumulative record. There was never any quarrel with quantification. The quarrel was with derived variables. Analysis one or more steps removed from and hence not directly verifiable by the data produced strong objections. Mathematical operations are typically geared to events that are either too small, too fast, too complex, or too numerous to be observed directly. A mathematical model attempting to achieve more than mere curve fitting or statistical summary typically leads to theorizing at least one step below the measurements. The data are then seen as examples of a process whose detailed description is not (or at least not yet) directly observable. Debates about theory usually reduce to disagreements over the appropriate level of analysis.

This philosophical barrier may have had an impact on Miller. At the time, he was working hard to perfect his mathematical skills. An important avenue of interest was barred to his curiosity. Moreover, he did not seem fully content with the breakup of the Psychology Department. Several of his closest colleagues were in Emerson Hall, and Miller seemed to spend considerable time there. But in the style of those times, frustrations, if they existed, were never discussed openly. It was probably also true that Miller's interests had already crystallized in the analysis of language. I never heard him speak either about the divided department or about the Skinnerians at the other end of Memorial Hall.

When I first saw the Psychological Laboratories in the late summer of 1948, Stevens was immersed in the last stages of editing his version of the *Handbook of Experimental Psychology*. It would be received with great critical acclaim when published in 1951.

The place seemed wall-to-wall with bright people: J. C. R. Licklider, Robert Galambos, Ira Hirsh, Walter Rosenblith, Floyd Ratliff, and Fred Frick, to name just a few. Some of the stars of the wartime research group had drifted away, notably Clifford Morgan, James Egan, and Wendell (Tex) Garner, but they were quickly replaced by outstanding Europeans: Von Békésy, Joe Zwislocki, and Gordon Flottorp.

In this remarkable cadre of talent, one of the youngest and brightest was George A. Miller, an assistant professor whose tiny office happened to be next door (a sure sign of high regard) to the headquarters of Professor Stevens at the east of Memorial Hall in the basement rotunda formed by the curved stage of Sanders Theatre above.

Miller's appearance was startlingly youthful. He was virtually beardless. His hair was dark and straight, exhibiting an unruly tendency to come down on his forehead. He was twenty-eight years old: tall, slim, and intense, with large, deep-set eyes, an actor's voice, and beautifully articulated speech hinting at Alabama. Later on, I felt uncomfortable working with him. He seemed so much younger than I. In fact I was twenty-six, but my face was already deeply lined, I tended to be overweight, and my hair was turning gray. Miller's only detectable vice was his chain smoking.

He made no effort to proselytize the graduate students, never buttonholing them in the corridors, telling tall tales about his research. He waited for us to come to him, and eventually many of us did. For our part, the graduate students were passing around excited accounts of Miller's research accomplishments. It was said that he had published no fewer than five major articles on auditory psychophysics during the twelve-month period just ended. I checked the story and found it to be true. The manuscripts included two first-rate experiments on energy integration at auditory threshold (Garner & Miller, 1947; Miller & Taylor, 1948). There was also a perfect little gem on incremental detectability of white noise (Miller, 1947). With the passage of time, this latter paper became a classic of the auditory literature because the main results are so pretty and so easily reproduced, even in an undergraduate laboratory (Fig. 1.1).

The student grapevine in the autumn of 1948 was abuzz with a story that Miller was now writing a book on language and communication. That did it! I vowed to introduce myself to him at the earliest opportunity.

Considering Miller's reputation, I prepared meticulously by subjecting the noise paper to exceptionally close study. One section was devoted to psychometric functions exhibiting marginal (I thought doubtful) evidence of the so-called neural quantum. The latter was a pet theory of Smitty Stevens, and I simply did not know what to make of it. How could one set out to prove that a phenomenon as intrinsically variable as the psychometric function is linear, with sharp corners? The argument seemed impervious to empirical testing, especially when Stevens claimed (as he usually did) that critics unable to reproduce the quantum failed because they were poor experimenters.

When I finally secured an appointment, I went to Miller's office prepared to do battle over the quantum; first to ask him about it and then to argue about it. Miller shocked me by brushing the entire topic aside. He said that his data had not really supported the quantum hypothesis and he did not care much about it. Even more devastating was the evidence, accumulating rapidly as he spoke, that Miller had lost interest in audition. His restless mind was taking him across terrain that I had not even discovered, leading him to contemplate vistas I could not begin to discern.

Specifically, he asked me what I knew about information theory. Nothing. He then gave me copies of Shannon's articles in the *Bell System Technical Journal* (Shannon, 1948). He told me to read them. What did I know about hill-climbing algorithms? Nothing. How much probability theory did I have? Some. Was I auditing Mosteller's course? No. What about Quine's courses in logic? No. What did I know about the various forms of Zipf's law? Nothing.

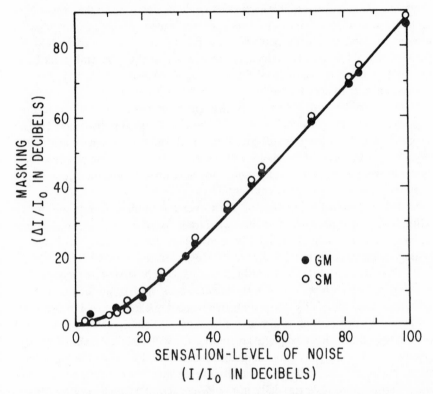

Figure 1.1   Discriminable increments in intensity of white noise plotted in a manner analogous to that of masking experiments. The solid line represents a function obtained by Hawkins for the masking of tones and speech by white noise. [Reprinted from Miller (1947) with permission of the American Institute of Physics.]

I came out reeling. It had been a nearly total disaster. Having gone in there to impress Miller with my command of his paper, I emerged feeling like an imbecile. He was not the least bit unfriendly. In fact he was very cordial, but comparing my intellectual interests with his in a face-to-face collision, no matter how cordial, was acutely depressing.

The single good outcome was that Miller invited me to join an informal reading seminar just finishing Von Neumann and Morgenstern's *Theory of Games and Economic Behavior* (1947). The group was soon to embark on a study of information theory. I resolved to try to recoup by mastering the theory that was revolutionizing the conceptual foundations of communication.

The reading group met once a week in the seminar room adjacent to the psychology library. Soon I did manage to impress Miller with an idea connecting transmitted information to partitioning of variance. It appeared to me that a multivariate form of information transmission could be devised and that it was conceptually similar to an analysis of variance performed on contingency tables. I worked out (and eventually published) the proof. The idea seemed to hold up, but in fact I did not really understand what was going on. Several years later, this analytical effort was revived during a summer spent with Tex Garner. He showed me how to do it correctly.

C. F. Mosteller and Robert R. Bush were charter members of the reading seminar. Mosteller, of course, was one of the world's great statisticians. He had attached himself to the Department of Social Relations, the new home of the other half of the divided Psychology Department. Bush, a young physicist, had come up from Princeton to study with Mosteller on a postdoctoral fellowship. They were interested in statistical learning theory.

Mosteller sketched his notions of linear operators applied to response probability following either reward or nonreward trials. Bush introduced me to Monte Carlo techniques via his wonderful little invention, the "stat rat," used in generating sequences obeying the rules of the Bush–Mosteller model.

We went on to read Birkhoff and MacLane's *Survey of Modern Algebra* (1948), followed by Feller's *Introduction to Probability Theory and Its Applications* (1950). I still own these old books. They are battered and dog-eared beyond recognition, but they are among my most precious possessions. Nothing has ever been read as closely as they were. The pages are interleaved with penciled notes on ghastly green paper. Recently, as I was thinking about Miller, I took the trouble to look at the backs of those old notes and discovered them to be throwaways from speech articulation tests run daily in the Psychoacoustic Laboratory by Miller. Probably we could not afford fresh notepaper.

Slowly the reading evolved into an informal but nonetheless demanding research seminar on Markov processes and statistical models for learning. Bush and Mosteller were generating continuous excitement with their linear operator model. They circulated dittoed manuscripts one after another, fresh weekly from their offices in Emerson Hall. The papers dealt with a variety of special cases and cute proofs.

The Bush–Mosteller scheme was quite simple. It addressed itself to sequences of responses and their possible consequences or outcomes. Imagine r mutually exclusive and exhaustive response classes, each with its appropriate probability. A particular outcome would take effect by operating on these probabilities, mapping each of them into a new value. The rule for this mapping was taken to be a simple, repeatable transformation, usually linear, in which case the outcome operator would be a matrix. The mathematical problem was to follow this reasoning through innumerable sequences of responses and outcomes in order to determine the terminal state of each response probability. Such processes rapidly fan out along intricate branching pathways from the states on a given trial to the states on subsequent trials. Mathematical tricks devised by Bush and Mosteller helped to track the branching and simplified the recordkeeping so that precise conclusions became possible.

One of the neatest cases had two response classes and two outcomes. Since response probabilities must sum to unity, we then need to follow only a single response class. The operators took the form

$$Q_1 p = a_1 + \alpha_1 p,$$
$$Q_2 p = a_2 + \alpha_2 p.$$

Evidently, Q_1 and Q_2 perform different linear transforms on p, the current probability of the response class under scrutiny. If the process involved regular reinforcement of some response and extinction of everything else, operator Q_1 (success) would be applied only on those trials in which the response did in fact occur; operator Q_2 (failure) otherwise. The model was able to forecast not only the asymptotic response probabilities but also the expected shape of the learning curve generated in achieving them.

One day in the midst of all this heady activity, someone acquired a preprint of William K. Estes's *Psychological Review* article on stimulus sampling theory (1950). A mild sensation was created in the seminar when Bush and Mosteller showed that their linear operators could be deduced from Estes's assumptions about stimulus elements.

The discovery led Miller and Mosteller to organize an interuniversity summer seminar under the aegis of the Social Science Research Council. The seminar was titled "Mathematical Models for Behavior Theory" and was scheduled to run from June 28 to August 24, 1951, at Tufts College in Medford, not far from Cambridge. Bill Estes and his collaborator, Cletus Burke, were invited from Bloomington, Indiana. So was Dave Zeaman of the University of Connecticut. They agreed to come. Miller spoke to Katherine Harris and me about helping out as graduate assistants.

For the first week or two at Tufts, Kathy and I sat in on the main seminar sessions during the mornings and ran stat rats for Bob Bush for the rest of the day. The group was settling into a predictable leisurely routine matched to the hot summer weather.

Then Miller shook things up by reporting an unusual problem in free-recall verbal learning. He and Jerry Bruner had been gathering data in Emerson Hall, using an extremely simple experimental format. Suppose, Miller said, a list of words is presented to a learner. The individual is free to recall them in any order he chooses. On each successive presentation, the list is scrambled and the learner writes down all the words he can remember. After n trials the words on the list are found to be in various states. Some have been recalled many times, others scarcely at all. Moreover, odd things happen. A word might intrude into the recall list and might then be recalled several times even though it was never presented.

The data were very orderly. They seemed to reflect a simple process that Miller thought might be a Markov chain, especially in view of the intrusions.

As the seminar discussed the free-recall data, it seemed likely that a Markov process might result if Q_2, that is, the "failure operator" in the Bush–Mosteller model, was an identity operator. An identity operator would leave all existing recall probabilities unchanged. Miller was encouraged to pursue this line of reasoning.

After the session, I told him that I was intrigued by the problem. Might I work on it with him? Miller replied that he would be delighted. Any help at all would be appreciated.

The next day, he came by the cubbyhole set aside as work space for the research assistants in the summer seminar. George had an idea. Suppose, he said, we identify the probability of recall after k previous recalls as τ_k and label the state of all such words as A_k. Suppose further, following the seminar's suggestion, success increases recall probability but failure leaves it unchanged. Then the entire process could be described by a single difference equation:

$$p(A_k, n+1) = p(A_k, n)\,(1 - \tau_k) + p(A_{k-1}, n)\tau_{k-1}.$$

The equation says that a word in state A_k (recalled k previous times) on trial $n+1$ was either already in state A_k on trial n and was not recalled, or was one step lower (state A_{k-1}) on trial n and was recalled with probability τ_{k-1}. Given the assumptions, this concise description covers everything.

Did I recognize the difference equation? Did I know how to solve it? "Solving" a difference equation means finding one or more expressions for $p(A_k, n)$ that obey the rule stated in the equation. When you succeed in solving a difference equation, you may produce a probability distribution no one has ever seen before or, perhaps more interesting, an application of a familiar distribution that no one knew existed.

In fact, the equation did look a lot like an expression for a pure birth process presented in Chapter 17 of Feller's *Introduction to Probability Theory and Its Applications*, but there were important differences. No, I did not know how to solve it. Would I like to work on the problem with him? You bet I would!

We agreed on how we would divide the work. George would struggle with the difference equation, attempting to find its solution directly. I would try to subvert it by considering special cases involving typical Bush–Mosteller restrictions on τ_k. For example, suppose

$$\tau_{k+1} = a + (1 - a)\tau_k.$$

This is a linear operator in the form proposed by Bush and Mosteller, but with a single parameter. Perhaps a few iterations might suggest a form for the solution.

We went our separate ways, checking in with each other every day to assess progress. Within a week, both of us had struck pay dirt. I had found a solution to the difference equation for the special cases involving one and two parameters. Miller had found the general solution.

He showed it to me on a blackboard. His method of attack involved a matrix analysis used in studying Markov processes. It was extremely elegant. I could follow each step of George's proof but could never have produced it myself.

Miller's solution for the probability $p(A_k, n)$, that a word is in state A_k on trial n, took a form that seemed tantalizingly familiar:

$$p(A_0, n) = (1 - \tau_0)^n \qquad \text{for } k = 0,$$

$$p(A_k, n) = \tau_0 \cdot \tau_1 \ \ldots \ \tau_{k-1} \sum_{i=0}^{i=k} \frac{(1 - \tau_i)^n}{\prod_{\substack{j=0 \\ j \neq i}}^{j=k} (\tau_j - \tau_i)} \qquad \text{for } k > 0.$$

My own solution for the two-parameter case was arrived at by applying rules for summing power series taught us by Bush and Mosteller in the reading seminar. Oddly, the expressions (Miller's and mine) were completely different. My result was much simpler, but we soon proved the two solutions to be identical. Evidently the Bush–Mosteller–Estes model cast Miller's result into an unusually simple form. Hence, the two solutions complemented each other neatly.

We then set about filling in the last piece of the puzzle, a three-parameter case in which the asymptotic probability of recall would be less than unity. Some of the recall lists had this property. The three-parameter series proved very difficult to sum, and we struggled with them throughout several afternoons. Finally, each of us took the problem home. The next morning, Miller had the answer, and I had a proof showing how to establish whether any given result is correct. They fitted together perfectly.

The problem was opening up like a summer flower. Miller set me to work figuring out estimation formulas based on the distributions we had devised. He himself began preparing figures comparing then unpublished data of Bruner, Miller, and Zimmerman (1955) with our theoretical distributions. The results were beautiful to behold (Figs 1.2, 1.3).

One of the most difficult and challenging features of any discovery is the exploration of its implications. We worked almost continuously to penetrate what we had found, trying to be sure that we understood it, preparing ourselves for every conceivable objection. Eventually all was in place, and we sprang our solutions on the other members of the Tufts seminar. Bush and Mosteller, Burke

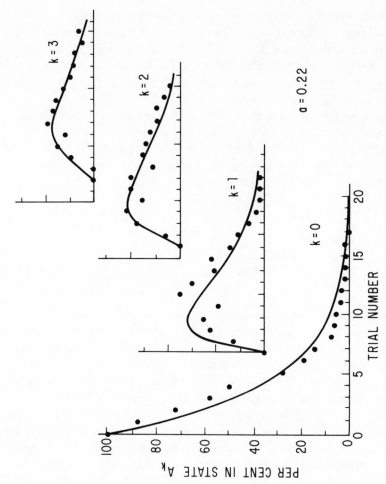

Figure 1.2 Observed and calculated distributions of words recalled exactly k times on successive trials. One-parameter case. Based on data of Bruner et al. (1955). [Reprinted from Miller and McGill (1952) with permission from *Psychometrika*.]

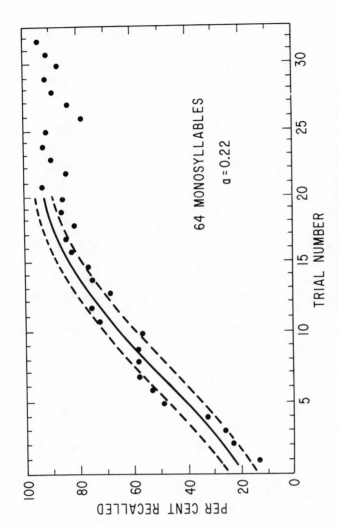

Figure 1.3 Observed and computed learning curve. One-parameter case. Based on data of Bruner et al. (1955). [Reprinted from Miller and McGill (1952) with permission from *Psychometrika*.]

and Estes were charmed. The Miller–McGill description of free-recall learning was not only perfectly in tune with their own work, but it also proved to be a rare case in which the complete probability distribution was known and could be written down in closed form. Mosteller encouraged us to publish it. He also invited us to read a paper at the upcoming winter meeting of the Institute of Mathematical Statistics (IMS).

When the summer seminar ended and we returned to Harvard, we found that word of our discovery had preceded us. Miller's solution of the difference equation and the news that we would present it to the IMS meeting in New York during the Christmas holidays further reinforced his reputation in Memorial Hall; the role I had played as his collaborator literally made my own reputation.

Miller read our paper before the IMS on December 27, 1951. It was very well received. Both of us were stunned when one of the discussants, Professor Max Woodbury of the University of Chicago, praised the paper and our results extravagantly – and then announced that he had put our distribution into the *Annals of Mathematical Statistics* two years earlier, in 1949. We checked and, of course, he was right. Neither of us had known anything of Woodbury's work.

I was completely dejected. Woodbury, on the other hand, was delighted. Until he encountered Miller–McGill, his distribution seemed to him nothing more than a mathematical curiosity. Now it might turn out to be something important. Woodbury told us that Feller had also published the solution in 1949.

I asked George whether we ought to continue working on our manuscript. He was very firm about it. We must get it done and get it published. The paper eventually appeared in *Psychometrika* in December 1952, almost exactly a year later. It was a few months after my dissertation had been submitted to the department (on an entirely different topic). I had moved, with Miller and Licklider, to MIT.

I dropped by George's office to pick up my share of our reprints and found him in an expansive mood. He concluded that we had worked well together. He urged me not to worry about Woodbury, whose prior claim was now carefully cited in the paper. "After all," George said, "nothing really good is ever entirely new."

I asked him whether he intended to take the work any further. George scowled his characteristic scowl reserved for doubtful propositions. "No," he replied. He had been intrigued by the problem posed in the Bush–Mosteller–Estes model when one of the learning operators is the identity operator, but that was all there was to it. The main thrust of his work remained in language and communication. He was beginning to dream of one day unraveling the intuitive logic of grammar.

Miller asked whether I would go on with it. Bob Bush was already organizing a new summer study in California involving Patrick Suppes, a brilliant young logician at Stanford. There might be a great opportunity for me. I too said "no."

I could never be happy far away from the MIT communication group in which both of us were now working.

Each evoked in the other a rough masculine affection fashioned by mixing nine parts admiration with at least one part competition. Still, I could not help feeling immensely grateful to George for letting me share the toil and the rewards with him. Perhaps some day, he said, we might find another problem, equally challenging, on which we could resume the collaboration. Alas, the opportunity never came again.

Looking back at it now, I realize that my efforts were greatly amplified by Miller's stimulation and by his hard-driving work habits. His sharp formulation of problems, his high intelligence, and his demanding personal standards made an extraordinary impression on me. They pushed me to levels I had never attained before. The collaboration left an indelible mental impression of Miller as a climber gone over the next hill while I struggled breathlessly to catch up. And when I finally made it, I found myself on a height I could never reach alone.

An experience with so many emotional overtones is difficult to put aside. I was never able to forget the difference equation, Miller's beautiful solution, or Woodbury's announcement to the December 1951 IMS meeting that he had solved the same problem two years earlier.

A decade later found me at Columbia, preparing a chapter on stochastic latency mechanisms for the *Handbook of Mathematical Psychology* (Luce, Bush, & Galanter, Vol. 1, 1963). A student of mine, John Gibbon, pointed out a connection between the Miller–McGill (Woodbury–Feller) formula and the general gamma distribution that I had never noticed before. It was amazingly simple. The general gamma describes the time up to the occurrence of an event whose probability changes with each successive occurrence. If you drop off only the last event, you produce an expression that is, in effect, a continuous approximation to Miller–McGill. Hence, the latter must be intimately related to the generalized Poisson distribution.

Gibbon and I decided to restudy the difference equation and the closely related differential equation describing the process in continuous form (McGill & Gibbon, 1965). We set about tracking down references to the generalized Poisson and the general gamma distributions, hoping to find something prior to Woodbury's (1949) solution. In fact, we managed to trace the solution back through a host of rediscoveries all the way to the early part of this century and a paper on radioactive decay by H. Bateman (1910). Bateman's formulation turns out to be remarkably similar to that of Miller–McGill. A radioactive substance emits a particle at random and then decays into a new substance with new parameters. The new substance emits another particle at random, becoming still another substance, and so on. Bateman wanted to calculate (among other things) the probability distribution of the number of particles observed in a fixed period of time.

It appears that Bateman was the first of more than a half dozen discoverers of the distribution identified in mathematical learning theory with Miller–McGill.

George Miller spoke wisely when he observed that nothing really good is ever entirely new. On the other hand, it is a rare privilege to be involved in anything genuinely good. I was given such an opportunity at the very beginning, just as I was starting out. Miller offered me that opportunity. Although we were never able to work side-by-side again, Miller played a formative role in all that I ever did afterward. I could never put aside either his visions or the standards he taught me.

References

Bateman, H. (1910). The solution of a system of differential equations occurring in the theory of radioactive transformations. *Proceedings of the Cambridge Philosophical Society, 15*, 423–7.

Birkhoff, G., & MacLane, S. (1948). *A Survey of Modern Algebra*. New York: Macmillan.

Boring, E. G. (1929). *A History of Experimental Psychology*. New York: Appleton-Century.

Bruner, J. S., Miller, G. A., & Zimmerman, C. (1955). Discriminative skill and discriminative matching in perceptual recognition. *Journal of Experimental Psychology, 49*, 181–92.

Estes, W. K. (1950). Toward a statistical theory of learning. *Psychological Review, 57*, 94–107.

Fechner, G. S. (1860). *Elemente der Psychophysik*. Leipzig: Breitkopf and Hartel.

Feller, W. (1950). *An Introduction to Probability Theory and Its Applications*, Vol. 1. New York: Wiley.

Feller, W. (1949). On the theory of stochastic processes with particular reference to applications. *Proceedings of the Berkeley symposium on mathematical statistics and probability* (pp. 403–32). Berkeley: University of California Press.

Garner, W. R., & Miller, G. A. (1947). The masked threshold of pure tones as a function of duration. *Journal of Experimental Psychology, 37*, 293–303.

Grassman, G. (1854). On the theory of compound colors. *Philosophy Magazine, 7*, 254–64.

Helmholtz, H. (1852) On the theory of compound colors. *Philosophy Magazine, 4*, 519–34.

Luce, R. D., Bush, R. R., & Galanter, E. (Eds.) (1963). *Handbook of Mathematical Psychology*. Vol. 1 (pp. 348–9). New York: Wiley.

McGill, W. J., & Gibbon, J. (1965). The general-gamma distribution and reaction times. *Journal of Mathematical Psychology, 2*, 1–18.

Miller, G. A. (1947). Sensitivity to changes in the intensity of white noise and its relation to masking and loudness. *Journal of the Acoustical Society of America, 19*, 609–19.

Miller, G. A., & McGill, W. J. (1952). A statistical description of verbal learning. *Psychometrika, 17*, 369–96.

Miller, G. A., & Taylor, W. (1948). The perception of repeated bursts of noise. *Journal of the Acoustical Society of America, 20*, 171–82.

Newton, I. (1704). *Opticks*. London: W. Innys.

Shannon, C. E. (1948). A mathematical theory of communication. *Bell System Technical Journal, 27*, 379–423, 623–56.

Skinner, B. F. (1948). *Walden Two*. New York: Macmillan.

Stevens, S. S. (Ed.) (1951). *Handbook of Experimental Psychology*. New York: Wiley.

Thurstone, L. L. (1935). *Vectors of the Mind*. Chicago: University of Chicago Press.

Von Neumann, J., & Morgenstern, O. (1947). *Theory of Games and Economic Behavior*, 2nd ed. Princeton: Princeton University Press.

Woodbury, M. A. (1949). On a probability distribution. *Annals of Mathematical Statistics, 20*, 311–13.

2 The contribution of information theory to psychology

Wendell R. Garner

What is information theory?

Before discussing in detail the contribution of information theory to psychology, a brief introduction to information theory will set the stage for my later comments about it. Information theory, at least for the purpose of understanding its role in psychology, consists of both a set of concepts and a system of measurement appropriate to quantification of the concepts. Although these two aspects are closely related in formal information theory, in at least some applications in psychology the concepts are more important than the measurement.

The concepts

As I note a bit later, although the initial appeal of information theory to psychologists came from its measurement properties, very quickly the stronger appeal came from the set of concepts. Therefore, of the two aspects of information theory (concepts and measurement), I will first describe the major concepts that have been used primarily in psychology. Later, I will argue that most of these concepts have been absorbed into cognitive psychology.

Information. The basic concept that comes from information theory is the definition of information itself. Information is specifiable not as the property of events themselves, but as a property of what events could have happened but did not. Thus information and uncertainty are closely related, with information being the reduction of uncertainty.

Amount of information. Not only is information a question of what could have happened but did not, the amount of information can be measured by how many things could have happened. Thus, even as a crude first approximation, amount of information is a function of the number of alternative events that could have occurred but did not.

19

Efficiency of communication. If the amount of information can be measured, then it is possible to measure how efficiently a communication system functions. As a simple example, the Morse code (long before formal information theory) used one dot for the letter *E* and one dash for the letter *T,* while using four dots or dashes for letters such as *X* and *Z.* Thus frequently used letters were efficiently transmitted with few symbols, and infrequently used letters were transmitted with more symbols. Such a system is obviously more efficient than one that requires an equal number of dots and dashes for all letters.

Redundancy. If more information is transmitted or used than is necessary for minimal communication, then the communication system is redundant. Furthermore, if desirable, the amount of redundancy can also be specified.

Communication channels. Information is transmitted through a communication channel. For engineers, the channel might be a telephone or telegraph system, but the important point for psychology is that the human came to be identified as a communication channel, which received information and then transmitted it to an output system. No longer was the human an organism that perceived a stimulus and emitted a response. Rather, it received and emitted information: It was a communication channel.

Channel capacity. Any communication channel, including the human one, has a maximum capability for transmitting information: It has a channel capacity. And again, given the ability to measure amount of information, this channel capacity can be determined quantitatively.

Coding. The form of an event may not be the same as the form in which information is transmitted. Thus the actual input to a communication channel must be encoded to be compatible with the properties of the channel and then decoded from the channel to be compatible with the receiver of the information.

A measurement system

The second aspect of information theory is as a measurement system, a statistical tool. Information theory constitutes an integrated set of statistical measures, and these measures, by being coherent, can determine not only the amount of information but also the amount of redundancy, channel capacity, and any related concept with a single unit of measurement. The unit used almost universally is the "bit" (contraction of "binary digit").

The initial appeal of information theory to psychologists was due to the fact that most experimental psychologists had long been quantitatively oriented, and the statistical properties of information theory were very appealing to them. Furthermore, this appeal was not to psychologists working on a single topic; rather, it was to many different kinds of psychologists working on quite different problems. It was probably this breadth of appeal that led to its rapid acceptance. If information theory touched only a single problem area, it would have been seen as an esoteric measure suitable for that problem, but not for too much else. However, the appeal was broad, and although its initial appeal may have been the mathematics, psychologists were actually absorbing the concepts along with the information measurement. So, although the two aspects of information theory could be separated, in practice they were not, and the concepts accompanied the measurement system.

A brief history

Shannon's contribution

Shannon in 1948 published a two-part paper, and in it he presented a full-blown theory of information with both a measure and the related concepts. The basic measure was logarithmic, a property already established by Nyquist (1924) and Hartley (1928), but Shannon added a probabilistic measure that could take care of unequal occurrences of particular signals, as well as unequal occurrences of different sequences of signals. So the measure of information was probability oriented (very comfortable for psychologists) and dealt readily with sequential issues. Shannon also discussed issues of redundancy and channel capacity, plus some other topics not of particular interest to psychologists. So here at last was what had been needed for so long, a complete theory of information, its definition, measure of amount, measure of redundancy, efficiency, channel capacity, and so on.

Its introduction to psychology by George Miller

Psychology must have been waiting, even eagerly, for such a theory, because it was introduced to the field almost immediately after Shannon's publication. Information theory was actually introduced to psychologists by Miller and Frick (1949), just a year after the original Shannon paper. The emphasis in that paper was on sequential behavior, and it used the Shannon measure of information as a measure of constraint or redundancy. Two years later, Frick and Miller (1951) published an experimental paper demonstrating the use of the information measure to describe the behavior of rats in an operant conditioning experiment. In that same year, Garner and Hake (1951) described how information measurement could be used to determine the number of categories that could be handled without error in an absolute judgment task.

Its rapid acceptance in psychology

The psychological world did not immediately accept information theory upon the publication of the Miller and Frick paper. Although experimental psychologists liked a quantitative and even formal approach to their problems, the initial concern (incidentally, shared by me) was that this measure was too restricted to have great generality. S. S. Stevens even commented at a conference that we would merely have to substitute one descriptive statistic for another, and what was gained by doing that? However, this reaction was very short-lived, as can be seen from the publication dates of the early papers. The change in attitude occurred as soon as psychologists saw that information theory was much more than just another statistic and that there was a fundamental theory behind the statistics, with a set of useful new ideas and concepts. In retrospect, I would say that the wait-and-see attitude lasted for little more than half a year, and after that it was accepted at what can only be called a phenomenal rate.

Some sense of the rapid growth of interest in information theory can be obtained by noting the number of conferences and symposia that occurred. The first of these was at Harvard in the spring of 1951, involving a miscellany of psychologists who had exhibited some interest in the topic. For myself, that conference was the culmination of my belief that information theory could easily solve a problem that I had been working on for at least a year. The problem was this: If people are asked to make absolute judgments on a sensory or perceptual continuum such as loudness or the position of a pointer on a line, what is the optimum number of categories to use? The answer is not that obvious, because the greater the number of categories, the more errors that will be made, but if the errors do not increase in proportion to the number of categories, it might be better to accept some level of error. I had been using a Thurstonian model to get an answer to this question, but there suddenly was information theory with its concept of channel capacity. That's what I needed. I threw away a year's worth of data and calculations, and shifted to the use of information theory. These ideas on the use of information theory were first published in the paper by Garner and Hake in 1951.

This conference also demonstrated that information theory was useful in quite different areas. George Miller and I had not only been graduate students together (even roommates), but had worked together during World War II. We had published several joint papers in those early years, but after the war I went to Johns Hopkins to work on perceptual and performance problems, while George stayed at Harvard and turned increasingly toward his long-lasting interest in language. He had even published a book, *Language and Communication,* in 1951. This conference at Harvard was as valuable to him as to me, but for him it was useful in clarifying how information theory could be used to study language, especially its sequential aspects.

Subsequent conferences were held in 1954 at the Massachusetts Institute of Technology and the University of Illinois, the latter resulting in a book (Quastler, 1955). Symposia were held at the International Congress of Psychology in 1954, 1957, and 1963. But the major impact on me, and I think on many others (including George Miller), had already occurred, so these events were more for the education of others about information theory than for our own learning. But there was one particular symposium at the meetings of the American Psychological Association in the early 1950s (I am unsure of the exact year), which I still remember with a certain irony. There were four speakers. Three of them extolled the virtues of information theory. I was the fourth, and gave an essentially cautionary, even negative, talk. My reason for doing so was that information theory had been accepted so wholeheartedly that psychologists expected more than it could provide. So I was warning that it was not a panacea for our problems; that frequently it only helped to answer problems rather than to generate questions; and that, if used wisely, information theory could be very valuable, but if used unwisely, it might lead to the kind of rejection that throws out the baby with the bathwater. Yet all this time I was myself merrily using information theory in my own work. But in my opinion, it was being accepted too rapidly.

Further evidence of its rapid acceptance came from the fact that Miller was invited to write an article on it for the *American Psychologist* in 1953. As the title of the article, "What Is Information Measurement?", indicates, Miller intended to explain information theory to a broader and perhaps less sophisticated audience. And this was just four years after the original Miller and Frick article. As I mentioned, psychologists were ready for information theory (almost too ready) and integrated it into their thinking very rapidly.

Statistic or concept? In the symposium at the International Congress of Psychology in 1957, two speakers presented their views on the future of information theory in psychology. Faverge (1957) stated that psychology had simply acquired another useful statistic. Broadbent (1957), on the other hand, argued that information theory had provided a fundamentally new point of view in emphasizing the importance of stimuli that could occur but did not. The two speakers differed on what had happened in psychology and what the future of information theory would be, one arguing for the concept and the other arguing about the statistic.

Which speaker was correct? When information theory was first introduced to psychologists, its statistical properties were prominent. In the original Miller and Frick (1949) article, the title of the paper used the term "statistical behavioristics," which clearly emphasizes the measurement aspect of information theory. Garner and Hake (1951) also emphasized its statistical properties (although also the channel capacity) in measuring the efficiency of an absolute judgment. In both cases, the statistics were being applied to a psychological problem that already existed. So, Faverge was reflecting reasonably accurately the very early uses of information theory in psychology, but by that time, the concepts were also established.

Broadbent, on the other hand, was perceiving something else: that along with the statistics and mathematics, the concepts were unobtrusively creeping into psychologists' ways of thinking. Miller and Frick in fact had described a measure of sequential constraint, which is redundancy. Garner and Hake had treated the human as a communication channel and were proposing a measure of channel capacity. Although the very earliest uses of information theory in psychology focused on the statistical aspect of the theory, the concepts were being accepted along with the statistics. Terms like "information transmission," "amount of information," "redundancy," "channel capacity," and "coding" were becoming part of the psychologist's vocabulary, even at times as jargon. Broadbent recognized the importance of the concepts, whereas Faverge reflected only the very early emphasis on statistical aspects of the theory. In other words, Broadbent was more nearly correct.

My own attitude by this time was also clear, and I made my statement at the conference (I was also a speaker) by simply reporting on a problem I was working on and using information theory on it. My failure to get into an argument was itself a statement of my point of view, since I felt that psychologists (at least in America) no longer were concerned about statistic versus concept. They simply used information theory if it was useful, and it could be useful as a statistic, a concept, or both. It didn't really matter. Although the formal measurement of information first grabbed the attention of experimental psychologists, the concepts were rapidly absorbed and used with little real concern for the nature of their use. Certainly George Miller's 1953 article was written in this mode. In order to explain information theory, the formal properties of its measurement had to be discussed, but these were not separated from the concepts. They went together.

Early applications in psychology

To provide further clarification of the extremely rapid rise in the use of information theory in psychology, I shall describe several problem areas in which it was employed. I will use a few examples for each of these areas, but obviously I must sample severely. I will use illustrations predominantly from the 1950s, primarily to emphasize the rapid acceptance of information theory in psychology.

Reaction time

In the latter part of the nineteenth century, reaction time had been a subject of some importance in experimental psychology. The examples are many, but Donders's use of it to determine components of a mental process was one of the more important. It was still an active area of research in the 1930s, but more as a subject in itself, with investigations of set, timing of warning signals, and so on being the kinds of variables used. Then it nearly disappeared, and accuracy was the primary dependent variable used in all kinds of experiments.

Information theory brought reaction time back to psychology, apparently on a permanent basis, but certainly at the present time as a major dependent variable. Hick (1952) first demonstrated that reaction time is linearly related to the logarithm of the number of alternative stimuli. This relation to the logarithm of the number of alternatives is exactly what the measure of amount of information required, and so demonstrated that reaction time is a function of amount of information. This linear relation of reaction time to the number of alternative stimuli has come to be known as "Hick's law." Hick had used an experimental situation in which different lights were the stimuli and finger pressings of telegraph keys were the responses.

Hyman, a student of mine at Johns Hopkins, demonstrated the same result in the following year (1953), using a display of lights again as the stimuli, but with a vocal identifying response to each stimulus as the response. In one condition, he, like Hick, used equal probabilities of occurrence of stimuli. Hyman went further, however, using different probabilities of occurrence of the lights and different sequential probabilities as well. His results showed that in all three experimental conditions reaction time was linearly related to the amount of information in the stimulus.

These two experiments quickly established the usefulness of reaction time in experimental psychology and led immediately to many studies within an information theory framework. For example, Leonard (1958) used six alternative lights, with the actual stimulus being the turning off of one of the lights. He broke the information into two stages by first presenting just three lights followed by turning one of them off. He found that with short times of such advance information, reaction time was the same as for all six lights, but that with advances of as little as 0.30 second, the reaction time was the same as for a three-choice condition.

Thus the total information required could be broken into two parts, and experimental subjects were able to use the advance information to reduce their reaction times appropriately.

Speech perception

As I mentioned earlier, George Miller's interest in information theory was related closely to his interest in language, and it is in these areas that most of his own publications occurred. He used information concepts and measures in the study of both speech perception and language redundancy, obviously very effectively in both. Once again, I want to stress the early dates on these publications. Remember that it takes two or three years from the beginning of a research project to its ultimate publication, and the date of the first Miller publication makes it clear that he began to do research on language problems almost as soon as he had had time to absorb the original Shannon paper.

Miller, Heise, and Lichten (1951) carried out an experiment on the auditory recognition of words heard in noise. The experimental variable was the number of words, on a list always available to the subject, so that the subject knew the nature and size of the test vocabulary. Two levels of noise were used, with test vocabularies of 2, 4, 8, 16, 32, or 256 monosyllables. The percentage of words correctly heard was the dependent variable. The result of importance, of course, is that accuracy of word identification decreased as a function of the logarithm of the size of the test vocabulary, in other words, as a function of the amount of information. This relation was essentially linear for the more difficult noise condition, although a ceiling effect occurred with the easier noise condition. Nevertheless, it was established that the amount of information in the stimulus was critical, not the actual word itself.

In a later study on this problem, Pollack (1959) was concerned with the question of whether the information effect was due to the number of possible stimuli (the input) or to the number of possible responses (the output). In most such experiments, including the Miller et al. research, the number of possible responses was equal to the number of stimuli, so it cannot be determined where the effect exists. Once again, auditory recognition of words heard in noise was determined. In one experiment most directly concerned with this question, Pollack used test vocabularies of two to sixty-four words. But instead of requiring just the usual single identification response, the subjects were told to make a second response, choosing between two words given by the experimenter, thus reducing the response uncertainty to just two, despite the fact that the initial "perceptual" uncertainty could have been considerably greater. The results were clear: The first response showed the same decline in accuracy with an increase in stimulus information, but the second response gave a flat function independent of the size of the initial test vocabulary. This result seemed to establish that the critical factor was the response uncertainty, not the stimulus uncertainty (or information).

Language redundancy

One of the research areas that information theory affected most strongly was that of language perception. The last section was concerned simply with the perception of words. But language has another important property, namely, that it is redundant. In simple terms, if a sequence of letters or words is known, the next letter or word can be predicted with far greater than chance accuracy. This ability to predict is due to redundancy.

Estimates of redundancy. Shannon (1948, 1951) had himself estimated the redundancy of printed English to be about 50 percent. He had used a technique in which a subject was given a passage of text and then required to guess the next letter until the correct response (i.e., that corresponding to the original text) was given. Redundancy was calculated from the distribution of the numbers of guesses required. Garner and Carson (1960) used another indirect technique, having many different subjects make the guess and then using the distribution of actual guesses to estimate the redundancy. They also estimated the redundancy of printed English to be about 50 percent. Newman and Gerstman (1952) used a direct technique by sampling actual text, determining the correlation between letters adjacent, one step removed, and so on, and then summing these correlations or contingencies to obtain a total estimate of redundancy. They estimated redundancy to be 52 percent.

Uses of redundancy. Although psychologists had some interest in estimating the redundancy of printed English as a problem in its own right, the more important point was to demonstrate that humans could make use of the redundancy. Such demonstrations were made in a variety of ways.

Chapanis (1954) and Miller and Friedman (1957) both showed that when text was mutilated by deleting different percentages of letters, subjects were able to restore the missing letters with a high degree of accuracy. Such restoration is made possible because of redundancy, so these experiments showed that redundancy was useful to humans.

In 1950 Miller and Selfridge (again, note the early date) used a procedure suggested by Shannon of producing word lists with different orders of approximation to English. To generate stimulus materials, some subjects were given one, two, three, or more words and were asked to add the next word. The orders of approximation were produced (up to order seven) by varying the length of the word list used. Details of the technique are less important than the result that the higher the order of approximation to real text, the easier it was for other subjects to learn lists of either twenty or fifty words. Thus redundancy aids memory for strings of words.

Two other illustrations should be sufficient. Miller, Bruner, and Postman (1954) used the technique just described to generate words of eight letters, except that the additional letters were found from actual text rather than by guessing. A word of first-order approximation might be "stanugop"; a word of fourth-order approximation might by "ricaning." The experiment showed that the percentage of correct recognitions with tachistoscopic presentation rose regularly with order of approximation. Miller (1958) also used constrained strings of letters in a free-recall learning experiment and found that lists of such strings of letters were learned much more rapidly when they resembled actual English words more closely.

In summary, printed English is redundant, and thus constrained, both in letter sequences within words and in sequences of words themselves. This redundancy is known to humans, who can use it to reconstruct mutilated text and to recognize and learn words and sequences of words that reflect varying degrees of this constraint. These were the sorts of issues that kept (and keep) George Miller interested.

Absolute judgments

As for myself, absolute judgment was the topic of main concern for many years, although pattern perception has also been a major interest. The study of absolute judgment most directly requires the use of the information measure, as well as the concept of channel capacity. Research in this area was quite common, both in the early years and in later ones.

Briefly, a number of possible stimuli from a stimulus dimension are used as the set, and the number of such stimuli is the experimental variable. Subjects are required to identify each stimulus, and a matrix of stimulus–response pairings is obtained. The measure used in this case is the information transmitted (measured in bits) by the stimuli through the human as a channel. Typically, no errors are made with small numbers of stimulus alternatives, so the information transmitted is the same as the stimulus information. As the number of stimulus alternatives is increased, errors are made, and the information transmitted is less than the stimulus information. This measure of information transmitted becomes constant above some number of alternatives, and a channel capacity – the maximum amount of information that can be transmitted through the human – has been measured.

Visual dimensions. Garner and Hake (1951) had shown how information theory can provide a measure of information transmission, and Hake and Garner (1951) carried out an experiment with stimuli consisting of pointer positions along a line. They obtained a maximum information transmission (the channel capacity) of a little over 3.0 bits, or eight stimulus categories. Eriksen and Hake (1955) carried out an equivalent experiment with judgments of visual size and obtained a channel capacity equivalent to about five stimulus categories. Hue and brightness were also used as stimulus dimensions, with roughly comparable results.

Auditory dimensions. Pollack (1952) carried out a comparable experiment with the auditory dimension of pitch and found a channel capacity equivalent to about five stimulus categories. The same result was obtained by Garner (1953) with the auditory dimension of loudness.

These are illustrative results of the earliest work done with absolute judgments within the framework of information theory. Many other experiments were carried out, and the problem area was extended to the use of multidimensional stimuli as well, but there are far too many studies to attempt any summary of them here. More complete summaries of these studies can be found in Miller (1956), a review that emphasized that, for single dimensions, about seven different levels are all that humans can use with essentially complete accuracy. Further summaries of these experiments, particularly those involving multidimensional stimuli, can be found in Garner (1962).

Pattern perception

In the study of pattern perception, the primary concept used was redundancy of patterns, especially, although not exclusively, to study pattern goodness. Attneave (1954), in a general article on this topic, suggested that the visual system attempts to describe or encode any pattern as economically as possible, that is, to encode those properties, such as boundaries, gradients, and loci of salient points, that are sufficient to identify a pattern. This argument basically states that there is redundancy in a pattern and that the visual system seeks those characteristics of a pattern that are the most important and least redundant. In an experimental paper, Attneave (1955) showed that for patterns generated from a fixed number of dots in cells of a matrix, fewer errors of identification were made with symmetrical dot patterns than with more random patterns. Thus redundancy aided identification.

Even earlier, Hochberg and McAlister (1953) had used reversible figures (Kopferman cubes, which can be seen as two- or three-dimensional). They found that the simplicity of the figure in its two-dimensional form was directly related to the amount of time the figure was seen as two-dimensional. By "simplicity," they meant the number of lines, angles, and intersections. Simplicity is easily related to the concept of redundancy, so the more redundant the figures were in two dimensions, the more readily they were perceived in that form.

Fitts, Weinstein, Rappaport, Anderson, and Leonard (1956) generated random and redundant patterns either by using random heights of six bars or by constraining them so that no two columns had the same height. They found, with a matching to sample procedure, that the random figures were discriminated more rapidly than the constrained figures, even though the constrained figures were more redundant. This result shows that redundancy may be useful in a discrimination task; that is, after all, the value of redundancy. Thus redundancy may contribute to the goodness of figures but may also make them more discriminable.

Once again, many studies on pattern perception were done, and continue to be done, using primarily the information theory concept of redundancy. A more complete summary of this work can be found in Garner (1962) and Garner (1970).

Motor skills

A last area of application to be discussed specifically is that of motor skills, and Fitts was the person primarily responsible for this work. The best example is his 1954 article. He carried out several experiments on the precision of movement. As one example, subjects were required to tap two plates back and forth, and the experimental variable was the width of the plates. In another example, subjects were required to transfer pins from one hole to another, and the experimental variable was the size of the holes with respect to the size of the pins. Fitts used the information measure by taking the logarithm of the ratio of the tolerance for the final placement to the total amplitude of movement. His reasoning was that the smaller this ratio, the more information required to carry out the task. Time per response was the dependent variable. He found that the more information required, the more time it took.

As a secondary consideration in work on motor skills, the issue of stimulus–response compatibility may be mentioned. Fitts and Seeger (1953), for example, altered the relation of a set of lights as stimuli and a set of key presses as responses. In measuring the reaction time as a function of the number of alternative stimuli, these researchers found that the simple relation between the logarithm of number of alternatives found by many researchers in addition to Hick and Hyman, whose work I described earlier, was lost with highly compatible stimulus–response relations. So motor skills are influenced by the amount of information, but efficiency of the motor skill also depends on the relation between the required motor act and the stimuli to which responses must be made.

It is of interest to note that Fitts and Seeger used reaction time in this work on motor skills and stimulus–response compatibility, just as Fitts et al. (1956) did in their work on pattern discrimination. In many of the problem areas described here, errors were still the basic measure used, but these examples make it clear that reaction time had indeed found its way back into experimental psychology.

Information theory in current psychology

What has been the long-term impact of information theory on psychology? Is it still influential, and if so, what is the nature of this influence? In discussing these questions, it is again useful to distinguish information theory as a statistical measure from the concepts that accompanied the theory.

As a measure

Amount of information. Although information theory first came into psychology with primary emphasis on its mathematical and statistical properties, it was soon clear that these more exact uses were not always of prime consideration. In many of the application areas I have discussed, data such as stimulus information were expressed in bits, yet the primary result of importance was that information was related to the number of alternative stimuli. As an *exact* measure, amount of information was not important because there was nothing in the theory that required any relation to the dependent variables used in the experiment other than that there be a monotonic relation. However, that there be some meaningful relation to the amount of information was important.

The one application area in which amount of information was crucial is the transmission of information in absolute judgment experiments to establish a channel capacity. This use has continued to the present time, although to a considerably reduced extent. Occasional research papers still occur in which bits of information are used to express a channel capacity. I review two or three such papers a year for journals even now.

Reaction time. In the initial studies of reaction time, once again, information measured in bits, or at least some logarithmic measure, was also important, because there was an expected exact relation between reaction time and amount of stimulus information. The fact of this linear relation is so well established that little research is currently being conducted on this issue.

This relation between reaction time and amount of information established so early in research using information theory brought reaction time back into human experimental psychology. A quick perusal of several recent issues of journals in what is now called "cognitive psychology" suggests that about half of the reported research uses some form of time measurement as the dependent variable. Even the now common term "information processing" connotes a time-related set of ideas. Although information measurement currently is sparsely used, its secondary consequence of the reintroduction of reaction time as a measure of great importance has made what is probably a permanent change in how experiments are conducted in cognitive psychology, and even in those areas of experimental research that would not necessarily be considered part of cognitive psychology.

As concepts

The concepts that accompanied information measurement have had a substantial effect on cognitive psychology, to the point where I would argue that the original paper on information theory by Miller and Frick (1949) could well be considered the birth date of cognitive psychology. The term "information" itself, as well as its information theory definition, is part of current cognitive psychology. Concepts such as "redundancy," "channel capacity," "coding," and so on have been so thoroughly absorbed into cognitive psychology that attribution of their origin is not even considered. To illustrate, consider a few examples:

Neisser (1966), whose book *Cognitive Psychology* probably is responsible for permanently establishing that term for the new approach to human experimental psychology (although the term had been used by others, to be discussed in other chapters of this book, before that time), used throughout the book two concepts from information theory: "coding" and "redundancy." Here we can see a direct connection between information theory and cognitive psychology, a connection that has only been strengthened by subsequent writers in cognitive psychology.

To illustrate further the insidious assimilation of the concepts from information theory, consider this quotation from a textbook on cognitive psychology by Lachman, Lachman, and Butterfield (1979, p. 68): "It is a striking fact that the word 'coding' does not appear in psychology textbooks or research papers before the publication of Shannon's theory, while since then there are entire books devoted to the topic." One such book is that of Melton and Martin (1972), which resulted from a series of papers given at a conference whose sole topic was coding. Note also the title of the Lachman et al. book: *Cognitive Psychology and Information Processing*. This conjunction of the terms "cognitive psychology" and "information processing" supports my argument that information theory was truly the forerunner of cognitive psychology.

Another concept from information theory that currently provides an active area of research is "channel capacity." That exact term is sometimes used; the term "resource limitation" is also frequently used, but it means the same thing. Furthermore, when topics such as resource allocation are studied, the allocation refers to what is going on in the human considered as a channel of communication. The concepts of information theory have indeed had a permanent impact on psychology, especially cognitive psychology.

One last example will suffice to demonstrate how diffuse has been the change in the way people think about psychological issues as a result of information theory. James Gibson, in his 1966 book, used the term "information," and a major issue for him was to distinguish information from stimulus. He continued to use the term "information" in his later writing, although it was not used in his early work or his first book, which appeared before information theory had arrived. Incidentally, Gibson denied that information in his sense is the same as that implied by information theory. Yet he also stated (p. 286): "Those features of a thing are noticed which distinguish it from other things that it is not." If ever a statement contains a definition of information in the information theory sense, that one does.

To conclude, the concepts from information theory are very much contained in current cognitive psychology. Sometimes their use is directly related to information theory, with direct attribution to it. More often, the concepts are used without awareness that they originated with information theory. At least some students of mine have been surprised to discover that concepts such as "coding," "channel capacity," and even "information" itself have not always been part of psychology. Yet, of course, they have not always been part of psychology – only since the advent of information theory. When a movement as strong as that provided by information theory occurs, it cannot help but have a pervasive influence. Information theory has had and continues to have, that influence.

References

Attneave, F. (1954). Some informational aspects of visual perception. *Psychological Review, 61,* 183–93.

Attneave, F. (1955). Symmetry, information, and memory for patterns. *American Journal of Psychology, 68,* 209–22.

Broadbent, D. E. (1957). Information theory and older approaches in psychology. *Proceedings of the 15th International Congress of Psychology* (pp. 111–15). Brussels.

Chapanis, A. (1954). The reconstruction of abbreviated printed messages. *Journal of Experimental Psychology, 48,* 496–510.

Eriksen, C. W., & Hake, H. W. (1955). Multidimensional stimulus differences and accuracy of discrimination. *Journal of Experimental Psychology, 50,* 153–60.

Faverge, J. M. (1957). Le modele de la theorie de l'information en psychologie. *Proceedings of the 15th International Congress of Psychology* (pp. 116–22). Brussels.

Fitts, P. M. (1954). The information capacity of the human motor system in controlling the amplitude of movement. *Journal of Experimental Psychology, 47,* 381–91.

Fitts, P. M., & Seeger, C. M. (1953). S–R compatibility: Spatial characteristics of stimulus and response codes. *Journal of Experimental Psychology, 46,* 199–210.

Fitts, P. M., Weinstein, M., Rappaport, M., Anderson, N., & Leonard, J. A. (1956). Stimulus correlates of visual pattern recognition. *Journal of Experimental Psychology, 51,* 1–11.

Frick, F. C., & Miller, G. A. (1951). A statistical description of operant conditioning. *American Journal of Psychology, 64,* 20–36.

Garner, W. R. (1953). An informational analysis of absolute judgments of loudness. *Journal of Experimental Psychology, 46,* 373–80.

Garner, W. R. (1962). *Uncertainty and Structure as Psychological Concepts.* New York: Wiley.

Garner, W. R. (1970). Good patterns have few alternatives. *American Scientist, 58,* 34–42.

Garner, W. R., & Carson, D. H. (1960). A multivariate solution of the redundancy of printed English. *Psychological Reports, 6,* 123–41.

Garner, W. R., & Hake, H. W. (1951). The amount of information in absolute judgments. *Psychological Review, 58,* 446–59.

Gibson, J. J. (1966). *The Senses Considered as Perceptual Systems.* Boston: Houghton Mifflin.

Hake, H. W., & Garner, W. R. (1951). The effect of presenting various numbers of discrete steps on scale reading accuracy. *Journal of Experimental Psychology, 42,* 358–66.

Hartley, R. V. L. (1928). Transmission of information. *Bell System Technical Journal, 7,* 535–63.

Hick, W. E. (1952). On the rate of gain of information. *Quarterly Journal of Experimental Psychology, 4,* 11–26.

Hochberg, J. E., & McAlister, E. (1953). A quantitative approach to figural "goodness." *Journal of Experimental Psychology, 46,* 361–4.

Hyman, R. (1953). Stimulus information as a determinant of reaction time. *Journal of Experimental Psychology, 45,* 188–96.

Lachman, R., Lachman, J. L., & Butterfield, E. C. (1979). *Cognitive Psychology and Information Processing.* Hillsdale, N.J.: Erlbaum.

Leonard, J. A. (1958). Partial advance information in a choice reaction task. *British Journal of Psychology, 49,* 89–96.

Melton, A. W., & Martin, E. (eds.). (1972). *Coding Processes in Human Memory.* Washington, D.C.: Winston.

Miller, G. A. (1951). *Language and Communication.* New York: McGraw-Hill.

Miller, G. A. (1953). What is information measurement? *American Psychologist, 8,* 3–11.

Miller, G. A. (1956). The magical number seven, plus or minus two. *Psychological Review, 63,* 81–97.

Miller, G. A. (1958). Free recall of redundant strings of letters. *Journal of Experimental Psychology, 56,* 485–91.

Miller, G. A., Bruner, J. S., & Postman, L. (1954). Familiarity of letter sequences and tachistoscopic identification. *Journal of General Psychology, 50,* 129–39.

Miller, G. A., & Frick, F. C. (1949). Statistical behavioristics and sequences of responses. *Psychological Review, 56,* 311–24.

Miller, G. A., & Friedman, E. A. (1957). The reconstruction of mutilated English texts. *Information and Control, 1,* 38–55.

Miller, G. A., Heise, G. A., & Lichten, W. (1951). The intelligibility of speech as a function of the context of the test materials. *Journal of Experimental Psychology, 41,* 329–35.

Miller, G. A., & Selfridge, J. A. (1950). Verbal context and the recall of meaningful material. *American Journal of Psychology, 63,* 176–85.

Neisser, U. (1966). *Cognitive Psychology.* New York: Appleton-Century-Crofts.

Newman, E. B., & Gerstman, L. S. (1952). A new method for analyzing printed English. *Journal of Experimental Psychology, 44,* 114–25.

Nyquist, H. (1924). Certain factors affecting telegraph speed. *Bell System Technical Journal, 3,* 324–46.

Pollack, I. (1952). The information of elementary auditory displays. *Journal of the Accoustical Society of America, 24,* 745–9.

Pollack, I. (1959). Message uncertainty and message reception. *Journal of the Acoustical Society of America, 31,* 1500–8.

Quastler, H. (Ed.). (1955). *Information Theory in Psychology: Problems and Methods.* Glencoe, Ill.: Free Press.

Shannon, C. E. (1948). A mathematical theory of communication. *Bell System Technical Journal, 27,* 379–423, 623–56.

Shannon, C. E. (1951). Prediction and entropy of printed English. *Bell System Technical Journal, 30,* 50–64.

3   Writing *Plans...*

Eugene Galanter

Almost as though my heart had stopped (I was always watchful of the states of my interior), the staccato of the small plane's engine ceased. The engine's sound was replaced now by the vagrant slashing of the propeller driven by the waning air speed. The silence at first induced a soothing sensation complementary to the usual irritability induced by the vicious engine. I snapped to attention, my right hand withdrawn from the crank of the radio I had been trying to tune. Without an engine at 3,000 feet above the southern reach of San Francisco Bay, there was little time for whatever it is that psychologists think people do when they think. A left turn would lead to the broken ground of the eastern shore; a right turn might carry me over the western shore, past El Camino Real to some pasture. The western shore meant a shorter hike to civilization. What nonsense! "Stop planning a landing and start reviewing the possible causes." Why had the engine stopped? I found the fuel tank selector surreptitiously deselected by my instructor and reset it to "on." The engine coughed to life. I returned unexceptionally to the ground and the Center for Advanced Study in the Behavioral Sciences. There the plans several of us were delineating were of less practical but, we hoped, of greater theoretical consequence. These aeronautically prompted forward jumps of thought that spanned large segments of action would have to be accommodated. We would find a way to include intentions that could lead to trouble.

On a low hill behind Stanford University lies the campus of the Center. It was at that time, and may still be, a sprawling, redwood-modern collection of ugly buildings, looking to the visitor like the up-scale motels that dot the California highways from San Francisco to San Jose. Coming from the East, one had the strong impression that these structures were impudently temporary; a bulldozer could rake them from the earth and leave nothing for the archeologist. Yet, in those late days of the first full decade since the Second World War, it was a symbol to most of us of the vigor and importance of our new science. We were on the threshold of deep insights into human nature.

I had been a visiting fellow at the Psychoacoustic Laboratory at Harvard,

36

working with Smitty Stevens on sensory scaling. Around me in that basement refuge were the young turks of the new experimental psychology, and over in the Yard in Emerson Hall, and in various warrens behind Mass Avenue and down as far as MIT were the "mathematikers," the theoreticians. All of us were busily enhancing the central ideas of psychology, ideas first promulgated by that bland British physician, David Hartley, who in 1746 had laid down the basis for a scientific investigation of mental life – the associative network. As methodological behaviorists, many of us were constrained by our principles to a theoretical position that we found uncomfortable. All, that is, except (mostly) George A. Miller, who believed that talk was the heart of the human mind, and Fred Skinner and his recent William James Lectures notwithstanding, talk was not an associative stochastic process.

George and I chatted in the halls occasionally, and once in a while we teamed up at lunch against Skinner, Stevens, or Jack Beebe-Center (a long-time Harvard psychologist who studied taste and smell, as well as sailboat hulls) on the side of the one who had the weaker position in the argument, whether about lobster pots, wide boat hulls, or sensory scales. But on the whole, our connection was primarily social. Smitty kept me seriously busy, and my philosophical biases – antiphysiological and proformalist – aimed me in other directions. Analysis, not synthesis, was my callow interest.

It was consequently unexpected when I received an invitation to the Stanford Center for the year 1959–60, tendered, I learned, at the request of George. I was part of a group of psychologists and near-psychologists that included, besides George, Jim Jenkins, Karl Pribram, Helen Peak, Charley Osgood, Michael Argyle, and frequent visits by the Stanford University psychologists. The agenda that was laid on was for the development of an experimental and theoretical capability to study natural language and communication. The bona fides for my inclusion were, I believe, my experimental and technical competence, my freeranging interests, and, perhaps most importantly, my willing suspension of disbelief. Also, by an odd accident, I understood some of the software aspects of serial (von Neumann) computers. That knowledge stemmed from associations with the philosophy and engineering academics in the postwar Philadelphia area. There, along with members of the local chapter of the Society of Industrial and Applied Mathematics, the Moore School of Electrical Engineering, and the Penn Philosophy Department, I was tutored, mainly by John Myhill, Murray Gerstenhaber, and Nelson Goodman in computational logic, Turing machines, and the implications of the Godel and Skolem–Lowenheim theorems. Although I had no name for it at the time, I believed that nonnumerical algorithmic procedures might be an alternative to closed-form analytical equations to express the structure of human behavior. Along with this computer analogy, I believed there was a potential for the use of symbolic logic as a structural or descriptive basis for psychological theory. These ideas stemmed in part from the powerful influences of Sidney Morganbesser, Zellig Harris, Betty Flower, and Noam Chomsky. We were all looking for nonnumerical representations of psychic structure.

As the glorious California autumn passed and I tired of watching the lizards shoot up the long spears of cactus outside my study window, I grew more and more tense and uncomfortable. I needed a purpose. My living quarters out on Old La Honda Road included a swimming pool, and so my role turned into that of social director and party organizer. The parties at the pool started at around 5 PM and ran normally until 10 or 11, when we all dispersed for dinner, supper really. In bed by 2 AM meant that I was up and functional by 10, with little to do until party time. I needed an active enterprise and found it – learning to fly at the Palo Alto airport. I made the physical act of piloting a plane an object of my own scientific concern. How could a person learn to do it, and more, how could a person do it at all? George, although enjoying the parties, must also have felt at loose ends about his own creative efforts. He had plenty of jobs to get done, but most of them were primarily administrative and organizational: seminars, conferences, and such. We took to meeting and brooding in his study after flying and before party time, along with Karl Pribram, our favorite neurosurgeon and physiological psychologist, who was always present to keep us in contact with bloody reality. The agenda of these discussions was never clear to me or, I think, to the others.

The moment at which we agreed to write a book (as an easier exercise than running experiments the way Jenkins and some of the other psychologists were doing) came as a surprise to the three of us, I think. It was certainly a surprise to me. George had recently finished reading Kenneth Boulding's *The Image,* which had been written at the Center, and said that we should do a similar speculative project. The aim, we all agreed, was to replace behaviorism (really our name for associationism) and trivial experimentation (the T-maze and the Skinner box) with the new insights and maybe even the new technology from computational logic, linguistics, and neurophysiology. The impetus for this direction of our effort came from a conference held at the Center, which I believe George organized.

It was a wild affair. The people who participated were mathematical psychologists and empirically oriented experimental psychologists who tore into each other with a viciousness I had rarely witnessed. The nub of the argument was a strange issue that might be summarized as psychological complexity. The argument from experimentalists like Doug Lawrence and theorists such as Leon Festinger proceeded along the following lines. Mathematical theories of psychological phenomena were, at best, only calculation schemes for an odd assortment of descriptive statistics. These statistics did no more than summarize data from trivial experiments. Not only did these theories fail to explicate the psychology behind the data, but by their attention to description they were deflecting us from understanding important processes and functions. In part the theories imposed this restriction by insisting upon a criterion for understanding (quantitative description and prediction) that constrained experiments to the limiting abstractions of these models. This resulted in making the more important psychological questions trivial.

Furthermore, the experimentalists screamed, these theories were an "attractive nuisance" that seduced bright young people into a dead-end endeavor. All the clever graduate students in experimental psychology wanted to dazzle their mentors by replacing thought and insight with slick little models. The crux of this argument could finally be appreciated by noting that the real problems of psychology were too complicated to be appropriately modeled by experiments that were simple enough to yield data that would crunch in the theoretical mill.

The mathematically committed theoreticians, like Bill McGill and Bob Bush, countered, of course, with the classic statement that "this is only the beginning; tomorrow our theories, like Heinz catsup, will be thick and rich." Others in their camp may have said, "people are not that complicated; it is only the random components of their behavior that make people seem difficult to understand." From our point of view, the experimentalists were correct. We were in the middle of a revision of our own theoretical leanings. This local state of affairs made us less sanguine with the technical theoretical aspects of some of our own previous work. However, there was a central, and to us a telling, point in the theoretician's argument. Without theory, data were of only accidental importance. The idea that the theoreticians at this conference failed to stress or even perhaps to acknowledge was that there might be other logical and internally consistent modes of theory construction besides the analytical and mathematical.

The energy for all of this agitation in psychology came, I believe, from outside. Five years earlier, biology, that forlorn science, had exploded into a coherent discipline with the vital promise of real elixirs to heal the body and mend the mind. The potential to deliver a box full of scientifically substantial products that advance the human condition is what gives any science its social justification. Without that implicit promise and eventual fulfillment, these enterprises are a secular retreat for amateur academics.

Psychologists, like the biologists earlier, also lacked a viable application of their science. Mental health had been announced as our object of application, with little in the way of theory or data to justify the cost of training practitioners. Engineering and human factors psychology, then as now, was a tatty collection of design data that could hardly be published, let alone sold at a profit. Only differential psychology in the form of tests and training devices had made a market impact, but the implications of these findings for packaging education had not (then or now) found an adequate and accepted theory to wrap the bundle.

We knew that without an empirically supported conceptual base the field of psychology would continue to drift from one set of technical observations to another.

A famous botanist, before the DNA revisions of his field, used to show me graphs relating exquisitely measured radiant energy incident to the green plants in his laboratory and their growth. He contrasted his science (evidence the graphs) with the work of his colleagues, who merely collected specimens. There was plenty of similar make-work in our field, and indeed the lashing recriminations at this conference illuminated the anxieties we all felt – anxieties that derived from the self-imposed limits of the classical behaviorist paradigm.

A few days later, the three of us were arguing about what the conceptual basis for a new theory of psychology could be. At one point, George proposed that we examine some intentional human act.

"Flying a plane," I suggested.

"No – too much. How about crossing a street? An equally dangerous act in the Bay area," Karl responded. I went to the blackboard and started a flow chart. The boxes, lines, and arrows snaked around the board as step after step was drawn.

"No," George said, "all that stuff on the board is only a string of reentrant reflexes. Let a whole piece of the action be repeated until it's finished."

"How will it know?" from Karl.

"With a cybernetic test," replied George.

"But how do I draw it?" I asked.

"Like this," said George, and the TOTE replacement for the reflex was designed.

Norbert Wiener's *Cybernetics* had already proposed feedback as a control system that may be represented in behavior larger than the vegetative. He also saw that the test sensors need not be built in as part of the original design, but could be added later as a product of experience. What George envisioned at that point was the potency of arranging feedback units hierarchically. These units of control consisted of a test protocol, a kind of perceptual sample against which behavioral consequences would be matched, and an operational element to control the activity. Test–Operate–Test–Exit: The TOTE was our prototype to replace the reflex. The nesting of lower-level TOTEs inside the operational phase of a functionally superior unit was a powerful explanatory mechanism. This design feature – the hierarchical organization of behavior – permitted us to bypass the perennial problem of levels of explanation and at a stroke made the need for molar and molecular analysis redundant. Our metaphor of action was complete almost from the start. We added little before launching into the task of revising the hoary associationist concepts of the accepted canon. You may recall that Tom

Kuhn was a fellow that year, busy writing his exciting history of science from the point of view of revolutionary paradigms.

With the gist of a theory of action in hand, we thought to turn to the input stage of the system. The test phase must surely have a perceptual input, but could we design it? We agreed quickly among ourselves that the serious question of examining how inputs from the external and internal environments were combined was beyond our competence, and probably beyond the available facts. The nature of the image as a distillation of many parallel coprocessors (as we might state it today) had to be shelved. Our way to bypass perception was to attend to the relation between images and plans. Although we had listened to Lashley, who first complained about gestalt psychology leaving the person unmoved by thought, we were unprepared to abandon the happy and active person reveling in a model world that needed no analysis. Even though the perceptual systems deliver much nonredundant information through parallel channels that may sometimes be contradictory (at least locally), we could not do more than say that they must combine somehow to form an image. For a start on a new metaphor, this was, we concluded, enough.

Although we could leave the image as an exercise to the interested reader, motivation and intention were nettles that had to be grasped. Our solution, which is not entirely unsatisfactory even today, was to attend to the brightly lit part of the mindscape: intentions. Here the idea of a plan offered a made-to-order solution to Zeigarnik's problem of the uncompleted task energizing recall and action. Intentions are merely uncompleted plans. Values, the magnitudes of desire and aversion associated with components of plans, were to be added to the test phases as needed to impute affective color to the observed behavior. What I think we all may have had in mind about value was a kind of utility measure that tinted the image. We could overwrite a super plan with a chroma of value, lodge it in the image, and so accommodate components of plans with values less than zero. The energy problem was left to the biologists and the measurement of utility to the decision theorists.

With these concepts in place, there still remained several other technical problems. The single most intractable one, now as then, was the experimental question. How do you study an unobservable phenomenon? Introspection is a possibility, but its history had given it a bad press. We turned to the natural adjunct of the practical scientist, the working model. There is no need here to rehearse the problems and pitfalls of simulation. We all respect the concepts of necessity and sufficiency, and yet a really clever robot is impressive. The self-guided torpedo or mechanical turtle had opened our thinking to the cybernetic model. We need only to attach these ideas to the digital computer to incorporate an empirical testing scheme into our armchair psychology. Of course, there was quite a bit of speculation that could be aborted by behavioral experiments, but testing alternative mediational mechanisms with common behavioral consequences was going to be the name of the cognitive science game – we conjectured.

Scientific psychology had not yet hatched that new generation of ingenious experimentalist-theoreticians who could, for example, study the rotation of mental images or the mode of access to remembered events by behavioral methods. As a consequence of such thinking, the computer would be our set piece. We were living during a period when the idea that fast, simple computers would be easily and affordably available in a few years was regarded as certain. Although we had considered the relevance and importance of powerful programming languages as a compelling necessity for the notions that we espoused, we could hardly produce a top-level flow chart for analysis, let alone the detailed code that would be necessary to simulate even the simplest act. We recognized the need for procedural languages to make such programs practical, and for sophisticated operating systems to support them, but they remained for us, temporarily at least, terra incognita. What we clearly failed to recognize at the time was the overriding importance of the computer as an experimental device. We did not catch its signal potential contribution to cognitive science. This machine, with its ability to control complicated input–output relations, would open the way to new and complex kinds of behavioral studies.

As the writing on *Plans* . . . progressed, we touched on many topics that had not been central to experimental psychology. Indeed, we anticipated that our contributions might be more appreciated in the outlands of the science. It was, consequently, with some hesitation and anxiety that we sent our first draft, complete with no citations, to our friends and colleagues. They hated it. Where were the footnotes? What were the references to X's (for X read "my") papers? Where were the data in support of such dream work? It was depressing as, each day, a new fusillade of criticism and derision arrived. Karl and I were for damning the torpedoes and publishing at once. George (thankfully) displayed a cooler hand.

"We will get the footnotes," he said.

We moaned and went about the task. This period of grace also allowed us to clean up some of the more egregious proposals and to lay in some more experimental-sounding text. Thank goodness for our pals at the Center. They held our hands and gave us the sympathy we needed to sustain us during this dark journey of the soul.

It came as some surprise to find that critical considerations that we now see as valid were, in that period, passed by. Our first substantive chapters on instincts and motor skills and habits received little comment. Yet in these sections we missed several opportunities to apply the computer metaphor. Inborn skills represent a strong analogy to the operating systems of a computer, as distinct from the programs they serve. The potential differences in such systems may suggest directions to search for individual differences in human information processing, as Broadbent's recent work could be taken to suggest.

In our discussion of motor skills, we failed to examine the role of ballistic strings of sophisticated, but essentially unguided, actions that had been neatly described by Lashley. These chunked behavior sequences must coexist within a system that tolerates TOTEs.

It also became clear within the decade that many purposes were served by behavior that could be characterized as ballistic: not merely the microacts of saccadic eye movements, but also such molar behavior as landing an airplane. These stripped-out sequential actions depended for their success on the running off of unguided chains of activity, the anathema of *Plans* . . . And yet the form of these ballistic endeavors, although clearly of an associationistic heritage, had been brought into being by paced experience with feedback processes. Indeed, much of the housekeeping that accompanied ballistic actions, the background acts that keep the wings level, were clearly servo-controlled.

With a new metaphor in hand and plausible stories about how things in the mind work, we undertook a review of topics that were normally absent from experimental texts. Of all of these excursions into uncharted kingdoms, two seem to have been most fruitful, one by its success: our discussions of memory and retrieval, and the other by its failure: motor skills and habits. The idea of a temporary "working memory" or buffer has succeeded in capturing an important distinction about how people store information of various kinds. Our ideas concerning retrieval from permanent memory, based on linguistic organizational structures, have also been taken up and shown to be (in part at least) central to long-term memory. This division of memory into short and long term, and the central importance of coding and retrieval, have quietly changed our conceptions of the central mechanism underlying human intelligence. As such, these notions may yet inform aspects of education and training, as well as serving to provide tools for testing procedures to enhance and restore faulty or damaged retention systems.

The analysis of motor skills and habits succeeded in concealing the essentially open-loop feature of much of motor behavior. What lay behind this notion was that motor skills were a servo-controlled system, even when the components were sufficiently habitual that the instantiating plan could not be recognized in the activity. The idea was that the scaffolding of the plan for skill acquisition remains as the matrix within which the actions are forever after performed. The recent interest in and new research on motor skills, slips, errors, and accidents has replaced the classic cybernetic picture of motor control, which earlier seemed the almost perfect rendition of the feedback loop. In his Foreword to the new edition of *Plans* . . . that has just appeared, Donald Broadbent makes this point quite effectively, and provides references to the new work that is reshaping many of our views on motor skills. My own experiments on extremely short interresponse times had shaken my faith in our original conception of motor habits. The more recent research in this area, depending as it does on micro-computer technology, promises to ignite a new interest in topics on motor control.

This then is a jaundiced look back, full of revisionist fervor, at the birth of cognitive psychology, as evidenced by the book that named the discipline. It serves, if nothing more, as a testament to the person we honor here who led many of us into the future.

4   George Miller's data and the development of methods for representing cognitive structures

Roger N. Shepard

According to a prevalent view, cognitive science is the science of systems for knowledge representation and information processing. Because the knowledge that must be represented and the information that must be processed come to us from a complicated world of haphazard events and arbitrary conventions, the internalized knowledge and processes that govern our mental lives and our behavior are similarly complicated, haphazard, and arbitrary. This view leads to an engineering approach to modeling the human mind by patching together specialized knowledge structures and ad hoc procedures to deal with various particular circumstances: features for recognizing the handwritten letter *a*, heuristics for terminating consideration of an alternative move in chess, scripts for dining out in a restaurant, and so on.

A less widely represented view, which I find appealing, is that cognitive science is the science of general principles governing mental processes, much as physical science is the science of general principles governing physical processes. In fact, the mind is guided by general principles, in this view, precisely because it has evolved in a world constrained by general principles. An individual who has internalized the enduring regularities of the world need not learn those regularities by trial and possibly fatal error. True, events in the mental world, just as in the physical world, often seem capricious: Because we cannot completely know the relevant boundary conditions, the trajectory of a chain of associations, like the trajectory of a falling leaf, may be quite unpredictable. Nevertheless, such trajectories may conform alike to abstract laws of thought or of mechanics, respectively. And the laws of thought may ultimately be rooted in the laws of mechanics (Shepard, 1984a, 1984b).

Beginning with my 1955 dissertation at Yale, I have been developing an ar-

Preparation of this chapter was supported by National Science Foundation Grant No. BNS 85-11685 to Stanford University. The research on which it is based was extensively supported, as well, by the Bell Telephone Laboratories (now the AT&T Bell Laboratories), where much of the work was carried out over the years by me and by my associates: Phipps Arabie, J. Douglas Carroll, Jih-Jie Chang, Stephen Johnson, Joseph Kruskal, and Myron Wish.

gument that general psychological laws can be obtained by formulating those laws in relation to a "psychological space," just as general physical laws are formulated in relation to physical space. Because we seldom if ever reencounter exactly the same situation, one of the most essential psychological laws must be a law of generalization – specifying how the probability that a response, originally learned to one stimulus, falls off with the dissimilarity between the test stimulus and the original stimulus. However, no invariant law of generalization is possible if the independent variable, dissimilarity, is defined in terms of the physical difference between the stimuli – for example, in terms of the difference of frequencies of tones (as with the whistles that Pavlov used in testing his dogs). The form of the obtained "gradient of generalization" then depends on the particular dimension of the stimulus difference used (frequency of tone, wavelength of light, etc.) and the particular species used (human, dog, pigeon, etc.), and can even be nonmonotonic (that is, can increase at certain larger distances, such as between frequencies differing by an octave, or between wavelengths at the opposite red and violet ends of the visible spectrum). (See Blackwell & Schlosberg, 1943; Bush & Mosteller, 1951; Lashley & Wade, 1946; Shepard, 1955, 1965, 1987.)

The approach that I have pursued is to determine a psychological representation of the stimuli such that psychological laws, when formulated in terms of this representation, take on an invariant form. Thus, I proposed that we represent the stimuli in an abstract psychological space determined just by the requirement that the law of generalization have the same functional form regardless of the dimensions along which the stimuli differ or the species tested. Although this sounds quite circular, I have demonstrated that it is not (Shepard, 1962b, 1965) and that it can yield information both about the proper psychological representation of the stimuli and about the functional form of the invariant psychological law – a law that closely approximates an exponential decay function in the case of generalization (Shepard, 1955, 1958b, 1984b, 1986, 1987).

In the years since 1955, my associates and I, first at the Bell Telephone Laboratories and then at Stanford, have developed a series of multidimensional scaling and clustering methods that yield informative psychological representations and, at the same time, permit the determination of general psychological laws. The development and testing of these methods would have been unmotivated and artificial in the absence of psychologically significant sets of similarity and confusion data. I have chosen to use this occasion to review the central roles played, in our development of these methods, by two of George Miller's exceptionally rich and challenging sets of psycholinguistic data – one from his earlier period of concern with the psychoacoustics of speech perception (Miller & Nicely, 1955) and one from his later period of concern with the semantic structure of the subjective lexicon (Miller, 1969).

A little background

Through a series of fortunate circumstances, George Miller's work came forcefully to my attention during the early stages of my career. My first exposure was through a graduate course on psycholinguistics at Yale that used his new textbook, *Language and Communication* (Miller, 1951). I had already been thinking about the representation of stimuli as points in a psychological space, and I was intrigued by the portrayals, in this book, of speech sounds in a parameter space – for example, the two-dimensional space of front-to-back and high-to-low articulation of vowels. When George later presented a colloquium at Yale, we were astonished to see that the author of our authoritative text was no more than a decade older than ourselves. I was electrified by this colloquium, which had the soon-to-become-famous title "The Magical Number Seven, Plus or Minus Two."

When the time then came to constitute my Ph.D. orals committee, the Yale Department of Psychology found that all of the mathematically oriented faculty members in the department were already on my dissertation committee and, hence, that the department could not satisfy the university's requirement that there be a member of the examining committee who was not a member of the dissertation committee. In taking the unusual step of seeking an examiner from another university, the department naturally found itself turning to their recent, mathematically sophisticated visitor, George Miller. A year later, George, who subsequently told me that he too had come to the conclusion that the problem of similarity was *the* central problem of psychology, invited me to join him at Harvard for a two-year postdoctoral fellowship.

That period (1956–8) was one of extraordinary intellectual challenge and ferment. Between Harvard, MIT, and the MIT Lincoln Laboratory, the Cambridge area was alive with young researchers making or soon to make major contributions to what was later to be called "cognitive science." In addition to George Miller (and his later close associate, Jerome Bruner), these included Bob Bush, Duncan Luce, Fred Mosteller, and Saul Sternberg (in mathematical psychology); Ulric Neisser and George Sperling (in experimental psychology); David Green and John Swets (in psychophysics); Bert Green and Warren Torgerson (in psychometrics); Marvin Minsky and Oliver Selfridge (in artificial intelligence and computer science); and Roger Brown and Noam Chomsky (in psycholinguistics and linguistics). A number of us regularly met at an informal evening discussion group held at MIT, known as the "Pretzel Twist."

It was during this period that George and I, through my association with George, came under the influence of two developments that were soon to redirect the evolution of cognitive science. One was Chomsky's formalization of grammar and the characterization of it as the manifestation of an innate schematism of the human mind. The other was Newell and Simon's development of a methodology, and an associated information processing language (IPL), for the computer simulation of complex human cognitive processes. I still remember the afternoon I came into George's office (then in the basement of Harvard's Memorial Hall) to find him on his hands and knees poring over the pages of the prepublication manuscript of Chomsky's (1957) *Syntactic Structures,* which he had spread across the floor. I remember, too, George's and my participation in the workshop on computer simulation (and IPL) that Newell and Simon conducted in Santa Monica, California, during the last summer of my two-year fellowship with George.

My own first attempt at computer programming occurred, somewhat earlier, during this same two-year period. (Yale, where I had recently completed my graduate studies, still did not have an electronic computer – though my principal advisor, Carl Hovland, confided to me that the university had formed an official committee to accept the gift of a computer, should one be tendered.) At this time, Harvard did receive the gift of a Remington Rand Univac 1. As I recall, it was about the size of an automobile (though considerably taller), held 1,000 words in active memory (in the form of recycling acoustic patterns in mercury delay lines), and had to be programmed laboriously in machine code. This first encounter with a programmable computer was, nevertheless, enough to open my eyes to its potential for attacking the problem, posed in my dissertation, of discovering structures hidden in generalization and confusion data.

So, in 1958, I welcomed the offer of a position at the Bell Telephone Laboratories, where I would for the first time have access to what by the standards of those days were powerful and rapidly expanding computing facilities (and where I was subsequently to be joined by my former Harvard colleagues, George Sperling and, later, Saul Sternberg). Taking advantage of the now available scientific programming language FORTRAN, I began in earnest the development of a computer-based method for extracting structures and functional laws hidden in psychological data. After demonstrating the effectiveness of the first method of nonmetric multidimensional scaling (Shepard, 1962a, 1962b), I was soon joined in the effort to refine and extend this general approach – initially at the Bell Laboratories, by the mathematicians Joseph Kruskal and Stephen Johnson and by the psychometricians J. Douglas Carroll and Jih-Jie Chang (both of whom I brought to the Labs); and later, at Stanford, by my co-workers Phipps Arabie and Jim Cunningham and, independently, by Amos Tversky and his co-workers.

Despite my geographical separation from George, he continued to exert a significant influence on this new line of work through the challenge that his extraordinarily rich psycholinguistic data provided for our development of new methods for the analysis of similarity data.

Representation of structures in Miller and Nicely's data on perceptual confusions among sixteen consonants

One of the many ways in which Miller has influenced the field of psychology has been by identifying and mastering formal theories and quantitative techniques newly developed in other disciplines, introducing them to psychology, and applying them himself to significant psychological problems with telling effect. The major role that Miller played in introducing Chomsky's transformational grammar to the psycholinguistic community is but one example. His study with his collaborator, Patricia Nicely, provides an earlier double example in which notions both of articulatory features taken from linguistics, and of information transmission, taken from the mathematical theory of communication, were jointly brought to bear on the problem of speech perception.

Overview of Miller and Nicely's consonants study

Miller and Nicely (1955) asked listeners to identify which of sixteen common English consonants initiated each auditorally presented syllable, consisting simply of the to-be-identified consonant uniformly followed by the single vowel /ɑ/, ("ah," as in *father*). The sixteen consonants included the voiceless stops /p/, /t/, /k/, ("pa," "ta," "ka"), the corresponding voiced stops /b/, /d/, /g/, ("ba," "da," "ga"), the voiceless fricatives /f/, /θ/, /s/, /ʃ/, ("fa," "tha," "sa," "sha"), the corresponding voiced fricatives /v/, /ð/, /z/, /ʒ/, ("va," "tha," "za," "zha"), and the two nasals /m/, /n/, ("ma" and "na"). The consonants differ also according to their place of articulation – in the orders listed, from those in which the constriction of the air passage is formed forward in the mouth (as in the bilabials /p/ and /b/, and the labiodentals /f/ and /v/) to those in which the constriction is formed toward the back (as in the glottals /k/ and /g/, and the sibilants /ʃ/ and /ʒ/). All of the back fricatives, or sibilants, /s/, /z/, /ʃ/, and /ʒ/ are also distinguished by their longer duration.

In order to provide evidence bearing both on the theoretical issue of the acoustic carriers of such articulatory features and on the practical issue of the design of speech communication systems, Miller and Nicely included seventeen different conditions – in which the signal-to-noise ratio varied over a range from +12 to −18 dB and in which low or high frequencies were differentially filtered out of the signal. For each of these seventeen conditions, Miller and Nicely obtained a 16 × 16 confusion matrix tabulating the frequency with which each particular consonant was misidentified as each other consonant.

On the basis of their information-theoretic covariance analyses, Miller and Nicely reached the following conclusions: (1) The total information about the consonants was, to a good approximation, transmitted as if through five channels corresponding to the five specified features: voicing, nasality, affrication, duration, and place of articulation. (2) The features of voicing and nasality accounted for the greatest portions of the information transmitted, and did so particularly when the high frequencies were masked (by adding noise or by decreasing the cutoff of a low-pass filter). (3) As the low frequencies were removed, however, information about voicing and nasality was lost, along with information about the other features – though least rapidly for the feature that Miller and Nicely called "duration."

Although an investigation of the perception of speech sounds would not have been out of place at the Bell Telephone Laboratories, I was principally attracted to the paper by Miller and Nicely as a source of data on which to test new methods of analysis. At the same time, though, the methods of multidimensional scaling on which I was then working did seem to offer some potential advantages even for the purposes of understanding speech perception. Miller and Nicely's covariance analysis would not necessarily reveal deviations from the framework of the five articulatory features assumed in that analysis. Possibly those particular features did not constitute the optimum set. Moreover, some unnoticed interactions could remain even among those five features. Multidimensional scaling does not require us to specify in advance what dimensions or even how many dimensions are to be used in accounting for the data.

Structure revealed by (two-way) multidimensional scaling

In multidimensional scaling, a spatial representation of the n stimuli as n points in a suitably low-dimensional space is sought such that the similarities between the stimuli (in the two-way $n \times n$ matrix of similarity data) are monotonically related to distances between the corresponding points– that is, such that points corresponding to more similar stimuli are closer together (Shepard, 1958, 1962a, 1962b). The hope is that the spatial configuration will tell us something about the underlying psychological structure and dimensions of the stimuli. Subcases include the so-called *nonmetric* multidimensional scaling of Shepard (1962a, 1962b) and Kruskal (1964a, 1964b), in which no further specification is made of the form of the monotonic function; and a type of *metric* multidimensional scaling, in which the function is specified to have a particular form – in the applications considered here, an exponential form (Chang & Shepard, 1966; and, for its precursors, Shepard, 1957, 1958b; Torgerson, 1952).

Preliminary analyses of the data that Miller and Nicely obtained from their six *unfiltered* conditions – in which they varied the noise level but imposed no differential filtering of high or low frequencies – indicated that the ratios of perceptual distances between the consonants and, by implication, the shape of the configuration of those consonants in psychological space, remained essentially invariant

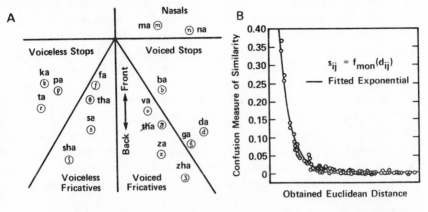

Figure 4.1 (A) Two-dimensional spatial representation for sixteen consonants obtained by applying multidimensional scaling to the confusion data combined from Miller and Nicely's (1955) six unfiltered conditions. (B) Plot showing the fit of Miller and Nicely's data to an exponential decay function of distances between points in the spatial representation. [Adapted, with permission, from Shepard (1972), copyright McGraw-Hill, and, in the present form, from Shepard (1980), copyright American Association for the Advancement of Science.]

over the whole -18 to $+12$ dB range of signal-to-noise ratio (Shepard, 1972). Accordingly, in order to obtain one maximally stable and representative solution, I combined the data from these six unfiltered conditions into a single 16×16 matrix of confusion data. To this single most representative matrix I then applied both nonmetric and metric multidimensional scaling.

The nonmetric analysis yielded a relation between the confusion data and underlying distances that approximated the expected exponential decay function. It also produced an interpretable spatial configuration with, however, some local "degeneracies," in which the points for some of the most confusable consonants collapsed on top of each other (see Shepard, 1974). The metric analysis (namely, that described by Chang & Shepard, 1966), by *assuming* an exponential shape for the function, avoided the degeneracies and furnished an even more fully interpretable two-dimensional configuration (Shepard, 1972, 1974).

Figure 4.1A displays this latter two-dimensional configuration in the orientation into which it was rotated for convenience of interpretation. The goodness of fit of the confusion data to an exponential function of Euclidean distance in this configuration is evident in Figure 4.1B. In fact, the configuration and exponential function jointly accounted for over 99 percent of the variance – a testimony both to the validity of the exponential function and to the impressive orderliness of Miller and Nicely's data.

However, if the sixteen consonants differ with respect to as many as the five distinctive features posited by Miller and Nicely, why was I able to account for 99 percent of the variance of their data by means of a configuration in a space with only two dimensions? By means of the various dividing lines and labels in Figure 4.1A, I have tried to indicate how this space, though only two-dimensional, actually accommodates all five of Miller and Nicely's proposed features.

Globally, the horizontal dimension separates the voiceless consonants, on the left, from the voiced consonants, on the right. The vertical dimension then orders the consonants essentially according to their place of articulation – such that the bilabials /p/, /b/, and /m/ and labiodentals /f/ and /v/, in which the constriction of the air passage is formed at the front of the mouth, appear toward the top of the configuration, whereas the back fricatives /ʃ/ and /ʒ/ and the voiced glottal /g/, in which the constriction is formed toward the back, appear at the bottom. Within the fricatives especially, there is a perfect ordering from front to back articulation, both for the voiceless fricatives, /f/, /θ/, /s/, and /ʃ/, and for their voiced counterparts, /v/, /ð/, /z/, and /ʒ/.

The other features included by Miller and Nicely also have orderly representations within this same two-dimensional space. The two nasals /m/ and /n/, in accordance with their voicing and relatively frontal articulation, are represented at the top right. The four long-duration sibilants /s/, /z/, /ʃ/, and /ʒ/, in accordance with their back articulation, are represented at the bottom. And the fricatives and stops are segregated into central and peripheral locations on the horizontal dimension, that is, with the eight fricatives arrayed in parallel voiceless and voiced columns down the center, and with the six stops horizontally separated into the voiceless stops, /p/, /t/, and /k/, at the far left and the corresponding voiced stops, /b/, /d/, and /g/, at the far right.

Thus all five of Miller and Nicely's features were preserved, but flattened out, so to speak, into a lower dimensional space – much as the sides of a box might be opened out onto a flat surface. The stops, rather than extending into a third dimension, opened out to the sides in the two-dimensional plane; the nasals, rather than extending into a fourth dimension, opened out into the top of the plane; and the long-duration sibilants, rather than extending into a fifth dimension, opened out into the bottom of the plane. Such a flattening into a two-dimensional plane is possible here because it is generally consistent with that plane's global dimensions of voicing and place of articulation. Moreover, any resistance to this flattening is reduced by the asymptotic leveling of the exponential function for large distances (see Fig. 4.1B), because the widely differing large distances, which primarily determine whether such flattening will or will not permit a good fit, all correspond to nearly zero similarity values.

However, this flattening may also reflect the influence of acoustic features of the stimuli that do not entirely correspond to Miller and Nicely's five articulatory features. The deviations are most evident in the case of the stop consonants. The wide separation between the voiceless and voiced stops, for example, may reflect the special distinctiveness conferred on the voiceless stops by the initial high-frequency noise burst that accompanies (initial) voiceless stops only. (This separation may also reflect subtle differences between the voiceless and voiced stops in the pitch transitions of their second formants to the following vowel ɑ; see Soli & Arabie, 1979; Wish & Carroll, 1974.)

These same acoustic factors may also explain two more local but, as we shall see, consistent deviations. First, although the front voiceless stop p grouped with the other voiceless stops, /t/ and /k/, in accordance with the distinctive feature scheme, the corresponding front voiced stop, /b/, did not group with the other voiced stops, /d/ and /g/, but instead with the front voiced fricative /v/. Second, the voiceless stops alone failed to exhibit the expected ordering from front to back articulation: /p/, /t/, /k/. Here an inspection of sound spectograms for these consonants (presented in Carroll & Wish, 1974) indicates that /t/, rather than the farther back /k/, manifests the highest-frequency initial noise burst. This may account for its relative downward displacement in the direction of the voiceless sibilants /s/ and /ʃ/, which are characterized by the presence of similarly high-frequency noise.

In sum, multidimensional scaling yielded results that are generally consistent with the conclusions reached by Miller and Nicely on the basis of their more structured analysis. But multidimensional scaling also provided the following new results: (1) The confusion data can be accommodated within a two-dimensional representation in which, as we shall see, the consonants are acoustically separated along the horizontal dimension primarily on the basis of their low-frequency content and along the vertical dimension primarily on the basis of their high-frequency content. (2) Latent patterns in the data implicate subtle interactions between features and/or the influence of additional (apparently acoustic) features not explicitly included among Miller and Nicely's five articulatory features. (3) Miller and Nicely's confusion data closely conform to the exponential decay function of psychological distance that I have proposed as a universal law of generalization (see Shepard, 1987).

Structure revealed by hierarchical clustering

In applying multidimensional scaling to Miller and Nicely's extensive set of data, I became aware of two limitations of the method. First, its computational cost and susceptibility to occasional problems of degeneracy or of entrapment in merely local optima discouraged its wholesale application to all seventeen of their matrices. Second, its representation of the stimuli as points in a continuous coordinate space left the identification of theoretically significant groupings, such as the nonparallel groupings of the voiced and voiceless stops, as a matter of subjective assessment. I therefore suggested to Stephen Johnson, then a graduate student in mathematics at Columbia University who was working with me at the Bell Labs for the summer, that he explore the possibility of developing a method for representing stimuli as members of explicit subsets or clusters.

With remarkable dispatch, Johnson conceived and programmed a nonmetric method of hierarchical clustering in which the stimuli, instead of being represented by points in a continuous coordinate space, are represented by the terminal nodes in an upside-down tree. A number is assigned to each internal node, specifying its height in the hierarchy, and the distance between any two terminal nodes is defined to be the number assigned to the highest node on the direct path in the tree between those terminal nodes. Johnson showed that the resulting distances are not Euclidean but *ultrametric*, having the property that the two largest distances between any three points are equal (Johnson, 1967). [It turned out that essentially the same idea was independently developed, at the same time, by Hartigan (1967) and by Jardine, Jardine, and Sibson (1967). Extensions to the fitting of nonhierarchical "additive" trees were subsequently achieved by Carroll (1976), Cunningham (1978), and Sattath and Tversky (1977).]

Figure 4.2A shows the hierarchical tree obtained when the matrix combined from Miller and Nicely's six unfiltered conditions was analyzed by the *diameter* variant of Johnson's hierarchical clustering scheme. [The diameter method – also variously called the "compactness," "maximum," or "complete link" method – follows Sørenson's (1948) procedure of merging clusters at each stage so as to minimize the diameter or largest distance between elements within the resulting cluster.]

Figure 4.2B portrays the same hierarchical clustering embedded in the two-dimensional scaling solution of Figure 4.1A. For representative levels of confusion, I drew closed curves around the consonants that are grouped together at each corresponding level in the tree. Such a combined representation offers the advantages of both types of representation within one picture. Thus, in the discrete clustering, the front voiced stop /b/ groups with the front voiced fricatives /v/ and /ð/ in a more explicit manner than in the continuous spatial representation. At the same time, the ordering of the fricatives from front to back articulation (namely, /v/, /ð/, /z/, /ʒ/ for the voiced and /f/, /θ/, /s/, and /ʃ/ for the voiceless) is more evident in the continuous spatial representation (where it is not contravened by the ultrametric inequality).

Beginning with the same two-dimensional spatial configuration, I also drew, for each of the six unfiltered conditions, a set of closed curves around the clusters resulting from a cut at a fixed 0.17 level of confusion through the hierarchical tree independently obtained for the data from that condition. The resulting curves

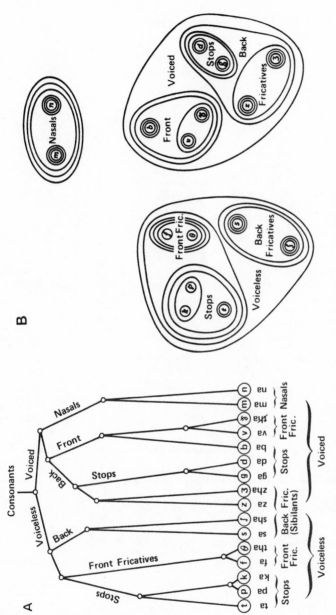

Figure 4.2 (A) Hierarchical tree representation of the sixteen consonants obtained by applying Johnson's hierarchical clustering method to the confusion data combined from Miller and Nicely's six unfiltered conditions. (B) The same hierarchical clustering embedded as a set of nested curves in the two-dimensional solution of Figure 4.1A. [Adapted, with permission, from Shepard (1972), copyright McGraw-Hill, and, in the present form, from Shepard (1980), copyright American Association for the Advancement of Science.]

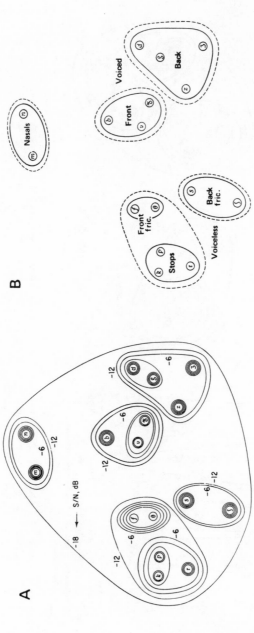

Figure 4.3 (A) Contours corresponding to a single cut (at the 0.17 level of confusion) through the hierarchical trees obtained from separate analyses of each of Miller and Nicely's six unfiltered conditions, for which the signal-to-noise ratios ranged from −18 dB (the outermost curve) to +12 dB (the innermost curves). (B) Contours corresponding to the invariant five- and six-cluster cuts through the trees for these unfiltered conditions. [Adapted, with permission, from Shepard (1972), copyright McGraw-Hill.]

are displayed in Figure 4.3A, along with the signal-to-noise ratios, in decibels, of the corresponding conditions. Because all of the trees were obtained by the diameter method, all consonants enclosed in the same curve were confused at or above the 0.17 level in the corresponding condition. We are here afforded a graphical depiction of which consonants are mutually confused at each noise level. For example, until the signal-to-noise level drops to -6 dB, the front voiceless fricatives /f/ and /θ/ are confused only with each other; then, at -12 dB, these voiceless fricatives become indistinguishable from the voiceless stops /p/, /t/, and /k/; and finally, at -18 dB, all sixteen of the consonants become indistinguishable.

The strict nesting of these curves supports the claim that despite a fiftyfold range in overall frequency of confusion for the different noise levels, the pattern of those confusions remained virtually invariant. Indeed, if we cut through each tree at the same number of clusters, rather than at the same number of confusions, the resulting five-cluster and six-cluster representations (displayed in Figure 4.3B) are exactly the same for all but the lowest and highest noise conditions, where the errors are either too sparse or too uniform, respectively, to support a reliable solution. The formerly noted departure from parallelism consistently occurs in which the voiced stop /b/ groups with the fricatives /v/ and /ð/ rather than with the other voiced stops /d/ and /g/.

Essentially the same clustering also emerged repeatedly in the low-pass conditions, except for the most extreme of those conditions. Only when all frequencies above 300 Hz were filtered out did the clustering finally reveal the originally anticipated parallelism between the voiced and voiceless consonants (Fig. 4.4A). Information about place of articulation, which is carried in the high frequencies, is then lost. That the resulting clusters are vertically elongated in the spatial representation indicates that the vertical dimension separates consonants differing primarily in high-frequency content.

Otherwise, as Miller and Nicely noted, the generally consistent pattern of confusions was markedly altered only by removal of the low frequencies. The character of this altered pattern is graphically indicated in Figure 4.4B, where the closed curves corresponding to a cut (again at the 0.17 level of confusion) through the hierarchical trees obtained from each of the high-pass conditions are displayed in a manner analogous to the preceding Figure 4.3A. As a result of removing the low frequencies, which carry voicing, each voiceless fricative now tends to be confused with its voiced counterpart. That these clusters are horizontally elongated indicates that the horizontal dimension separates consonants differing primarily in low-frequency content. (As already noted, the voiceless stops may remain relatively distinguishable by virtue of their initial high-frequency noise burst.)

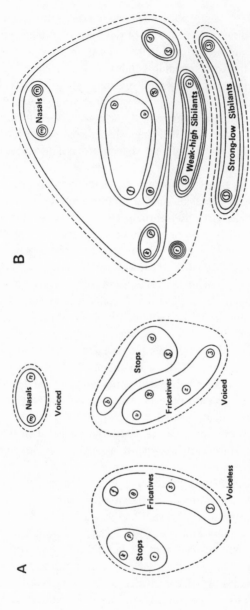

Figure 4.4 (A) Contours corresponding to cuts through the hierarchical tree obtained from an analysis of Miller and Nicely's most extreme low-pass condition. (B) Contours corresponding to a single cut (again at the 0.17 level of confusion) through the hierarchical trees obtained from separate analyses of each of Miller and Nicely's five high-pass conditions. [Adapted, with permission, from Shepard (1972), copyright McGraw-Hill.]

Structure revealed by additive clustering

A limitation of hierarchical clustering, made clear by Miller and Nicely's data, is the method's preclusion of overlapping clusters. Thus, once the front voiceless fricatives /f/ and /θ/ have been grouped with the front voiceless stops /p/, /t/, and /k/, neither of those front fricatives can be grouped with either of the back voiceless fricatives /s/ and /ʃ/, until all of these voiceless consonants are indiscriminately merged together (see Fig. 4.2B). Yet there are reasons to believe that listeners are simultaneously sensitive to the distinctive features of affrication and place of articulation.

The additive clustering model was conceived in order to provide for the recovery of precisely such overlapping features (Shepard, 1974; Shepard & Arabie, 1979). In this model, the similarity between two stimuli is accounted for not as a monotonic function of any sort of distance between them but rather as the sum of the weights associated with properties that the two objects are inferred to have in common. Additive clustering becomes equivalent to hierarchical clustering only when the obtained clusters are strictly nonoverlapping or nested. [For a full description of the original additive clustering method, ADCLUS, see Shepard & Arabie (1979), and for a subsequent method that uses a different numerical procedure to fit the same model, see Arabie & Carroll (1980).]

Figure 4.5A displays the clusters obtained by applying the original ADCLUS method to the combined data from Miller and Nicely's six unfiltered conditions. As before, the clusters are represented by closed curves drawn around the points in the previously obtained two-dimensional scaling solution. The number within each closed curve is the rank of the weight estimated by ADCLUS for that subset (with 1 indicating the greatest weight). These sixteen subsets, together with their estimated numerical weights (listed in Shepard & Arabie, 1979), account for over 94 percent of the variance in the data from the combined matrix for the unfiltered conditions.

The obtained clusters, unlike the strictly nested ones obtained by hierarchical clustering (Fig. 4.2B), do overlap. Thus, for the voiceless consonants, the front fricative /θ/ groups both with the front stop /p/ and with the farther back fricative /s/; and, for the voiced stops, the back stop /g/ groups both with the back fricatives /z/ and /ʒ/ and with the farther forward stop /d/. And, once again, the front stop /b/ groups with the front fricative /v/. (Fig. 4.5B will be discussed later.)

Structure revealed by three-way multidimensional scaling

The two-way methods of multidimensional scaling or clustering can be applied to only one matrix at a time. When, as in the case of Miller and Nicely's data, we have many matrices obtained for the same set of stimuli under different con-

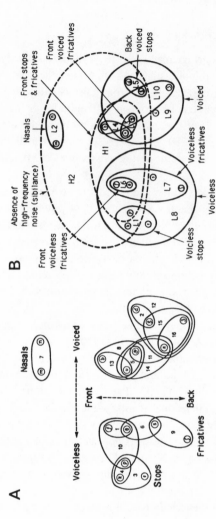

Figure 4.5 (A) Contours coresponding to the subsets obtained by applying two-way additive clustering (ADCLUS) to the combined data from Miller and Nicely's six unfiltered conditions (with enclosed numbers indicating the ranks of the weights assigned to the subsets). (B) Contours corresponding to the subsets obtained by applying three-way additive clustering (INDCLUS) to the data for all seventeen conditions (with L-numbers indicating the ranks of the weights important in the low-pass conditions and H-numbers indicating the ranks of the weights important in the high-pass conditions). [Part A is adapted, with permission, from Shepard (1974) and, in the form presented here, from Shepard and Arabie (1979), copyrights Psychometric Society and American Psychological Association. Reprinted by permission of the publisher. Part B is based on results reported in Soli, Arabie, & Carroll (1986).]

ditions, we should be able to gain additional information by simultaneously analyzing the entire set of three-way data (stimuli × stimuli × conditions). Carroll's individual differences scaling model, INDSCAL, does this by assuming that the psychological space of the stimuli has a fixed set of preferred dimensions and that differences in the similarity data in different conditions arise solely as a result of differential weighting (equivalently, stretching or shrinking) of those dimensions under the different conditions (see Carroll & Chang, 1970, for a fuller description).

Because it takes account of more data, a three-way analysis often permits the extraction of more dimensions than is possible using only two-way analyses. Higher dimensions that were flattened out into a low dimensional space by two-way multidimensional scaling (Fig. 4.1A) may emerge as orthogonal dimensions in a three-way analysis. Moreover, according to the INDSCAL model, such dimensions should be directly interpretable without rotation. Three-way multidimensional scaling can also yield results having some of the properties of a discrete clustering. Instead of taking on many different values on a very few dimensions, the stimuli may take on very few values on a larger number of dimensions.

For example, Wish (1971), applying INDSCAL directly to Miller and Nicely's seventeen matrices of confusion data, obtained a six-dimensional solution in which the sixteen consonants, which had been spread out in the earlier two-dimensional solution (Fig. 4.1A), tended to form relatively tight clumps (see Carroll & Wish, 1974; Wish & Carroll, 1974). The projections of this six-dimensional representation onto the planes of dimensions 1 and 2, dimensions 3 and 4, and dimensions 5 and 6 are displayed in panels A, B, and C, respectively, of Figure 4.6. This representation, together with the different weights for the dimensions in each condition, accounted for 78 percent of the variance in the entire set of seventeen matrices.

The configuration in the plane of dimensions 1 and 2 resembles that originally obtained by two-way scaling (Fig. 4.1A) but, as a result of the marked clumping together of the consonants that differ only in affrication or place of articulation, provides a purer representation of the dominant features of voicing and nasality. Instead of being flattened out into this same plane, the other features now emerge as higher orthogonal dimensions: dimensions 3 and 4, which sharply separate out the back, long-duration fricatives into two tight clusters, the strong-low sibilants (/ʃ/ and /ʒ/) and the weak-high sibilants (/s/ and /z/); dimension 5, which widely separates the voiceless consonants on the basis of their manner of articulation (with the stops at the far left, fricatives at the far right); and dimension 6, which orders the voiced consonants (for each manner of articulation) according to place (with front articulation at the top, back articulation at the bottom).

Three-way analysis is uniquely informative concerning the relative psycholog-

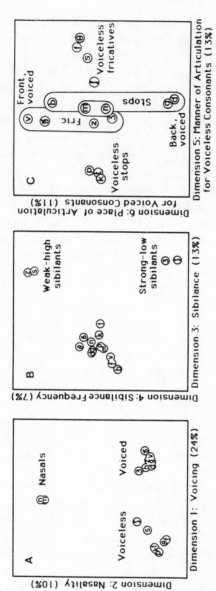

Figure 4.6 Six-dimensional representation obtained by applying three-way multidimensional scaling (INDSCAL) to the data from all seventeen conditions. The three panels (A, B, C) show the projections of the six-dimensional structure onto the orthogonal planes of different pairs of dimensions (with the percentage of the variance explained by each dimension indicated in parentheses). [Adapted, with permission, from Wish & Carroll (1974), copyright Academic Press.]

ical weights of the dimensions under the different conditions. These weights (tabulated in Wish & Carroll, 1974) indicated the following: First, the separation of the three clumps of consonants in the plane of dimensions 1 and 2 diminishes as the low frequencies are filtered out. This agrees with the notion that voicing and nasality are carried by low-frequency energy. Second, the separation of the three clumps of consonants in the plane of dimensions 3 and 4 diminishes as the high frequencies are filtered out. This agrees with the notion that sibilance is carried by high-frequency energy. Third, the separation of the consonants in the plane of dimensions 5 and 6 is reduced by the removal of both high and low frequencies. Closer examination of the corresponding sound spectograms suggested to Wish that dimension 6 distinguished whether the transition of the second formant to the following vowel /ɑ/ (a formant that is in the middle of the frequency range) was rising or falling (see Carroll & Wish, 1974).

Although these results were based on a very different multidimensional scaling method, they are generally consistent with the various clustering results exhibited in Figures 4.2 through 4.5. (For another INDSCAL solution for these data, see Soli & Arabie, 1979; see also Shepard, 1980.)

Structure revealed by three-way additive clustering

Three-way multidimensional scaling (INDSCAL) succeeded in overcoming the limitation that two-way scaling could be applied to only one matrix at a time. It also tended to yield somewhat more well-defined clusters. Still, like two-way scaling, it did not provide the explicit categorization of the stimuli obtainable by either hierarchical or additive clustering. As soon as Arabie and I had verified the effectiveness of two-way additive clustering, ADCLUS, Carroll and Arabie proceeded to develop a three-way extension of additive clustering analogous to Carroll's earlier three-way extension (INDSCAL) of multidimensional scaling. Their method, called INDCLUS, extends the ADCLUS model of Shepard and Arabie in allowing the weights associated with the clusters to take on different values for the individual matrices in order to achieve the best fit to the entire set of matrices (Carroll & Arabie, 1983).

In Figure 4.5B, the set of clusters that Soli, Arabie, and Carroll (1986) obtained by applying INDCLUS to Miller and Nicely's matrices for all seventeen conditions is juxtaposed to the set of clusters that Arabie and I obtained by applying ADCLUS to the single matrix combined from only the unfiltered conditions (Fig. 4.5A). As before, I have represented the clusters by drawing closed curves around the appropriate points in my original two-dimensional scaling solution for those unfiltered conditions (Fig. 4.1A). For visual clarity of Figure 4.5B, I have, however, omitted the last two of the fourteen clusters, which had appreciably lower weights than all of the other clusters and which Soli et al. had classified as uninterpretable. The INDCLUS solution accounts for nearly 83 percent of the total variance in the seventeen matrices. This result compares favorably with the 78 percent accounted for by the six-dimensional INDSCAL solution and attests to the essential validity of the additive model of similarity underlying both ADCLUS and INDCLUS.

Moreover, all but the two omitted clusters produced by INDCLUS are readily interpreted, as indicated by the labels attached to the corresponding closed curves. The weights (whose numerical values are tabulated in Soli et al., 1986) are also interpretable: In a manner analogous to the numbering in Figure 4.5A, the symbols L1, L2, and so on indicate the rank order, by their weights in the low-pass conditions, of the clusters that had the heaviest weights for the low-pass conditions; and the symbols H1 and H2 indicate the rank order, by their weights in the high-pass conditions, of the clusters that had the heaviest weights for the high-pass conditions. These latter clusters, which are represented by the dashed curves in Figure 4.5B, do not appear in the ADCLUS solution (Fig. 4.5A) because that earlier solution (like those in Figs. 4.2 and 4.3) did not take any account of the data from high-pass conditions. Those two clusters are similar, however, to the large horizontal clusters in Figure 4.4B, which I previously obtained from two-way clustering analyses of just the high-pass conditions. But the grouping of each voiced fricative with its voiceless counterpart, which was clearly revealed by those previous analyses (Fig. 4.4B), failed to emerge in the INDCLUS analysis. Again, the alternative analyses, being differentially responsive to different latent patterns, can complement each other.

Despite their differences, all of the clustering results are uniformly consistent with my original two-dimensional scaling solution (Fig. 4.1A). True, when embedded in this solution, the clusters obtained under the different conditions vary in shape. Nevertheless, they are virtually always representable as smooth, generally convex, and roughly elliptical curves that differ primarily in being vertically elongated in the low-pass conditions, horizontally elongated in the high-pass conditions, and roughly circular in the unfiltered conditions. The two dimensions of the multidimensional scaling solution, even though based solely on the unfiltered conditions, evidently provide for the separation of consonants differing primarily in their higher or lower frequencies. Although the various hierarchical and nonhierarchical clusterings have brought many significant patterns into sharper relief, the two-dimensional spatial configuration has provided a convenient and meaningful framework in which these clusterings can be uniformly displayed, compared, and interpreted.

Representation of structures in Miller's data on semantic relations among twenty body-part terms

Over the years, the flow of psycholinguistic data that George Miller and his co-workers have generated has followed his own shift in primary interest, from the perception of speech to the cognition of language. I would not do justice to his later period if I did not say something about the analyses that my associates and I have carried out on a particularly interesting set of semantic data with which Miller had challenged us, namely, data that he collected on the conceptual relations between terms referring to parts of the body. The challenge of semantic data in general, and of data concerning body-part terms in particular, is that some terms, such as *body* itself, are superordinate with respect to other, relatively subordinate terms such as *arm* or *ear*. Yet none of the scaling or clustering methods considered in the preceding sections provide for explicit super- or subordination of the elements represented. (For a discussion of other far-reaching cognitive significances of body-part terms, see Miller & Johnson-Laird, 1976, pp. 298–300; and for a discussion of the clinical relevance of what the perceived relations among such terms tell us about body image, see Mayer and Eisenberg, 1986.)

Overview of Miller's body-parts study

Miller had fifty people sort twenty names of body parts into groups of terms that seemed to belong together. (For a more complete description of this sorting task, see Miller, 1969; and for more about this particular set of Miller's data, see Carroll, 1976; Carroll & Chang, 1973.) For any two terms, the number of persons who assigned those two terms to the same group can be taken as a measure of the conceptual relatedness of those two terms. Accordingly, the various (two-way) methods for the analysis of similarity data can be directly applied to the resulting 20 × 20 matrix of these measures. I shall describe the results obtained by just three of these methods.

Structure revealed by hierarchical clustering

As I noted, some sort of hierarchical representation would seem to be particularly appropriate here because, for example, "elbow" seems subordinate to "arm," and "arm" seems subordinate to "body." However, in the hierarchical clustering methods so far considered, including the one developed by Johnson (1967), all objects are assigned alike to the terminal nodes at the lowest level of the tree. To accommodate semantic data of the sort collected by Miller, therefore, Carroll and Chang (1973) devised a method for assigning objects to internal nodes of the tree when this permits a better fit to the data (also see Carroll, 1976). Figure 4.7A shows (in the rearranged form presented in Shepard, 1980) the results that Carroll and Chang obtained by applying their method to Miller's body-parts data. This hierarchical representation accounted for nearly 93 percent of the variance in the similarity data by the adjustment of only five continuous parameters, namely, the heights of the five internal nodes, as indicated in the figure. Moreover, the expected semantic hierarchy seems to be well recovered, with "body" dominating "leg," "arm," "head," and "trunk," and with each of these dominating the appropriate set of still more subordinate terms.

Structure revealed by multidimensional scaling

Figure 4.7B, reproduced from Shepard and Arabie (1979), shows a two-dimensional projection of a three-dimensional solution that Arabie had obtained by applying Kruskal's version, MDSCAL, of nonmetric multidimensional scaling to the same set of body-parts data, using the so-called city-block metric (see Kruskal, 1964a, 1964b; Shepard, 1964). For these data, the city-block metric afforded an appreciably better fit than the Euclidean metric and yielded a three-dimensional solution that should be interpretable without rotation. As is evident in the figure, the three orthogonal axes, I, II, and III, do pass directly through the clusters of leg, arm, and head terms, respectively. The remaining trunk and body terms are more widely scattered in a large cluster, which falls around the origin of the coordinate system and, in this projection, farther back in depth. My principal reason for presenting this scaling solution here, however, is to furnish a convenient pictorial framework in which to display the results of the additive clustering.

Structure revealed by additive clustering

As before, the closed curves in Figure 4.7B encircle the items that were grouped together in the solution obtained by ADCLUS, and the arabic numeral within each such closed curve indicates the rank of that cluster according to the estimated weight. These ten clusters, together with their associated weights (listed in Shepard & Arabie, 1979), account for over 95 percent of the variance in the similarity data.

In comparison with the hierarchical representation obtained by Carroll and Chang (Fig. 4.7A), the ADCLUS representation fails to provide an explicit representation of the superordinate status of some of the terms, such as "body" and "trunk." Unlike the hierarchical representation, however, it does provide an explicit representation of the overlap of certain of the subsets. Most significant among the overlapping subsets are subset 10, which connects the arm and leg

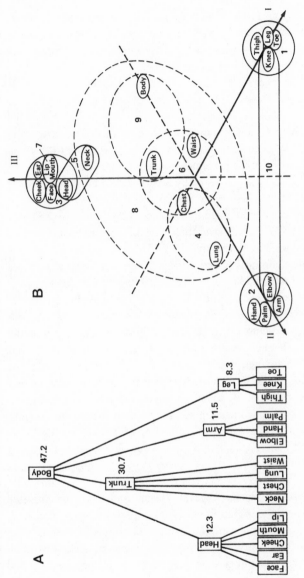

Figure 4.7 (A) Hierarchical representation of Miller's twenty body-part terms, obtained by Carroll's method, which assigns some terms to internal nodes of the tree. (B) Two-dimensional projection of a three-dimensional scaling solution for the same set of data, with embedded contours corresponding to an additive clustering solution for those data. [Part A is adapted, with permission, from Carroll & Chang (1973) and, in the form presented here, from Shepard (1980), copyrights Bell Telephone Laboratories, Inc. and American Association for the Advancement of Science. Part B is reproduced, with permission, from Shepard & Arabie (1979), copyright American Psychological Association.]

subsets through the analogous terms "elbow" and "knee;" and subset 5, which connects the head and body subsets through the term "neck." This is yet another illustration of the complementary roles that different methods of analysis can play in revealing structures hidden in a matrix of data.

Concluding remarks

Knowing that George Miller's many far-reaching theoretical contributions to cognitive science will have been brought out by other contributors to this volume, I have focused on his role as a generator of extraordinarily rich data. Even though I have considered only two of his many sets of data, I hope I have made clear the influence that even these have exerted on the development of methods that are now widely used throughout cognitive science. I think it remarkable that the Miller–Nicely data, collected well over three decades ago, are still providing a challenge for seekers after buried treasure.

I began this chapter by contrasting two views of cognitive science: one that emphasizes complex and often ad hoc or conventional knowledge structures and one that emphasizes general psychological laws. The methods that I have reviewed here accommodate both views. By means of these methods, we can uncover complex cognitive structures in such diverse forms as continuous spatial configurations, hierarchical trees, or sets of discrete, overlapping attributes. At the same time, we can obtain evidence for general (e.g., metric) principles that underlie these diverse forms and for general laws that specify how behavior and thought are guided or constrained by them. Examples of such general laws include the exponential law of generalization verified by multidimensional scaling and the additive composition of similarities verified by additive clustering.

Thirty years ago, when I was beginning my postdoctoral fellowship with George Miller, he was still feeling the effects of his own earlier association with Princeton's Institute for Advanced Study. Immured there with world-class mathematicians and theoretical physicists, he had evidently been prompted to ask himself, as he now asked me, whether *our* chosen field could rightfully be regarded as a science. With the increasing demonstration of the orderliness of its data, the quantifiability of its underlying structures, and the existence of general psychological laws, I now feel confident in giving my answer: Yes, George, and thanks not only to your stimulation and theoretical guidance but also to your data, cognitive science, having earned its name, is now indeed a science.

References

Arabie, P., & Carroll, J. D. (1980). MAPCLUS: A mathematical programming approach to fitting the ADCLUS model. *Psychometrika, 45,* 211–35.

Blackwell, H. R., & Schlosberg, H. (1943). Octive generalization, pitch discrimination, and loudness thresholds in the white rat. *Journal of Experimental Psychology, 33,* 407–19.

Bush, R. R., & Mosteller, R. (1951). A model for stimulus generalization and discrimination. *Psychological Review, 58,* 413–23.

Carroll, J. D. (1976). Spatial, non-spatial, and hybrid models for scaling. *Psychometrika, 41,* 439–63.

Carroll, J. D., & Arabie, P. (1983). INDCLUS: An individual differences generalization of the ADCLUS model and the MAPCLUS algorithm. *Psychometrika, 48,* 157–69.

Carroll, J. D., & Chang, J.-J. (1970). Analysis of individual differences in multidimensional scaling via an N-way generalization of Eckart–Young decomposition. *Psychometrika, 35,* 283–319.

Carroll, J. D., & Chang, J.-J. (1973). A method for fitting a class of hierarchical tree structure models to dissimilarity data and its application to some "body parts" data of Miller's. In *Proceedings, 81st Annual Convention, American Psychological Association,* 1097–8.

Carroll, J. D., & Wish, M. (1974). Models and methods for three-way multidimensional scaling. In R. C. Atkinson, D. Krantz, D. Luce, & P. Suppes (Eds.), *Contemporary Developments in Mathematical Psychology,* Vol. 2 (pp. 57–105). San Francisco: W. H. Freeman.

Chang, J.-J. & Shepard, R. N. (1966). Exponential fitting in the proximity analysis of confusion matrices. Presented at the annual meeting of the Eastern Psychological Association, New York (April 14).

Chomsky, N. (1957). *Syntactic Structures.* The Hague, The Netherlands: Mouton.

Cunningham, J. P. (1978). Free trees and bidirectional trees as representations of psychological distance. *Journal of Mathematical Psychology, 17,* 165–88.

Hartigan, J. A. (1967). Representation of similarity matrices by trees. *Journal of the American Statistical Association, 62,* 1140–58.

Jardine, C. J., Jardine, N., & Sibson, R. (1967). The structure and construction of taxonomic hierarchies. *Mathematical Biosciences, 1,* 173–9.

Johnson, S. C. (1967). Hierarchical clustering schemes. *Psychometrika, 32,* 241–54.

Kruskal, J. B. (1964a). Multidimensional scaling by optimizing goodness of fit to a nonmetric hypothesis. *Psychometrika, 29,* 1–27.

Kruskal, J. B. (1964b). Nonmetric multidimensional scaling: A numerical method. *Psychometrika, 29,* 28–42.

Lashley, K. S., & Wade, M. (1946). The Pavlovian theory of generalization. *Psychological Review, 53,* 72–87.

Mayer, J. D., & Eisenberg, M. G. (1986). Mental representations of the body: Cognitive and affective dimensions studied across four clinical groups. Unpublished manuscript. (Available from J. Mayer, Department of Psychology, Division of Natural Science, State University of New York at Purchase, Purchase, NY 10577.)

Miller, G. A. (1951). *Language and communication.* New York: McGraw-Hill.

Miller, G. A. (1969). A psychological method to investigate verbal concepts. *Journal of Mathematical Psychology, 6,* 169–191.

Miller, G. A., & Johnson-Laird, P. N. (1976). *Language and Perception.* Cambridge, Mass.: Harvard University Press.

Miller, G. A., & Nicely, P. E. (1955). An analysis of perceptual confusions among some English consonants. *Journal of the Acoustical Society of America, 27,* 338–52.

Sattath, S., & Tversky, A. (1977). Additive similarity trees. *Psychometrika, 42,* 319–45.

Shepard, R. N. (1955). Stimulus and response generalization during paired associates learning. Unpublished Ph.D. dissertation, Yale University.

Shepard, R. N. (1957). Stimulus and response generalization: A stochastic model relating generalization to distance in psychological space. *Psychometrika, 22,* 325–45.

Shepard, R. N. (1958a). Stimulus and response generalization: Deduction of the generalization gradient from a trace model. *Psychological Review, 65,* 242–56.

Shepard, R. N. (1958b). Stimulus and response generalization: Tests of a model relating generalization to distance in psychological space. *Journal of Experimental Psychology, 55,* 509–23.

Shepard, R. N. (1962a). The analysis of proximities: Multidimensional scaling with an unknown distance function. I. *Psychometrika, 27,* 125–40.

Shepard, R. N. (1962b). The analysis of proximities: Multidimensional scaling with an unknown distance function. II. *Psychometrika, 27,* 219–46.

Shepard, R. N. (1964). Attention and the metric structure of the stimulus space. *Journal of Mathematical Psychology, 1,* 54–87.

Shepard, R. N. (1965). Approximation to uniform gradients of generalization by monotone transformations of scale. In D. J. Mostofsky (Ed.), *Stimulus Generalization* (pp. 94–110). Stanford, Calif.: Stanford University Press.

Shepard, R. N. (1972). Psychological representation of speech sounds. In E. E. David & P. B. Denes (Eds.), *Human Communication: A Unified View* (pp. 67–113). New York: McGraw-Hill.

Shepard, R. N. (1974). Representation of structure in similarity data: Problems and prospects. *Psychometrika, 39,* 373–421.

Shepard, R. N. (1980). Multidimensional scaling, tree-fitting, and clustering. *Science, 210,* 290–8.

Shepard, R. N. (1984a). Ecological constraints on internal representation: Resonant kinematics of perceiving, imagining, thinking, and dreaming. *Psychological Review, 91,* 417–47.

Shepard, R. N. (1984b). Similarity and a law of universal generalization. Presented at the annual meeting of the Psychonomic Society, San Antonio, Texas (November).

Shepard, R. N. (1986). Discrimination and generalization in identification and classification: Comment on Nosofsky. *Journal of Experimental Psychology: General, 115,* 58–61.

Shepard, R. N. (1987). Toward a universal law of generalization for psychological science. *Science, 237,* 1317–23.

Shepard, R. N., & Arabie, P. (1979). Additive clustering: Representation of similarities as combinations of discrete overlapping properties. *Psychological Review, 86,* 87–123.

Soli, S. D., & Arabie, P. (1979). Auditory versus phonetic accounts of observed confusions between consonant phonemes. *Journal of the Acoustical Society of America, 66,* 46–59.

Soli, S. D., Arabie, P., & Carroll, J. D. (1986). Discrete representation of perceptual structure underlying consonant confusion. *Journal of the Acoustical Society of America, 79,* 826–37.

Sørenson, T. (1948). A method of establishing groups of equal amplitude in plant sociology based on similarity of species content and its application to analyses of the vegetation of Danish commons. *Biologiske Skrifter, 5,* 1–34.

Torgerson W. S. (1952). Multidimensional scaling: I. theory and method. *Psychometrika, 30,* 379–93.

Wish, M. (1971). An INDSCAL analysis of the Miller–Nicely consonant confusion data. *Journal of the Acoustical Society of America, 49,* 85 (abstract).

Wish, M., & Carroll, J. D. (1974). Applications of individual differences scaling to studies of human perception and judgment. In E. C. Carterette & M. P. Friedman (Eds.), *Handbook of Perception,* Vol. 2 (pp. 449–91). New York: Academic Press.

5 The magical number seven: information processing then and now

George Sperling

The magical hypotheses

George Miller read an invited address to the Eastern Psychological Association on April 15, 1955: "The Magical Number Seven, Plus or Minus Two: Some Limits in Our Capacity for Processing Information." He complained: "I have been persecuted by an integer." The article was published the following year in the *Psychological Review*. Both the spoken version and the written version (here referred to as 7 ± 2) were immediate successes. A survey conducted twenty years later found that 7 ± 2 was the single most often cited paper in cognitive psychology (Garfield, 1975). Every student of cognitive psychology has been exposed to it, and many cognitive psychologists, including myself, have been profoundly influenced by it.

The central thesis of 7 ± 2 is that the number 7 occurs in two contexts. The first context is absolute judgments of brightness, loudness, pitch, extent, and so on. In absolute judgments – that is, classification of sensory stimuli into categories – 7 ± 2 *is* the effective number of categories that the subject can maintain. This number is derived from what was then a novel statistical computation: the 2 to 3 bits of *information transmitted* by an observer in these tasks.

To transmit more than 3 bits of information in an absolute judgment, a subject requires sensory stimuli that vary in more than one dimension. The transmitted information in each component dimension suffers somewhat as new dimensions are added; nevertheless, subjects can transmit enormously greater amounts of information about multidimensional stimuli than about one-dimensional stimuli.

The second context in which 7 ± 2 occurs is memory. In short-term recall (the classical immediate memory test), 7 ± 2 describes the number of items that a subject can recall. In contrast to the absolute judgments, the number of recallable items does not depend on their information content, so the information-transmitted statistic does not predict performance. Although binary digits contain less than one-third the information of decimal digits, a subject can recall only very slightly more binary digits than decimal digits. However, by recoding sev-

71

eral separate elements (e.g., binary digits) into a unitary "chunk" (e.g., an octal digit), the subject can enormously increase his or her recall capacity for binary digits.

George Miller classified many of the experimental procedures that had been used to study information processing into two categories (absolute judgments and immediate recall) and invented twin hypotheses, one to characterize the human performance limit in each category. One-dimensional absolute judgments could transmit up to 3 bits of information; immediate recall was limited to 7 ± 2 chunks. All of the experiments that George Miller advanced in support of these twin hypotheses had been performed by others. The contribution of 7 ± 2 is entirely theoretical – its succinct classification of a great deal of data and its clear formulation of two hypotheses that demanded theoretical explanations.

Professor George Miller

In the spring of 1958, Professor Miller offered a seminar in information processing for the graduate students in the Psychology Department at Harvard. I enrolled in that class and volunteered to give the seminar presentation on 7 ± 2. How I got to this point is a story in itself.

The previous spring, I had been a student in the neighboring Department of Social Relations. Professor Miller conducted the last sessions of the required proseminar (offered jointly with Jerome Bruner, Richard Solomon, and George Mandler). I presented a class report on a paper by Lawrence and Laberge (1956). After describing their experiments, I proposed a partial report experiment that could better address the same issues. Professor Miller was sufficiently interested in this proposed experiment to offer to support it. Thereby began our association.

In the summer of 1957, Professor Miller obtained permission for me to use Jerry Bruner's tachistoscope during Bruner's absence, and he supported my application for a transfer to the Psychology Department. In the fall, just as I entered the Psychology Department, my draft board officially notified me that they now expected me to turn my attention to their needs. This was obviously to be my last chance in graduate school. Fortunately, during the summer, with the encouragement of Roger Shepard (Professor Miller's postdoctoral fellow, whom he designated to oversee the research), I had completed the experiments for my Ph.D. thesis on what Ulric Neisser (1967) later dubbed "iconic memory."

In those days, from the students' point of view, Harvard's Psychology Department was clearly divided on ideological grounds that were reflected in its geographical layout. Fred Skinner was located at the north end of the basement of Memorial Hall, Smitty Stevens was entrenched at the opposite end, and George Miller, Phil Teitelbaum, Edwin Newman, and everyone else who had not chosen sides was thrown together in the middle. At the opposite ends of Memorial Hall, students attended competing discussion groups offered weekly by Stevens and Skinner. Cognitive science was centered in the middle.

In Professor Miller's seminar, each student was to present an extended two-hour seminar on an important paper. I chose 7 ± 2 because it was supposed to be a very important paper. On first reading, 7 ± 2 seemed to offer the student an opportunity for a dazzling display of critical acumen. Its assertion that the span of absolute judgment could be so low was patently absurd. Simply searching out the references would uncover their procedural artifacts. For visual judgments of spatial extent, this nitpicking paid off. The displays were tiny (subtending less than ½ degree) and, even so, 3.25 bits of information were transmitted (corresponding to 9.5 alternatives). I imagined that larger displays would undoubtedly produce still better performance and thereby significant violations of 7 ± 2. In all of the other modalities, however, the data withstood scrutiny, and they firmly contradicted my intuition. I almost began to feel persecuted, too.

Miller had noted that, with multidimensional stimuli in absolute judgment experiments, the additional dimensions enable the subject to surpass the 7 ± 2 restriction on the number of effective categories. I intended to propose using this property in reverse to discover what the underlying dimensions of judgments were. Since this seminar was often attended by postdoctoral fellows (such as Roger Shepard) and students from Social Relations (such as Saul Sternberg), as well as by the Psychology Department students, it was an occasion for lively exchanges. However, on this occasion, another psychology student, Jerry Shickman, objected so vehemently and persistently to my use of the concept of dimension that I was unable to proceed. By the time Professor Miller intervened to get things going again, so much tension had built up that subsequent discussion was totally inhibited.

The seminar meeting was a failure. However, the intellectual seed had been sown. The particular set of problems and the issues surrounding them have remained with me ever since. And although I have been persecuted by editors and critics for many more than seven years, my experiments and the data they generated have been a source of much comfort.

The challenge of a theory

What was it about 7 ± 2 that made it such a milestone in cognitive psychology? As usual, it was not just one thing but a propitious combination of many factors. The framework of the presentation was masterful: the provocative challenge of the theoretical approach. Like Sherlock Holmes, the theoretician demonstrates that the evidence is already at hand. One need only be clever enough to perceive it. By implication, of course, the data-bound experimenters and the rest of us in the audience were not up to the task. It was unnecessary for George Miller to proclaim ponderously that there must be a role for theoreticians in a discipline dominated by experimentalists; the demonstration was a better proof. A cognitive psychologist could be a theoretical psychologist proposing simple hypotheses that organized large amounts of data.

The classical period and the dark ages of information processing

To understand why George Miller's twin hypotheses – his theory – had such an impact, we must examine the field as it was when 7 ± 2 burst forth upon it. The three main textbooks of the time were Woodworth and Schlosberg's *Experimental Psychology* (1954), Osgood's *Method and Theory of Experimental Psychology* (1953), and Stevens's *Handbook of Experimental Psychology* (1951).

Osgood offers no treatment whatsoever of any of the paradigms, data, or issues raised in 7 ± 2. In Stevens's *Handbook,* C. H. Graham's chapter on visual perception has a subsection suggestively entitled "Span of Perceptions," but its four pages are devoted entirely to Hunter and Sigler's (1940) study of estimated dot numerosity as a function of luminance and exposure duration in brief displays. The chapter on cognitive processes by Leeper is utterly astounding in terms of how the field is defined today. The beginning is bogged down in a discussion of consciousness, and the remainder is devoted to concept formation in monkeys.

Not only George Miller's interests in 7 ± 2 (information transmitted in perceptual judgment and in short-term recall) were given short shrift in Osgood's and Stevens's compendia of the 1950s. Attention, in the context of human performance, is entirely absent. Yet, in classical psychology, attention is the heading under which the paradigms of 7 ± 2 would be treated. Related subjects were also ignored. For example, even a subject with sensory as well as cognitive implications – saccadic eye movements as our means of acquiring visual information – is not mentioned in either text. Anyone who thinks that 7 ± 2 did not represent a leap forward in our conceptualization of the important issues of psychology need only look at the primordial ooze from which it sprang.

Woodworth and Schlosberg's views of the important issues in psychology fare better by today's standards. Most of the topics previously mentioned are considered. The treatment is dust bowl empirical; many experimental procedures are summarized and the results stated matter-of-factly. If one already knows what the interesting questions are, the data speak for themselves. But there is not a trace of theory.

The treatment of spans in Woodworth and Schlosberg derives directly from the earlier edition of Woodworth (1938). And this book, in turn, owes much to Woodworth's long internship in Wundt's laboratory.

The debt to Wundt

Wundt was concerned with precisely the issues that 7 ± 2 raises and devoted considerable attention to them immediately in Chapter 1 of his popular *Introduction to Psychology* (1912), a condensation of his longer *Outlines*. Wundt asks, how many elements can be maintained simultaneously in consciousness? When the elements are ticks of a metronome, the answer depends on how the subject groups them. Subjectively grouping ticks by twos (imagining 2/8 time) yields sixteen conscious clicks grouped into eight "chunks" (to use Miller's term). Grouping by eights (imagining 4/4 time) yields only five chunks, although chunking increases the total number of ticks from sixteen to forty. Similar advantages of chunking appear in the visual domain when viewing clearly visible tachistoscopic flashes of unrelated letters or words. Viewers report they can perceive as many unrelated words as unrelated letters (about four). In the auditory modality, observers can report back six spoken nonsense syllables. Braille characters are designed to use only six tactile dot positions. Basically, Wundt proposes the magical number 6 ± 2, and indeed, for immediate memory, this describes the situation.

Unlike his mentor, Helmholtz, whose procedures are as timely today as they were one hundred years ago, Wundt's usual methods are entirely subjective. This was by Wundt's design. When he thought the occasion required it, Wundt could be quantitative and rigorous by today's standards. For example, his *Physiological Psychology* is full of examples of the comparative structure of sense organs in various species and of mathematical formulations of significant relations. Wundt was versed in biology and mathematics. In trying to forge a distinctive science of psychology, different from physiology, Wundt wanted to use distinctively different procedures. Thereby, he chose the wrong path. The new psychology was not then, and still is not, ready for Wundt's introspective methods. Cognitive psychology still succeeds best with experimental procedures that place the complexity in the stimulus and leave the response simple and constrained. Wundt's reverse procedures, such as presenting the subject with a simple red patch and asking him to introspect at length about what he sees, are still beyond our reach.

Helmholtz and Wundt raised many questions that we regard as core issues of cognitive psychology. Helmholtz concentrated primarily on perception, and his methods were universal. Wundt went further, to information processing, thinking, and beyond, but his methods too often were introspective. Many of Wundt's followers were less well versed in scientific protocol than he. In their hands, the introspective methods ultimately stimulated psychologists to create the behavioral revolution. Unfortunately, as in many revolutions, the good was overthrown with the bad. For almost half a century, not only the methods but even the questions were discarded by most American psychologists.

Traces of interest in cognition survived in a new empirical garb, as noted, for example, by Woodworth and Schlosberg. Although casting cognitive questions in empirical, behavioral terms was an improvement, in the absence of theory the spark was lost. Aside from observing empirical relationships, as in the span of apprehension experiments, there was no inkling of how to cast theories.

The renaissance

When Shannon's (Shannon & Weaver, 1949) information theory came on the scene, it was quickly adapted to a variety of paradigms because it was the only systematic framework psychologists had for dealing with information. [At the same time, Wald's (1950) statistical decision theory blossomed in psychology as signal detection theory.] But the routine application of information theory to psychological paradigms was unfruitful. In the morass of information-oriented experiments, 7 ± 2's contribution was the clear delineation of a domain in which information theory was useful (absolute judgments) and a complementary domain (short-term list recall) in which it was not. This was an important and necessary step in moving forward. In a larger scale, in relation to its time, 7 ± 2 redefined the classical subject of span experiments in terms of information processing, an area of cognitive psychology with clearly phrased problems and the possibility of significant theoretical approaches.

The baroque era and the age of computers

The classical past offered the fascinating cognitive issues posed by Wundt and, in the United States by James but completely lacked an adequate methodology. In the post–World War I period of unmitigated empiricism, the intellectual thread was lost. A post–World War II flurry of information theoretic studies culminated in 7 ± 2. What was and is yet to come?

In outline, the path ahead looks straightforward. The 7 ± 2 theory is a descriptive macro theory. That is, it offers mathematical descriptions of stimulus–response relations at a very global level. The descriptive formulations of 7 ± 2 will eventually be supplemented with process theories – models that embody the step-by-step computations carried out in the cognitive microprocesses that underlie performance. Eventually, the process models will be fleshed out with neural components that represent the biological structures that carry out the cognitive microprocesses. The early stages of this process of scientific evolution can already be discerned.

Acoustic confusibility

The first important progress following 7 ± 2 came with the observation that not all items were equivalent, even when they conveyed precisely the same information. It was discovered that the number of items recalled from visual or auditory presentations depends on the acoustic structure of the items. Items that are acoustically confusible (such as the letters *b, c, d, g, p, t,* and *v*) are not recalled as well as items that are less confusible (Conrad & Hull, 1964; Sperling, 1963; Sperling and Speelman, 1970). Thus, all chunks are not equivalent; how well a chunk is remembered depends on its sound.

That acoustic structure is critical suggests an acoustic basis for short-term memory (Sperling, 1968). Articulatory coding is an alternative possibility (Hintzman, 1967). There are severe difficulties with any purely structural theory – acoustic or articulatory – since familiarity, which is not easily embodied in any of these theories, has an enormous role in short-term recall (Sperling, Parish, Pavel, & Desaulniers, 1984). Any contemporary theory of short-term recall must deal in much more detail with much more detailed cognitive processes than Miller was forced to do. For example, we know that the phonemic and acoustic structure of the to-be-remembered chunks matters; that recoding, rehearsal strategies, and grouping have specifiable mnemonic effects; and that prior learning experiences with the items are critical. These are some of the presumed components of process theories.

Neural models for immediate memory have been proposed by Grossberg (1980), bypassing the functional process description. However, in the absence of a functional model to explain recoding, rehearsal, grouping, and other strategic options available to the subject, neural specification is probably premature.

Memory noise in absolute judgments

The limiting factor in absolute judgments seems to be that subjects cannot remember the precise boundaries of their categories. There is some uncertainty (noise) in coding stimulus intensity, but the main bottleneck seems to be limited capacity memory (Durlach and Braida, 1969).

One particular formulation of the memory bottleneck (Heinemann, 1984) has been extensively tested on pigeons as well as humans. Chase (1984) and Heinemann find that pigeons make absolute judgments of auditory intensity that are qualitatively quite similar to human judgments. They model the limited capacity memory by assuming that, in memory, the outcome of a trial is represented by a record containing the stimulus, the response, and the feedback on that trial. Memory contains about 1,000 locations. Each new trial is stored independently at a random location of memory, overwriting the previous contents of the location. When it comes time to make a judgment of a new stimulus, some records, typically estimated to be about seven, are extracted from the 1,000-location long-term memory and placed into a short-term working memory. The judgment is made by comparing the unknown stimulus to the contents of working memory.

Heinemann's model accounts nicely for a number of second-order effects relating to absolute judgments, such as how discimination in various parts of the stimulus dimension depends on the spacing of stimuli and how a relabeling of the stimuli is gradually learned. Although Heinemann avoids the inference, for me the attractive aspect of this kind of process model is that the working memory that holds the records of previous trials of the judgment experiment may be the same memory that holds the chunks in the immediate memory experiment. This kind of theory is representative of the exciting kinds of models of mental microprocesses that cognitive psychology offers. It also illustrates the incompleteness of theories in which the complex control processes needed to utilize limited-capacity memories are axiomatically assumed rather than explicitly modeled.

The coming era

Physiologically, it is unlikely that formatted records of the sort described in Heinemann's model are written in a memory with a fixed number of locations. This description of a process is best regarded as a convenient, workable conceptualization of a neural network. Indeed, it is easy to design neural networks that behave like the stack memory previously described. Whether the network that actually performs the stacklike memory function in the brain is describable in simple terms is not known. It may or may not be simply organized. However, a complete functional description that can be applied to any particular experimental situation will undoubtedly be very complex.

One of the remarkable emerging properties of the many recently proposed neural networks is that they are quite similar in their overall learning properties, even though their structures are profoundly different. These networks can be used interchangeably to fill the black boxes of the functional process models in much the same way that computer memory chips of different manufacturers can be interchanged on a central processing unit board. At least, that is how one aspect of the future of cognitive models appears to me in the 1980s.

The future

What is the future of 7 ± 2? It offers a descriptive theory of two classes of phenomena. We look forward to better process theories and eventually, to physiologically plausible neural theories. Does this mean that 7 ± 2 will become outmoded and replaced? Not necessarily. Predicting the fate of any psychological theory requires a careful consideration of the more general role of the theory.

The goal of theory in experimental psychology is to provide the best possible description of a class of phenomenon at a given level of complexity (Sperling, 1978). Subsequent theories may be more complex and detailed, but they will not replace earlier theories unless they can explain more with equal or less complexity. Insofar as a theory offers the best description at a given level of complexity, it is eternal and will not be replaced, though it certainly will be supplemented. There are many difficulties with this formulation of the goal of theory, not the least of which is the continuously changing nature of complexity. But the magical cognitive powers of the number seven make 7 ± 2 a probable candidate for the best theory at its chosen level of complexity. If so, 7 ± 2 will endure. That is the ultimate achievement of any theory.

References

Chase, S. 1984. Pigeons and the magical number seven. In M. L. Commons, R. J. Herrnstein, & A. R. Wagner (Eds.), *Quantitative Analyses of Behavior: Discrimination Processes* (pp. 36–47). Cambridge, Mass.: Ballinger.

Conrad, R., & Hull, J. A. (1964). Information, acoustic confusion, and memory span. *British Journal of Psychology, 55*, 429–32.

Durlach, N. I., & Braida, L. D. (1969). Intensity perception. I. Preliminary theory of intensity resolution. *Journal of the Acoustical Society of America, 46*, 372–83.

Garfield, E. (1975). Highly cited articles. 19. Human psychology and behavior. In E. Garfield, *Essays of an Information Scientist* (pp. 262–8). Philadelphia: Institute for Scientific Information.

Graham, C. H. (1951). Visual perception. In S. S. Stevens (Ed.), *Handbook of Experimental Psychology* (pp. 868–920). New York: Wiley.

Grossberg, S. (1980). How does a brain build a cognitive code? *Psychological Review, 87*, 1–51.

Heinemann, E. G. (1984). A memory model for decision processes in pigeons. In M. L. Commons, R. J. Herrnstein, & A. R. Wagner (Eds.), *Quantitative Analyses of Behavior: Discrimination Processes* (pp. 3–19). Cambridge, Mass.: Ballinger.

Hintzman, D. L. (1967). Articulatory coding in short-term memory. *Journal of Verbal Learning and Verbal Behavior, 6*, 312–16.

Hunter, W. S., & Sigler, M. (1940). The span of visual discrimination as a function of time and intensity of stimulation. *Journal of Experimental Psychology, 26*, 160–79.

Lawrence, D. H., & Laberge, D. L. (1956). Relationship between accuracy and order of reporting stimulus dimensions. *Journal of Experimental Psychology, 51*, 12–18.

Leeper, R. (1951). Cognitive processes. In S. S. Stevens (Ed.), *Handbook of Experimental Psychology* (pp. 730–57). New York: Wiley.

Miller, G. A. (1956). The magical number seven, plus or minus two: Some limits on our capacity for processing information. *Psychological Review, 63*, 81–97.

Neisser, U. (1967). *Cognitive Psychology.* New York: Appleton-Century-Crofts.

Osgood, C. E. (1953). *Method and Theory in Experimental Psychology.* New York: Oxford University Press.

Shannon, C. E., & Weaver, W. (1949). *The Mathematical Theory of Communication*. Urbana: University of Illinois Press.

Sperling, G. (1963). A model for visual memory tasks. *Human Factors, 5,* 19–31.

Sperling, G. (1968). Phonemic model of short-term auditory memory. *Proceedings, 76th Annual Convention of the American Psychological Association, 3,* 63–4.

Sperling, G. (1978). *The Goal of Theory in Experimental Psychology*. Bell Telephone Laboratories Technical Memorandum 78-1221-12.

Sperling, G., Parish, D. H., Pavel, M., & Desaulniers, D. H. (1984). Auditory list recall: Phonemic structure, acoustic confusibility, and familiarity. *Bulletin of the Psychonomic Society, 18,* 36.

Sperling, G., and Speelman, R. G. (1970). Acoustic similarity and auditory short-term memory: Experiments and a model. In D. A. Norman (Ed.), *Models of Human Memory* (pp. 149–202). New York: Academic Press.

Stevens, S. S. (Ed.). (1951). *Handbook of Experimental Psychology*. New York: Wiley.

Wald, A. (1950). *Statistical Decision Functions*. New York: Wiley.

Woodworth, R. S. (1938). *Experimental Psychology*. New York: Holt.

Woodworth, R. S., & Schlosberg, H. (1954). *Experimental Psychology* (rev. ed.) (pp. 90–105). New York: Holt.

Wundt, W. *An Introduction to Psychology*. (1912). (R. Pintner, translator, from the second German edition). London: Allen & Unwin. (Reprinted 1924.)

6   Cognitive recollections

Ulric Neisser

It was the spring of 1950 at Harvard, and George Miller was my faculty adviser. I was doing my senior honors project at the Psychoacoustic Laboratory, running subjects in a big, creepy, lightless room called the "anechoic chamber." The whole room was covered with odd-looking triangular baffles designed to eliminate echoes – an ideal place in which to study "The Effect of Visual Stimulation on the Auditory Threshold." (I liked odd and paradoxical-sounding effects, even then.) You entered it through a large control room, impressively lined with the electronic instruments that George had taught me to use but that I never learned to love. When the big ice-cream-freezer door had clanged shut, you were in a special kind of space – echoless, airless, motionless, utterly quiet. It was just the right environment in which to attend to one's own auditory sensations, an enterprise that seemed very important in those days. Psychophysics was the scientific core of scientific psychology, and the Harvard anechoic chamber was the inner temple of that psychophysics.

George was often in the control room, which in any case was right next door to his office. One day – I had come in to do some of the endless calibrations necessary to my project – he had just finished setting up an interesting and little-known auditory effect. Would I like to hear it for myself? I would. When I had entered the chamber and put on the earphones (in this case the chamber was being used simply as a sound-shielded room), I heard a faint, high-pitched tone that soon faded away into what seemed to be complete silence. (The effect is now called "tone decay.") The apparent silence continued for a while, and then – suddenly – I heard the tone *stop*. Or perhaps it would be better to say that when the tone finally did stop, I suddenly realized that – in some sense – I had really been hearing it all along. "Oh, *that* was the tone!" I said to myself. And although tone decay itself no longer seems very interesting, my memory of that demonstration makes a point worth keeping in mind: I often picked up George's signals without realizing it until later.

All through the 1950s and 1960s, George Miller heard the sound of things getting under way: new ideas, a new psychology, cognitive science. But he did more than just listen to those things; he was in the control room helping to make them happen, trying to get the rest of us to hear them too. The redundancy of the speech signal, distinctive features and phonemes, information measurement, the magic number seven, transformational grammar, the mental lexicon, the idea of Cognitive Studies, giving psychology away – the list of things that George has persuaded us to listen to is a long one. They have all been interesting and they have all made a difference. Perhaps some of them can be heard with a special clarity now that their beginnings lie well in the past and now that cognitive psychology is finally coming out of the anechoic chamber.

For about five years beginning in the late 1940s, George Miller taught a course at Harvard called "The Psychology of Speech and Communication." Even at the time – which for me was the spring of 1949 – I couldn't help noticing that it covered some pretty unusual topics. Where the other courses in my chosen major had focused almost exclusively on psychology itself, the scope of Psychology 165 extended to such esoteric disciplines as linguistics, acoustics, articulatory physiology, and engineering mathematics. George taught us about decibels and filters, phonemes and morphemes, Shannon's theorem and Zipf's law, coding principles and the redundancy of English. Naturally there was no standard textbook for such a course, so he was writing one himself. In 1949, we worked from mimeographed copies of the first draft. We didn't know then that it was a first draft of the future.

I do not want to represent George as an infallible prophet. His enthusiasm for mathematically formulable ideas led him into some odd corners – odd then and (to me) odder now. In the spring of 1950, for example, he joined with Fred Frick to offer a course called "Statistical Behavioristics." The topics included Markov chains, fundamentals of information measurement, aspects of set theory, and other mathematical models that I have now forgotten. But even to-be-forgotten models can have their uses: If Miller had not been so interested in Markov processes, he might not have realized the importance of Chomsky's proof that no such process – no set of conditional probabilities defined from left to right across a sequence – can ever encompass the grammar of English.

Although the sound of the future must have been at least moderately audible in Psychology 165, I did not yet know what I had heard. Instead, my undergraduate sympathies lay with the ideas of the gestalt psychologists – Köhler, Wertheimer, and Koffka – who had only recently emigrated to the United States. Gestalt theory was no longer quite new, but it seemed to offer the most generous and coherent account of human nature to be found anywhere in psychology. I was not so much interested in choosing a particular field of research – perception or learning, for example – as in finding a theoretical position I could live with. Since I vastly preferred gestalt psychology to all forms of behaviorism, as well as to functionalism and psychoanalysis (there wasn't anything else), I decided to begin graduate work at Swarthmore College, where I could study with Köhler and his colleagues. Miller was less than enthusiastic about my decision but couldn't talk me out of it.

After two years at Swarthmore – where I learned many things that do not come into this chapter – my commitment to gestalt psychology had faded a little. I still believed that a good theory would have to begin with "organized units" rather than "meaningless elements," but Köhler's interpretation of those units as electrical fields in the brain was obviously not going to work. As I mulled over what to do next, the ideas I had encountered in "The Psychology of Speech and Communication" seemed increasingly important. George Miller had taught me more than I had realized; perhaps my destiny lay with information theory and psychoacoustics after all. At that time, Miller had just moved from Harvard to MIT, where the new Psychology Section (in the Sloan School of Economics, of all places) also included J. C. R. Licklider, Herb Jenkins, and others. I decided to go there too.

As it turned out, MIT in 1952 was not yet quite ready for psychology. The Psychology Section didn't last very long, and Miller himself was back at Harvard in two or three years. (A permanent Psychology Department was not established at MIT until about a decade later, and then under quite different auspices.) My own graduate year at MIT was a mixed experience; I learned a lot, but somehow it wasn't quite what I had wanted to know. Following George Miller's lead (again!), I went back to Harvard myself in the fall of 1954. Unfortunately, although George was doing wonderful work in those years – on phoneme perception, on the magical number 7 ± 2, on recoding – I was not yet wise enough to see its importance. (I eventually did my Ph.D. thesis, with S. S. Stevens, on a problem in psychoacoustics.) George himself went right on working, and by the middle of the 1950s a lot of other people were working the same side of the street.

Not all of those people were psychologists. In the mid-1950s I attended a symposium on information theory at MIT where most of the participants seemed to be – or at least sounded rather like – mathematicians. Nevertheless, some of them were very impressive, especially a brash young man named Oliver Selfridge, whom I couldn't fit into any professional category at all. Nowadays Selfridge would be called (and is in fact called) a "computer scientist" or a theorist in the field of artificial intelligence. Then he was just a very bright person with a mathematical background who worked on something he called "pattern recognition." There was a consensus that it was time to establish a real science of human behavior, and that those present at the symposium were going to do just that.

This was probably the same symposium – perhaps even the same day – that George Miller (1979) has since described as "the birthday of cognitive science." He went away from it convinced that "human experimental psychology, theoretical linguistics, and the computer simulation of cognitive processes were all pieces of a larger whole, and that the future would see a progressive elaboration and coordination of their shared concerns'' (p. 9). He was right, as usual: That is indeed what happened, although some other things have happened too. But (also as usual) I didn't get the message myself until some time later. My own impression of the symposium was not nearly as positive as George's.

From where I sat (behind the slide projector, which I ran during one of the afternoon sessions), there was rather too much mathematics at the symposium and not nearly enough psychology. Part of my reaction was perhaps predictable in a fresh psychology Ph.D.: To call so blithely for ''a new science of behavior'' was to cast aspersions on the honorable discipline I had just worked so hard to join. And although the new mathematical formulations were clever, it was a specialized kind of cleverness that I didn't much appreciate. My own preference has always been for clever *experiments*. An important part of the identity of cognitive psychology today is based on the ingenuity of its outstanding experimenters – on the ability of people like George Sperling, Roger Shepard, Saul Sternberg, Lee Brooks, or Eleanor Rosch to devise surprising new laboratory methods that reveal surprising new facts. But in the 1950s their work was yet to come. So far as I can remember, no important empirical research was reported at the MIT conference.

Something else was missing too, although I didn't understand what it was until much later. Most of the speakers I heard at the symposium seemed to think of living organisms as essentially equivalent to electronic systems; their discussions were about computation, not adaptation. Partly for that reason, there was little emphasis on describing the *environment* in its reciprocal relation to the organism, and no one cautioned us that principles valid under laboratory conditions might not always be applicable in more natural settings. In retrospect, these omissions are a little surprising: Tinbergen's *The Study of Instinct* (1951) had appeared five years earlier, and the ethological movement was already well established. If the first cognitive scientists had realized that the specific information processing mechanisms of organisms must have evolved in relation to equally specific information structures in the environment, the subsequent development of the field might have followed a somewhat different course.

To be sure, this is all hindsight. My own discontent with the MIT conference had nothing to do with ecological validity. The tone was just too computational for my taste, not human or wholistic enough. Could these arcane mathematical formulations really be the wave of the future? As it turned out, they were not. It was not to be the mathematics of information but just the concept of information, as an entity in its own right, that would shortly transform psychology. With that concept, it became possible to think about cognitive processes in an entirely new way – to dispense with both the hypothetical implicit responses of the behaviorists and the sensations and images of the introspectionists, focusing on the vicissitudes of information itself. The proper study of cognition became possible as soon as we understood what it was the study *of*. George Miller understood that as early as anyone. By the end of the 1950s he had joined with Jerome Bruner to found the Harvard Center for Cognitive Studies, and – with Eugene Galanter and Karl Pribram – was writing *Plans and the Structure of Behavior* (1960).

Although things were moving fast, several key ingredients of modern cognitive psychology were not yet in place when *Plans* was published. The seminal experiments were only beginning to appear: Sperling's (1960) discovery of the icon, for example, and Peterson and Peterson's (1959) demonstration of very rapid forgetting in short-term memory. (It was George himself who first told me about the Petersons' experiment in a casual conversation at the Center for Cognitive Studies. By that time, I was teaching at Brandeis University.) The idea of making "an information-flow diagram for the organism," as Donald Broadbent put it (1958, p. 299), was not yet widely understood. American psychology was still nominally in the grip of behaviorism: At the end of their book, Miller et al. described themselves not as cognitive psychologists but as "subjective behaviorists."

Plans and the Structure of Behavior was itself a plan – a second draft of the future, successor to "The Psychology of Speech and Communication" (Miller, *Language and Communication,* 1951). The authors envisaged a dynamic as well as a cognitive psychology; their book was organized around the idea that actions require hierarchical plans. Its topics included not only language and memory and thought (and computer simulation and speculative neuropsychology) but also intention, conflict, and hypnosis. There was also a chapter devoted to ethology, but not as a basic paradigm for understanding adaptation to the environment: The point was just to show that plans could be innate. Other topics that would soon become central to the study of cognition are now conspicuous by their absence. There was no mention of vision, no discussion of pattern recognition, and not a single reaction-time study! But *Plans* was thoughtful, lively, and consistently interesting; most important, it showed that the new computer-influenced psychology could wear a human face.

Meanwhile, I was finally becoming a cognitive psychologist. Oliver Selfridge, the young man I had met at the MIT symposium, turned out to be interested in my gestalt-prompted musings about visual perception; we soon became friends and collaborators. The principles on which Selfridge's pattern-recognition programs were based – redundancy, parallel processing, effective order emerging from what looked like sheer pandemonium – seemed eminently applicable to human cognition. I began to operationalize them in a series of experiments on visual scanning. A number of other ideas were in the air at the same time: I read Bartlett and Piaget and Freud, heard Noam Chomsky speak, watched the development of so-called artificial intelligence with a skeptical eye, and was regularly reminded by A. H. Maslow – my chairman at Brandeis – of the importance of human values in psychology.

By 1964, it had come together in my head. In principle, I thought, one could follow the information inward from its first encounter with the sense organ all the way to its storage and eventual reconstruction in memory. The early stages of processing were necessarily wholistic (an idea I borrowed from Gestalt psychology) and the later ones were based on repeated recoding (an idea borrowed, even more obviously, from George Miller). But the processing sequence was by no means fixed; at every point there was room for choice, strategy, executive routines, individual constructive activity. Noam Chomsky's linguistic arguments had shown that an activity could be rule governed and yet indefinitely free and creative. People were not much like computers (I had already sketched out some of the differences in a 1963 *Science* paper), but nevertheless the computer had made a crucial contribution to psychology: It had given us a new definition of our subject matter, a new set of metaphors, and a new assurance.

I took a leave from Brandeis and spent the next two years writing a book. *Cognitive Psychology,* which appeared in 1967, had both a theoretical and a tutorial purpose. At the theoretical level, it tried to integrate the facts of cognition into a purposive and coherent account of human nature, drawing heavily on the metaphor of "constructive processes" to do so. As a tutorial, it presented what I took to be the state of the art in the mid 1960s – an art that was just establishing its own identity. That identity was partially defined by the concept of information, but also by a particular set of laboratory methods: tachistoscopic presentation, reaction-time measurement, pattern identification, short-term recall, speech perception, linguistic analysis, and so on. Both vision and hearing were important, not as information-seeking perceptual systems (at the time, I assumed that cognitive processes could be studied independently of perception proper) but simply as channels for input. The several chapters of *Cognitive Psychology* devoted to acoustic and linguistic issues were markedly influenced by what I had learned, years earlier, in George Miller's "Psychology of Speech and Communication."

Despite its relatively broad scope, something was missing from *Cognitive Psychology* (indeed, from cognitive psychology): the same ecological ingredient that had been missing from the MIT symposium ten years before. The argument of the book relied almost exclusively on experiments in which the stimulus information had been deliberately impoverished. The possibility that the structure of the normal environment might play a key role in cognition – that there might be organization in the objectively existing information itself – had not occurred to me. Neither "adaptation" nor "environment" is listed in the index. Again, the omission is surprising: J. J. Gibson's ecological manifesto *The Senses Consid-*

ered as Perceptual Systems (1966) had appeared the year before. Gibson insisted that the study of perception must begin with a description of the environment in which the perceptual systems had evolved and an analysis of the information that that environment makes available. In his view, all of the standard laboratory methods of cognitive psychology were suspect – along with the models based on them – because they were not based on such an analysis. Gibson argued (correctly, I think) that it is fruitless to speculate about the processing mechanisms inside a system without a good description of the information to which the system itself is tuned. Once we have that description, we will be able to give a more purposive and coherent account of human nature – one in which perception appears not as constructive and inferential but as adaptive and direct.

It is now 1988, twelve years since I first tried to reconcile the ecological and information-processing approaches in a book called *Cognition and Reality* (1976). In that time, both approaches have flourished. Many theorists now believe that cognitive psychology itself is only part of a broader and more important enterprise, "cognitive science," which also includes artificial intelligence, linguistics, neuropsychology, and the philosophy of mind. Taken as a whole, that enterprise is surprisingly close to what George Miller has had in mind all along. But it has also been increasingly influenced by ecological considerations, especially in certain subfields: perception (Marr's [1982] influential book *Vision* relies explicitly on detailed environmental analysis), perceptual development (see the review by Gibson & Spelke, 1983), movement (e.g., Kelso, 1982), categorization (Rosch, 1978; Neisser, 1987), and memory (Neisser, 1982; Bruce, 1985). The study of cognition has finally come out of the anechoic chamber, and is making not only echoes but waves.

References

Broadbent, D. E. (1958). *Perception and Communication*. London: Pergamon Press.

Bruce, D. (1985). The how and why of ecological memory. *Journal of Experimental Psychology: General, 114*, 78–90.

Gibson, E. J., & Spelke, E. S. (1983). The development of perception. In P. H. Mussen (Ed.), *Handbook of Child Psychology*, 4th ed. New York: Wiley.

Gibson, J. J. (1966). *The Senses Considered as Perceptual Systems*. Boston: Houghton Mifflin.

Kelso, J. A. S. (Ed.). (1982). *Human Motor Behavior: An Introduction*. Hillsdale, NJ: Erlbaum.

Marr, D. (1982). *Vision*. San Francisco: W. H. Freeman

Miller, G. A. (1951). *Language and Communication*. New York: McGraw-Hill.

Miller, G. A. (1979). A very personal history. *Occasional Paper #1*. Cambridge, Mass.: MIT Center for Cognitive Science.

Miller, G. A., Galanter, E., & Pribram, K. (1960). *Plans and the Structure of Behavior*. New York: Holt, Rinehart, & Winston.

Neisser, U. (1963) The imitation of man by machine. *Science, 139*, 193–7.

Neisser, U. (1967). *Cognitive Psychology*. New York: Appleton-Century-Crofts.

Neisser, U. (1976). *Cognition and Reality*. San Francisco: W. H. Freeman.

Neisser, U. (Ed). (1982). *Memory Observed: Remembering in Natural Contexts.* San Francisco: W. H. Freeman.

Neisser, U. (Ed.) (1987). *Concepts and Conceptual Development: Ecological and Intellectual Factors in Categorization.* New York: Cambridge University Press.

Peterson, L. R., & Peterson, M. J. (1959). Short-term retention of individual verbal items. *Journal of Experimental Psychology, 58,* 193–8.

Rosch, E. (1978). Principles of categorization. In E. Rosch & B. B. Lloyd (Eds.), *Cognition and Categorization.* Hillsdale, NJ: Erlbaum.

Sperling, G. (1960). The information available in brief visual presentations. *Psychological Monographs, 74,* No. 11.

Tinbergen, N. (1951). *The Study of Instinct.* London: Oxford University Press.

PART II The Center for Cognitive Studies

Plans was written while George was on leave from Harvard at the Center for Advanced Study for the Behavioral Science. The interdisciplinary environment of this Palo Alto, California, institution whetted his appetite, and after a few months of discontent following his return to Harvard, he sat down with Jerry Bruner and gave birth to the Center for Cognitive Studies. As George writes:

We called our new enterprise the Harvard Center for Cognitive Studies. . . . Jerry's group at Bow Street had been calling themselves the Cognition Project for some time, so we had a precedent for using the term to name the Center. To me, even as late as 1960, using "cognitive" was an act of defiance. It was less outrageous for Jerry, of course; social psychologists were never swept away by behaviorism the way experimental psychologists had been. But for someone raised to respect reductionistic science, "cognitive psychology" made a definite statement. It meant that I was interested in the mind – I came out of the closet. (Miller, 1987, p. 24)

Jerome Bruner tells of this journey out of the closet in his chapter. Donald Norman and Willem Levelt offer their recollections of the Center from a student's perspective.

7 Founding the Center for Cognitive Studies

Jerome Bruner

Writing about events that you have known close up or that you have participated in, and particularly writing about the people involved, forces you into an historiographic stance. You resist, of course, clinging as long as you can to the illusion of objectivity. Besides, letting your stance show diverts you from the real purpose; it is not easy to be brief in justifying historiographic stances, particularly when you are an amateur. But there you are. Does one, for example, embrace a Great Man theory (the topic of this chapter deserves it!) or a Shaping-Events theory, or, in some Woody Allen fashion, does one opt for a Crazy Quilt theory? Of course, it is also possible (though exceedingly sneaky) to go the constructivist way and argue that each writer of history has his own version and none is the aboriginal one. I must confess that I am alternately pulled one way, then another: a victim of our age of radical epistemological doubt. Or maybe history *is* like that. Or maybe it has to do with being brought up, as George and I both were, by E. G. Boring, who made history sound just a little too much like an account of who was there and who said what to whom.

So, when I find myself trying to write a chapter about the founding of the Center for Cognitive Studies and George Miller's role in it, I am like Buridan's ass in a multidimensional space, tempted simultaneously by a very large number of bales of hay, all a little out of reach. Yet, there are some matters that seem self-evident to me, even if they are contradictory. I have no doubt (1) that there would have been no Center without George Miller, (2) that George and the other actors in the events surrounding its establishment were corks on the waves of history, (3) that there were a crucial number of idiosyncratic rogue waves and rogue people around at the time to constitute a Crazy Quilt, and (4) that it is all in my own head. And I would add one more for good measure: (5) that what brought the Center into existence was not necessarily what shaped its growth. But more of that later.

The Center for Cognitive Studies was founded in 1960. That much is clear and true. Immediately, one wants to write a lot of sentences with causal constructions containing topic phrases like "the spirit of the 1960s." There was plainly

90

something going on in the early 1960s, and it has been written about at some length by people who date the cognitive revolution from the year 1960. Things like foundings are hard to account for in terms of their necessary and sufficient conditions. I think that both George and the spirit of the 1960s were in the former category. But what constitutes the range of the sufficient conditions eludes me. I know it is broad-spectrum. How *do* historians cope with all of the gristly counterfactual conditionals? I'll come back to some of them later.

The causes of the Center's founding are typically complex. They inhere in events and in long-term trends; in personalities and in abstract ideas; in enthusiasms and in despondencies. Perhaps if psychology had not split into sociotropic and biotropic extravaganzas at Harvard, there would not have been a Center founded within a decade of the Great Fission. If, perhaps, George Miller and Jerry Bruner had not been so temperamentally prone to act out their intellectual dissatisfactions institutionally, it would not have occurred. And if there had not been an activist dean of the faculty who distrusted the compartmentalism of Harvard departments and saw interdepartmental centers as the means of diluting departmental power, Miller and Bruner would not have found so ready an ear for their institutional fantasies about a Center. But then again, the particular acting-out tendencies of the two founders *and* the ready ear of McGeorge Bundy, the dean in question, might only have been the historical surface of deeper cultural changes in the organization of human knowledge. And so too the cordial welcome we received from the psychologist-administrator, John Gardner, then president of the Carnegie Corporation, when we broached the idea of the Center on a visit to him in New York. Like our dean, he felt that departments were becoming corsets on learning. There was undoubtedly a suspicion abroad that the old disciplinary boundaries, though they had once been useful in shaping the division of scholarly labors, were now no longer the natural joints of the enterprise. In circles where this general view prevailed, psychology was believed to be too narrowly focused on a few traditional problems to deal interestingly with the nature and uses of the human mind, a view shared by many inside psychology, who felt that the old behaviorism was a hopelessly wrong epistemological base from which to view the higher functions of the mind. Besides, there were, so to speak, such nearby figures as Von Neumann, Shannon, Nelson Goodman, Norbert Wiener, and the vigorous young Noam Chomsky who were making such claims loudly and convincingly.

But already the account is becoming too linear, too patently causal. There were those rogue events as well. Take, for example, the very particular personality of J. Robert Oppenheimer. In the years preceding the founding of the Center, both Miller and Bruner had not only spent sabbatical leaves at the Institute for Advanced Study, where he presided, but had served on an Advisory Committee on Psychology there, where it had become an emblematic truth that psychology by itself was not enough of an instrument to probe the mysteries of the human mind, that there were even central problems in physics that had a cognitive dimension, and that even historians were not immune from doubts about the knowledge-acquiring processes on which their craft depended. Did that have an effect? Well, it certainly made each of us aware of the epistemological troubles in the scholarly world – their depth, their pervasiveness, their relation to the psychology of the higher mental processes.

The first definite causal thing that I would have to say is that George Miller's genius (whatever else may constitute it) rests upon an uneasy susceptibility to troubles in the domain of the epistemic. It is like an allergy. Let there be a pollen of doubt in the epistemological atmosphere, and he sneezes. But that does not capture it: It isn't that he sneezes. He moves to where the action is; he takes up arms; he flings himself into the fray. Indeed, he even searches out the places where the pollen is thickest, as if to keep his spirit properly exacerbated. In all of my long academic life, I have never known a man more productively activated by the turbulences in epistemology than George Miller. It is some magic mix of elation and dejection that seizes and drives him.

About the story of the actual founding of the Center, several versions have already been written – by George (1979), by me (1983), and by Howard Gardner (1985). As with all new departures, some genuinely comic things led up to it. Like finally deciding to do it after months of shilly-shallying, when George and I (according to *my* memory) consumed a splendid bottle of port in the course of one evening and had to cope with residual doubts the next day against the ravages of two terrible and interacting hangovers. George, I think, believes that it was claret; if he is right, the hangovers were less ravaging, but the doubts were still there. What we had decided was that psychology was too complicated a field to leave to the psychologists, and that what we needed was an alliance with colleagues in other disciplines who were, each in his or her own context, concerned about how humans acquired and used knowledge. When eventually we tried out our new credo on our dean, McGeorge Bundy, he smiled and asked how that differed from what Harvard as a whole was trying to do!

George had just turned forty. It is a bold time in life for a successful intellectual, and he had tasted enough success to be prone to activism about his convictions, an activism further fueled by his dissatisfactions with the state of psychology at Harvard. But here I must pause and say a word about the status of psychology at Harvard in those days. For it is, I think, an important part of the story.

The fission in psychology that had led in 1946 to the establishment of two departments, Psychology and Social Relations, created plenty of fuming and ferment. In its wake, there was a "postrevolutionary" vigor that led eventually (and perhaps inevitably) to a narrowing and sharpening of foci in the two departments. Psychology (housed in the basement of Memorial Hall) became increasingly monopolized by two unconnected preoccupations – sensory psychophysics and operant conditioning, and the rest thrown in for good measure. Social Relations (housed in Emerson Hall), though it had its share of psychologists, nonetheless had as its principal goal the integration of the empirical social sciences – sociology, anthropology, and "sociotropic" psychology. (It was E. G. Boring who had introduced the distinction between "biotropic" and "sociotropic" psychology, and although it did not quite capture the actual difference between the two departments, it did much to create a cultural reality.) There was not much of a support system in the two departments, given that aim, for the study of those higher mental processes that interested George and me. He felt as marginal in Memorial Hall as I did in Emerson. We had for some years been giving a joint course, Psychology 148, "The Cognitive Processes," that we had conceived as a bridge between the two departments. But bridges are not places where one lives. I had set up a Cognition Project located "offshore" at 9 Bow Street. And George had students working on psycholinguistics at Memorial Hall. He missed the linguists and the computational theorists at MIT. Both of us longed for a locus in which to trade easily in ideas about cognitive processes.

The Center that we envisaged would at a stroke relocate the study of higher mental processes both in psychology and in the university. It would have a more autonomous existence that would make it easier to connect with others in the university who were in fact, if not departmentally, dealing with cognitive issues. And by the good luck of our grant from the Carnegie Corporation, we would be able to bring in as visitors the kinds of intellectual companions who shared our enthusiasms, regardless of the label on their disciplinary hat. In a sense, then, we started with a dual aspiration: to go more broadly afield in order to make common cause with whomever was concerned with problems of knowledge, and to go more deeply into the specialties each of us was developing as a probe into the nature of cognition.

I must say that both in those early days of planning and throughout the decade of the Center's life, I have never had a colleague and friend to match George for open-mindedness, good humor, and loyalty. He is the great practitioner of intellectual accountability: If you have an idea and can argue its virtues convincingly, he will be with you all the way. In all of our years of close collaboration, I have never known him to have a secret agenda or to harbor a secret grudge. And when there was an intellectual issue at stake that he did not know about, he would "read it up."

Well, as George once put it, we nailed our flag to the door and wondered what would happen. At the end of the first year, these words appeared near the opening of our Annual Report:

Cognition seems suddenly to be a matter of great interest to many people in different walks of life. Businessmen are asking how to stimulate invention and creativity. Engineers are wondering if their computers really think. Anthropologists, after years of relating culture and personality, are beginning to show an interest in the cognitive and linguistic bases of culture. Educators are asking how these new ideas might be applied in the classroom. Psychologists all over the world are attacking the complex mental functions with new theories and new methods of observation.

Neurophysiologists are having extraordinary luck in uncovering mechanisms of attention and memory. All these developments and more converge to make the study of cognitive processes one of the most active and exciting areas of modern science. This is clearly not an enterprise that can be entrusted to any single discipline, that can be developed from any limited or specialized point of view. Harvard's Center, planned from the beginning as a cooperative, interdisciplinary enterprise, has a precious opportunity to provide coherence and leadership for this sudden swell of new interest.

The roster of the Center reflected this ideal. Lists are boring, but they tell a story in a stark way. Among the Fellows in those opening years were the linguists Roman Jakobson, Noam Chomsky, and Ruth Weir; the psychiatrist Joseph Jaffe; the philosophers Nelson Goodman and Robert Schwartz; the anthropologist David French; and the applied mathematicians Benoit Mandelbrot and Zoltan Dienes. And we tried to get visiting psychologists who would enjoy the mix – like Bärbel Inhelder and Paul Kolers, David McNeill and Masanao Toda, Donald Norman and Albert Bregman, Norman Mackworth and Peter Wason. I think it had a profound effect on our students – young scholars like Patricia Greenfield and Jacques Mehler, Christopher Alexander and Harris Savin, Susan Carey and Dan Slobin. Even our advisory board reflected the spirit: a philosopher (W. V. Quine), a linguist (Roman Jakobson), a mathematical statistician (Fred Mosteller), an historian (H. Stuart Hughes), an educational psychologist (John Carroll), and a most wide-ranging psychologist-linguist (Roger Brown). They were our advisers and our talent scouts.

There never was a preformulated program of research on Kirkland Street, where the architect Robert Woods Kennedy had refashioned President Eliot's old house for the Center's use (with the top floor a warren of carrels for graduate students in the style of the Academie Julien in Paris, where our architect had spent a happy postgraduate year). Rather, we collected a group of interesting people each year, each with his or her own research and graduate students, and the intellectual life of the Center revolved around the seminars, the Thursday lunches, and the weekly colloquia. The visitors were chosen on the sole (and risky) ground that they interested either George or me, with each holding (but never using) a blanket veto power. It was in the seminars, the colloquia, and at lunch that the exchanges took place. A good taste of what the atmosphere was like is provided (again with apologies for the bareness of its list structure) by a simple count-off of the late Thursday afternoon colloquia in that opening year of 1960–1.

Jerome Bruner. Similarity and difference: two approaches to knowing.

Ernst Mayr. The phylogenetics of information processing.

Daniel Berlyne. Epistemic curiosity.

Roger Brown. The acquisition of grammar.

Roman Jakobson. Infants' and aphasics' testimonies on language and thought.

Walter Rosenblith. Computer-aided electrophysiological studies in sensory communication.

Richard Held. Exposure to strange environments and an ordering principle in perception.

Raymond Bauer. Rational versus emotional appeals.

Eric Lenneberg. The biological matrix of speech.

Zoltan Dienes. A theory of learning mathematics.

Frederick Frick. Pattern recognition.

Ulric Neisser. A theory of intuitive thinking.

Gordon Allport. Intuition revisited.

David Page. On teaching mathematics.

Walter Mischel. Cognitive activity and delay of gratification.

I. A. Richards. Film sequences in the investigation of learning.

Noam Chomsky. Grammatical factors in the perception of sentences.

Harold Conklin. The cultural relevance of cognitive contrast.

Jules Henry. Cultural factors in elementary school readers.

Gerard Salton. Automatic information retrieval.

David French. Anthropology, ethnoscience, and cognition.

The next year, the horizon broadened still further: Stuart Hughes on "What does the historian think he knows?", Frederick Deknatel on "On looking at contemporary painting," and Kevin Lynch on "The image of the city." There was, of course, plenty of psychology as well. But I think we gauged our good luck by how well we did in casting a wider net. And the colloquia – with "outreach" speakers or regulars – drew an audience well beyond what, today, we would think of as the usual "cognitive sciences crowd." George and I were always a little astonished at the sprinkling of art historians, philosophers, law professors, and even mathematicians and physicists, who showed up on Thursday afternoons. After a while, we even began getting a share of those e. e. cummings "Cambridge ladies who are interested / In oh so many things including God and Longfellow / Both of whom are dead." I think the Center may even have served the function, in those years, of getting psychology out of the closet and into the Cambridge community. The British playwright-cognitivist Jonathan Miller said, on the occasion of the BBC series on the cognitive sciences that he hosted, that the Center had been the first in our times to use the dirty, four-letter word "mind" in public.

I must digress to introduce a more abstract point. It is about a distinction that the political theorist Gabriel Almond once made between what he called the "intrinsic" and the "extrinsic" appeals of social and intellectual movements. The former is what welds the in-group of the movement; the latter, of course, is the extended appeal. Structuralism provides a nice illustration. Its linguistic in-group was formed around an intrinsic program of purely technical analysis – of utterances, texts, and so on. The broader out-group saw structuralism first as a metaphor and eventually almost as an intellectualized ideology: a way of looking at literature, at culture, indeed almost at life itself. Intrinsically motivated in-groups and extrinsically driven out-groups don't always get on with each other; nor do the two impulses always rest happily inside the same breast.

In retrospect, it seems obvious that the Center at Harvard was, at the outset, attempting to espouse both intrinsic and extrinsic ideals for cognitive studies. For although Miller and Bruner were genuinely devoted to the extrinsic ideal – their manifesto was, in effect, *all* about that – they were both seriously committed as well to a much more intrinsic and specific program of revisionism within their own particular disciplines. And I think both of them felt that the two ideals would nourish and reinforce each other. But it was not easy to keep a balance over those years – either in terms of time spent or even visitors invited. One can spend all of one's waking life and more discussing such plainly cognitive issues as the nature of interpretation in law, psychoanalysis, anthropology, literature, and so on. Or the issue of applying cognitive ideas to education can easily take a lifetime. Or matters that arise when one thinks of the interface between humans and machines. Once, we even had to reject the offer of a thoughtful philanthropist to double the size of the Center in order to extend our research to the study of cognitive defects.

I am totally convinced that the "double" atmosphere of the Center – the inward and the outward perspectives – was enormously stimulating. For all of that, it was also sometimes distracting. But perhaps distractions serve a good function if you are lucky in your choice of distractors. George once said in jest that when he got anxious he "hit the formalism bottle" for relief. But I think the occasional anxiety-arousing breadth of our activities at the Center made George's intrinsic research richer and broader than perhaps it might have been – even granting his natural scope.

At the center of his interests, I think, George was concerned not only with creating a psychology of language that did justice to the structure of language itself, but with establishing a theory of language processing that did not lean on the dogmas of association and learning theory. He was then (and has always remained) dedicated to formulating a theory of computation that could serve not only as a basis for describing language comprehension and use but also for elucidating the operations of mind and of mindlike artifacts. I was deeply involved at the same time in theory and research on mental development, work that I hoped might encompass structural description in the manner of Piaget's theory, while at the same time providing a functional account of how development adapted our species to the demands of a language-dependent culture.

So although we were both committed to the broader extrinsic conception of cognitive studies, it was a little like what the French call *un violin d'Ingres* – Ingres having had aspirations as an amateur musician while practicing painting as a real painter's painter. George more than did his duty to the broader extrinsic ideal – spending much time with our visiting philosophers, anthropologists, and with anybody who had an honest doubt about the status of knowledge in their discipline. Indeed, it was in those opening years of the Center that Volney Stefflre was in pursuit of the Whorfian hypothesis, when Conklin and Frake and many other anthropologists were trying to found ethnoscience, when Eric Lenneberg was in search of the neural substrate of language. I think George did more than any scholar of his generation to launch and support those efforts.

Typical of those opening years at the Center was a seminar in which George was involved. It was led by a graduate student in applied mathematics, Fischer Black, and it worked at writing programs in Information Processing Language (IPL)-V simulating various cognitive processes. The debate centered on the issue of why particular programs succeeded in some ways while failing in others. Was there anything structural or necessary about the relation between simulative successes and failures? I mention the example here to give some sense of the range that existed at Kirkland Street between the detail of cognitive studies and its scope. Wasn't that the same year when we had a wild visit and lunch presentation from the French psychoanalyst Jacques Lacan, who tried to convince us of the linguistic basis of the unconscious?

In retrospect, I think that as time went on, fatigue pushed us toward more intrinsic problems. George was soon at work with Noam Chomsky on a formal description of grammar, and particularly on a theory of the language user and on the manner in which context affects the interpretation of language – or more accurately, the manner in which rules for the formation of higher-order linguistic units dominate the interpretation of lexical and other units encompassed by those higher-order units. And so it went in other corners of the Center. The task of intrinsic revision was sufficiently demanding to shoulder aside much of the more extrinsic, interdisciplinary preoccupation that had initially inspired us. That extrinsic work took on the character more of avocation than of vocation.

I think that it was bound to be so. For the shift came not just from temperament and the economy of work, but also from the structure of a university community where specialism is where the proof lies. The cognitive point of view needed working out in detail if it was to be convincing. Mies van der Rohe once said about architecture that "God is in the details." And it is just as true in scholarship and science. So we and our visitors and our students banged away at the details – eye movements, the difference in signal-to-noise ratios for words heard in and out of context, and the rest. Or maybe it simply had to do with the fact that the cognitive revolution was succeeding, that historians and anthropologists and educators and the others with whom we had hoped to cohabit were picking up the message on their own and in their own way.

I don't know. In many ways, one can argue, the cognitive sciences (as they are now so blithely called) would have benefited from broader contacts. The old psychological chestnuts seem to have returned, and one senses an emergence of what I am tempted to call "computational realism." Only that is real (and fundable) that is demonstrably simulated by a computational program. Perhaps the reason why the old chestnuts of learning theory and rote memory are back, just perhaps, is that computational models in the hands of psychologists are often not much richer than the old stimulus – response theories that used to animate much of psychological research. But that surely is not fair. Yet it is a worry. And it is still true, I think, that psychology is a subject of such gravity and complexity that it should not be left to the psychologists. And the cognitive scientists? Might they not better consort with some distractors?

Some of the most important things that happened at the Center were not planned at all and, I suppose, could never have been foreseen. George saw the founding of the Center as an act of rebellion against the state of psychology at Harvard and at large, and I felt much the same way. The Center was at Harvard on sufferance as far as our two departments were concerned. When William James Hall was in the process of completion, we were asked to look at plans for the eleventh and twelfth floors, where we were to be housed, and a few years after our founding, we were out of our quaint headquarters and down the street in the new highrise home of the behavioral sciences – though better housed than we had been before. The opposition never did quite stop, but it may nonetheless have added to the mystique of the "new" cognitive approach. And it surely added to the attraction we had for graduate students and young scholars from all over the place who wanted to come and have a year's visit. That was the hidden, unexpected impact of the Center.

It could not have been predicted. I do not think, in fact, that either of us was aware of it when it was happening. In fact, a new generation of cognitive psychologists, psycholinguists, and cognitive developmentalists was spawned at the Center. And while the likes of George Miller, Roger Brown, and I were teaching our heads off in courses, seminars, over lunch, and in the corridors, the testimony one picks up in traveling the circuit where the research is being done tells a richer story. When you talk to Masanao Toda or Pim Levelt, to Ino D'Arcais or Dan Kahnemann, to Don Norman or Molly Potter, to David McNeill or Amos Tversky, the story you hear is about a "culture" or a "self-instructing community." And whenever there is such talk, there is always a part of it given over to George. "He was such an elegant thinker that it was unthinkable to be a slob." "He was so demanding yet so open to what you had to say." Or "he took such fantastic pleasure in playing around with an idea that it was infectious.'' Or ''I never knew what clarity could be until I heard George give a lunch talk.'' So, in the end, you do have to worry about your historiographic stance. About Great Men in History. About the relation of the Individual and Culture. I said at the start that it was inconceivable that there would have been a Center without George. I don't know whether ''more inconceivable'' gets a linguistic asterisk, but I would still say that it is even more inconceivable that the Center would have been what it was without him.

References

Bruner, J. (1983). *In Search of Mind*. New York: Harper & Row.

Gardner, H. (1985). *The Mind's New Science: A History of the Cognitive Revolution*. New York: Basic Books.

Miller, G. (1979). A very personal history. *Occasional Paper #1*. Cambridge, Mass.: MIT Center for Cognitive Science.

8   Life at the Center

Donald A. Norman and Willem J. M. Levelt

In Chapter 7, Jerry Bruner tells of his vision of the Center for Cognitive Studies, one that complements ours in this chapter. His is the view from the top, the view of a founder and director who knew the context, the goals, the aspirations. Ours is the view from below, the view of the young researchers let loose to do as they would. The global context and purposes were foreign to us, not to be realized until much later (and for some things, not until now, when we read them in Bruner's chapter). Bruner states that "the intellectual life of the Center revolved around the seminars, the Thursday lunches, and the weekly colloquia." Perhaps. But that is not our memory. For us, the intellectual life was in the routine daily activities, in the offices and halls, in the labs late at night, and in the social interactions. The excitement was in the personal interaction and the private discussions and arguments. The formal seminars and lunches and colloquia were, well, formalities: the public display of the refinements. Formal presentations of ideas and results after much of the initial excitement had been polished, prettied up. We were the saplings, struggling to become trees. It is no wonder that we did not perceive the forest, or, for that matter, perceive how or even that we had been planted, nurtured, and cultivated. Such is the view from below.

The Harvard Center for Cognitive Studies. Ah, the good old days. The heady days of the cognitive revolution – when we were all much younger. But, as any modern psychologist will tell you, the good old days were never quite the same as memory would have them be. As for the revolution, there were really two different revolutions in progress, one in psycholinguistics, one in information processing, cognitive psychology. Both were probably revolutionary from the local, American perspective, but not so from the more global, historical perspective.

It is always difficult to know what goes on in another person's mind, especially when the person is George Miller. Quiet, tactful, reticent. A thoughtful thinker and writer, not given to quick responses and dashes of rhetorical comeback. That role was reserved for others. Actually, it was quite easy to know what was on some people's minds. Well, perhaps not to know, but to be told. Thus for Noam Chomsky, we always knew. Not that Chomsky said that much, but there were always people eager to tell us what he meant or what he would have meant had he said something. The prototypical lunchtime seminar – or at least, prototypical in our memory – is of everyone assembled around the large wooden

100

seminar table with an active, young cast of protagonists (perhaps Mehler, Bever, Fodor, and Katz), each paraphrasing and explaining to the lunchtime audience what the one had tried to explain to us what another had just said what yet another had just previously said that Noam would have said in retort to whatever the issue was at the time. All the time, Chomsky sitting and listening to the others explaining his mind. George did not go for flocks of interpreters. He stood on his own. One had to read his writings, attend his lectures, and re-create his thinking to figure out what was being thought.

In retrospect, what was accomplished at the Center was quite remarkable. At the time it seemed natural, nothing special. Now, some twenty-five years later, we can evaluate the impact of the Center from a distance, with some understanding of the historical perspective. Psychology was in a period of rapid change. Chomsky had started his work on transformational grammars, changing the face of linguistic theory. The field of artificial intelligence had just begun. Mathematical psychology was blooming. The concepts of information processing were pervading everything: computation, philosophy, communications, engineering, biology, linguistics and, of course, psychology. In the midst of these happenings, the Center for Cognitive Studies gathered together a vibrant group of people with unconventional knowledge and interests, stuck them together in one place, gave them excellent research, meeting, and support facilities, and then allowed what was to happen to happen. There were frequent meetings and seminars, a continual stream of visitors, and, for the members of the Center, no responsibilities. All of the ingredients were present: facilities, people, an active spirit, and critical mass. The Center offered a true demonstration of the critical mass theory of research, the notion that work proceeds best when there are enough people interested in the same or closely related topics so that there is always an audience for new ideas, an audience that can criticize in depth, suggest, and help generate the next generation of ideas.

Was there a cognitive revolution? Norman points out that he didn't even know what "cognitive" meant. "I remember asking Miller one day while we were out walking just what the word *cognitive* meant," recollects Norman. "Whatever it was that he replied, it didn't make much of an impression. My memory is that he told me a few things it was not, and concluded by saying that it meant whatever one wanted it to mean." Ah, the Center for Cognitive Studies, populated by folks who didn't even know what the name meant. The point probably was that the Center at Harvard was not set up to be *for* anything in particular; it was set up to be *against* things. What was important was what it was not: not psychophysics (at the time, a major, mainstream activity in psychology), not animal studies, certainly not Skinner's operant psychology (whose world headquarters were just down the street). Basically, not contemporary American 1950s psychology. Late 1800s or early 1900s psychology, perhaps, but certainly not the contemporary American psychology of the 1950s. The enemy was the present. Whatever we were to do, it was not to follow contemporary trends. The innocence of ignorance.

The common enemy was an especially interesting creature for somebody brought up in a European psychological tradition. Levelt remembers:

When I came to the Center, it was quickly made clear to me (but not by George Miller) that, by and large, all psychologists are behaviorists – even if they might deny that themselves – and that the Center was in the business of demolishing behavioristic doctrine and replacing it by a mentalistic approach. The polemic excitement was, of course, largely lost on someone who had been educated on an eclectic mixture of gestalt psychology, phenomenology, psychophysics, and ethology. All of these are either mentalistic or nativistic or both, and behaviorism had been so completely absent from my horizon that I didn't even know the difference between classical and operant conditioning. What had been the unmarked nativist background of most psychology that I had learned at Leyden University and with Michotte in Louvain now became the marked foreground issue. It was somewhat like experiencing the American excitement over Heineken beer, which I had always thought to be just beer.

Both Miller and Bruner were well aware of the historical and European roots of psychology, but that awareness was rather more the exception than the rule at Harvard. For sure, some of the major landmarks of European psychology were known and discussed: Piaget, Broadbent, Vygotsky, Craik, Luria. European psychophysicists were widely known and admired, but that seemed different, not really relevant to cognitive functioning. The fact is that much thought directly relevant to the interests of almost the entire crew at the Center was conveniently ignored. In retrospect, the excitement about the common enemy can be understood only if one takes into account the loss of continuity that had taken place in American academic psychology. A loss that took place even within Harvard itself. Art Blumenthal, who decided to use his time at the Center to study the history of psycholinguistics, discovered one psycholinguistic classic after another in Harvard's own Widener Library: major works by Preyer, Wundt, the Sterns, Buehler, Guillaume, and many others. And according to the library slips, basically none of these books had ever been loaned out before. At the time that Roger Brown and his co-workers were doing their magnificent work on the psycholinguistic development of the two children they called "Adam" and "Eve," the Widener Library contained the complete Stern Archives, including the most detailed and extensive longitudinal records of child language development ever made. Yet these records had never been consulted in the almost thirty years they had been there. It was therefore easy for Eva (not a pseudonym this time!), one of the Stern children, to convince the library to give the Archives to the Hebrew University of Jerusalem on permanent loan.[1]

Miller's scholarship wasn't sufficient to beat this ignorance. He was careful not to dominate, not to impose his views upon others. He provided the catalyst and the facilities. It was up to us to do our own work, to make our own discoveries.

The Center started in a pleasant old house on Kirkland Street, separated from all other parts of Harvard. Later the Center was to move to William James Hall, which combined in one building all of the heretofore disparate groupings of the two psychological departments at Harvard: Psychology and Social Relations. A sleek white building: modern architecture in full folly. Cutting up research groups into arbitrary groupings determined by floors and, worst of all, by the speed of response of the elevator, a speed so slow that it led to debates and experiments about response times, trade-offs (stairs versus elevator), and much discussion. On the middle floors, the Psychology Department with its three reigning professors: Skinner, Stevens, and Miller. Boring and Newman on the sidelines. Von Bekesy down below, existing on research grants, just a quiet-spoken psychophysicist, interested in prehistoric art, studying the details of the most sound-sensitive device in existence, next to the ventilation equipment for the entire building. No faculty position, no tenure. No students. Just a Nobel Prize. Soon to retreat to the University of Hawaii. Social Relations upstairs, a combination of social and clinical psychology, anthropology, and sociology. Social Relations and Psychology were separate departments at the time because of an academic feud that predated our existence. (Recombined again once the major protagonists had passed from the scene, but that was after our time, after the active days of the Center.) The Center had its roots in both departments – Miller was from Psychology, Bruner from Social Relations – and its location in the building was symbolic of these roots, with Psychology just below, Social Relations just above. The location did serve a purpose, easing communication with those just above and those just below. The course of science controlled by architecture and elevators.

The members of the Center interacted in groups, not by any purposeful arrangement but by the accidents of time, space, and organizational structure. One arrived, was assigned an office, told where to get supplies, where the lunchtime seminars were held, introduced to whomever was standing around at the time, and that was it. Except that that really wasn't it. The spirit of the Center did not reside within anything one could be introduced to or shown: the spirit came from the intense intellectual climate. Norman puts it this way:

In my memory there were immediate and vociferous debates from the moment I entered the Center, especially with the people I first encountered: Al Bregman, Paul Kolers, Jacques Mehler, Nancy Waugh. Debates that in every case led to collaborative and productive ideas, experiments, and creativity on language, memory, attention, perception, and thought (although to publishable results only in the case of Waugh). Did it start the first day? My memory has the heated discussions with Bregman starting in the first hour, as he helped me carry my books to our joint office. The experimental studies with Nancy Waugh that led to the work on primary memory started almost immediately after my arrival at the Center.

So it was with many of us. We all did whatever we were interested in. George Miller asked whether we could use a digital computer to control experiments. Norman and Bregman answered "yes," and before we knew what had happened, Miller had written a proposal, shipped it off to Washington, gotten approval, and purchased a DEC PDP-4: 8,000 words of memory, a paper tape reader, and special digital and analog input and output channels. We squeezed it all into a tiny office on the first floor (shared with Dave McNeil). The PDP-4 provided computational power, unheard of in any other psychological lab, and a full 8,000 words of memory. Today even the smallest computer one can purchase has more computational power than that early thing. At the Center, and especially once we moved into William James Hall, the computer worked faithfully. This was one of the first uses of a laboratory computer in psychology.[2]

What really did go on at the Center? The study of language was at the core, but the range of topics was immense. Both Miller and Bruner had wide-ranging interests. This led to an eclectic selection of visitors to the Center and active research that covered more areas than any individual could follow. It led to novel interactions and to continual groupings and regroupings as research interests fluctuated. What were the topics? There was work on memory, perception, concept formation, thinking, developmental psychology, decision theory, and especially the development of language in children. Miller was continually searching for new paradigms, a search that started in psychoacoustics, speech, information theory, mathematical models, computer simulation, and, at the Center, transformational grammars. Each new approach richer and more powerful than the previous, each with its own set of limitations. Miller had a reputation for being the first to show how each approach might enrich our understanding of psychological phenomena, but also the first to point out the fatal flaws.

Was it revolutionary? Chomsky certainly spoke of a revolution, and there can be no doubt that Chomsky intended to create a revolution in linguistics. But was it a revolution for us psychologists? The answer depends upon the perspective one takes. Consider first Miller's psycholinguistics. Historically speaking, its significance and impact are huge, with the only competition coming from Wundt's psychology of language. Around the turn of the nineteenth century, every study in the psychology of language had to take account of Wundt's views, either for or against. Similarly, during the Center's years and long after, every major psycholinguist had to take account of Miller's views or the views of Miller's co-workers and students. There were even public conversions or, in some cases, public announcements that no conversion would be forthcoming.[3]

So, at least in psycholinguistics, the air was revolutionary. But now compare Miller's psycholinguistics to that of Wundt. Three major features characterize Wundt's position: His psychology of language was, first, mentalistic (and quite

Humboldtian, for that matter). It was, second, strongly linguistically inspired (by a group of young turks in Leipzig, the *Junggrammatiker*). And, third, it was nonexperimental (this coming from the father of experimental psychology himself!). How does Miller's psycholinguistics compare? Clearly it shares mentalism, and even a Humboldtian kind of mentalism, with Wundt. Miller's mentalism was pretty revolutionary from the perspective of the then current American scene, but it is not so revolutionary from the wider historical perspective in psycholinguistics.

Miller's psycholinguistics was, like Wundt's, deeply affected by a revolutionary kind of linguistics. In fact, this feature was probably the most distinguishing characteristic of Miller's psycholinguistics: a "transformational psycholinguistics." From a historical perspective, the fact that the psychology of language was affected by linguistic theory was not new. What was new was the transformational grammar and the effort to test its "psychological reality" by experimental means.

This brings us to the third feature: Miller's psycholinguistics was experimental. This marked a departure from the work of Wundt. But, of course, this was not seen as revolutionary. Psychologists were supposed to do experiments, so it was only natural that the psychologists of language would do experiments with verbal materials. There was no disagreement here with the tradition of behavioral psycholinguistics, except that the unit of study was now the sentence, not the isolated word or meaningless nonsense syllable. Still, from the historical perspective, this *was* a pretty revolutionary feature of Miller's work. More precisely, it was Miller and his co-workers who, for the first time in the history of psycholinguistics, developed at any scale experimental procedures for studying the mental processes underlying sentence parsing, memory, and generation. It was exactly these kinds of mental processes that Wundt had declared to be inaccessible to experimental study, and before Miller, there had been no more than scattered and occasional attempts to approach these issues experimentally. In this particular case, the experiments defeated the linguistic theory: It was precisely the psychological reality of transformations that could not stand experimental tests. But whatever will survive of the psycholinguistic theories from the Center (such as the derivational theory of complexity and the coding hypothesis), the methodology has become the foundation of modern experimental psycholinguistics.

And what of those of us not in psycholinguistics? Did we perceive the Center as revolutionary? No. We simply did our work, pushing forth in whatever direction seemed most promising. To most of us, the work wasn't revolutionary; we were simply working on new areas of research, areas in which nobody else was working. We were studying how the mind operated, what its structure was, what the nature of information processing might be, what the flow of processing looked like, and what mechanisms might be involved. It is true that the work was novel to the then contemporary psychology, but it followed its own rich heritage.[4]

From the time of the very first computational machines constructed of gears and cogs, scientists have tried to determine how machines might be made to imitate humans. Developments in the mid-1900s gave major impetus to this work, which to a large extent was summarized in the various conferences on "thought processes" held in the late 1950s. Information theory and theories of computation gave a formal mathematical structure to the work, as did the evolution of a formal model of computational approaches, from developments in formal logic to McCullough and Pitts, who showed how it might all work with neurons, to Shannon, who applied it to computing machinery. And to Lettvin, Maturana, McCullough, and Pitts, who showed how specialized circuits might be implemented in the frog's eye. Rosenblatt's work on the perceptron was in the air. Minsky and McCarthy were beginning at MIT. Newell, Simon, and Shaw had started their work on problem solving, following a long European tradition going back to Selz and de Groot (a heritage that has now been explicitly acknowledged).

The research directions being explored at the Center were natural follow-ups to the thrust of information and computational sciences. To those of us who had been brought up on this approach, nothing was more natural than to pursue the question of how the human brain processed information. In this sense, from this historical perspective, we can say that there was nothing special about the application of ideas about information processing and computation to the understanding of psychological issues: It followed a long tradition. The work could be considered revolutionary only from the perspective of American psychology of the time. From a more global, more historically oriented perspective, the work was evolutionary, not revolutionary.

Note that the term "evolutionary" can be applied in two senses. First, the work was evolutionary in that it had developed in a natural way from a rich heritage. The basic ideas could each be traced to their natural, logical predecessors. Second, the work was evolutionary in the sense that when a new species takes over a niche that has not yet been occupied, it drives out the inhabitants of the surrounding niches. This is a somewhat revolutionary style of evolution. And this is what did happen at the Center. We occupied ground that others in psychology did not care about. Contemporary psychologists did not perceive us as revolutionaries. They probably thought we were irrelevant. But because we succeeded in our endeavors, the work came to dominate psychology, driving out much that had come before. (Driving out the good as well as the bad, but such is the way with evolution.)

The approach of the Center, focused as it was on doing new things, things thought never to have been done before, led to insularity and arrogance. Insularity in that, since it was assumed that nobody in psychology had ever had these ideas before, we could afford to ignore all else that was going on. Arrogance in part because we assumed that these were the only ways to approach psychological issues and in part because this was a long-established Harvard tradition. Full professors did not speak to junior professors. Junior professors were told at the time of hiring that "Harvard is a good place to be from," being promised from the beginning that they had no future at Harvard (unless they had received their Ph.D. there). And everyone at Harvard was either a competitor or irrelevant. It actually wasn't all that bad, but this description captures the spirit.[5]

The success of the Center

The Center brought together the leaders of a new generation of psychologists. It fostered an atmosphere of creativity. It helped to establish the cognitive revolution in psychology. Miller's influence was pervasive. His quiet presence was a powerful force on the work. First, in his own writings and seminars he pushed back the boundaries of psychology. Second, by the policy of letting people alone, free to push their work in their own directions, he helped to create the excitement at the Center. And finally, he served as a role model of the research scientist.

For some, he had another influence: subtle education about the rest of the world. He achieved this gently, without force, without direct confrontation – these are not Miller's ways. But by gentle conversation, subtle hints and suggestions, and through the examples of his own writings. Norman describes the impact upon his own development this way:

I arrived at Harvard relatively untutored in psychology. Yes, I had a Ph.D., but it was in a very specialized area of mathematical models, with a thesis in psychoacoustics (working on a problem discovered by von Bekesy, then developed by, among others, Stevens and Miller – for that matter, a topic upon which Neisser had done his doctoral dissertation). Most of my training had been in electronics, and my three years in the Psychology Department at Pennsylvania had not done much to broaden my views: Psychoacoustics and mathematical models of learning were, after all, very much in the engineering tradition. I guess I fitted in well at the Center, for I was one of the arrogant, thinking that the work we were doing was unique, that there was no need to read what others had done.

Miller showed the falsity of that. He produced two books while I was at the Center that demonstrated how wrong this view was. One, a review of mathematical psychology *(Mathematics and Psychology,* 1964), the other an introduction to psychology *(Psychology, the Science of Mental Life,* 1962). Both revealed the literature. But it was most especially the latter book, *Psychology, the Science of Mental Life,* that opened my eyes. It introduced me to the early literature of psychology, showed that there was life in the field, that there were ideas from the past that still exceeded the present capacity to bring them to fruition. My fascination with William James started then.

Consider the impact of Miller's book *Psychology, the Science of Mental Life.* Today, although it is still a very nice introduction, it does not seem courageous or particularly special in its choice of subject matter. Consider the title – *The Science of Mental Life*. The title is nothing to wonder at. You would have had to be there to understand. At the time, such a title was unheard of. Skinner, just down the street, exerted an amazing influence. He had banished the word "mental" from the vocabulary of psychology. Therefore, Miller's choice of title was a political statement. Yes, the title was borrowed from William James; that was just the point. The behaviorists had thought that they had banished mentalism from psychology forever, especially William James. And here it was back again, right under their own noses. We don't know what battles Miller and Bruner must have gone through to create the Center, what problems it caused for them in their departments. It must have been difficult.

The Center worked because it created a high-tension atmosphere of creative, ambitious people coupled with good research support. The interaction was intensive, critical, powerful. It was not a relaxed place. One always had to produce ideas and then defend them against the onslaught of critical, informed opinion. It didn't matter how good your work was last year or even last week: What have you done today? Such an atmosphere will not work for all, but for the particular group assembled at the Center, it did. Mostly. And at this particular time in American psychology, a time when behaviorism still dominated everything, the Center turned out to be a critical force.

From the point of view of the young researcher, everything seemed perfect. The continual intellectual challenge, the research facilities, even the lack of responsibilities, save to create and produce. The administrative burden of running such a large operation was borne completely by George Miller and Jerry Bruner, their efforts invisible to the rest of us. Perhaps too invisible. Getting research facilities seemed so easy. If we wanted a computer, George would get it. Give him a week to write a grant proposal. If we wanted a this or a that, it would happen. Now that we are out in the world getting our own support, we can see what a tremendous amount of work must have been involved. In retrospect, it was amazing that Miller and Bruner got any of their own work done.[6]

What was bad? The insularity, the narrowness, the naïveté and arrogance. But maybe that was necessary, necessary to push the field into uncharted waters. To move psychology from the dark ages of behaviorist traditions into the modern age, in which "mental" and "mind" and "consciousness" were words that could be used without apology, without quotation marks.

Notes

1 The Stern records have now been transcribed and stored in the computer files at the Max-Planck-Institut in Nijmegen. They are available in the United States at CHILDES, the Carnegie-Mellon/ Max-Planck Child Language Archives.

2 As far as we can tell, this was the second digital computer to be used specifically for the control of psychological experiments, the first in a university setting. The first laboratory computer for psychology was probably the DEC PDP-1 used by Rubenstein, Hayes, Nickerson, and others at the Air Force Decision Science Laboratories at Hanscom Field in Bedford, Massachusetts. (See Miller, Bregman, and Norman, 1965.)

3 An example of a conversion is the 1969 article by Deese, "Behavior and Fact." An example of the public refusal to convert is Osgood's (1968) article "Towards a Wedding of Insufficiencies."

4 It is important to note that we are concentrating upon the work done by the people with whom we interacted, which means primarily those centered around George Miller. There was another major focus of the Center, that of infant perception and motor development, centered around Jerry Bruner. Our efforts focused upon the linguistics and information processing developments. The resulting lack of involvement in the work of those studying infants means that we cannot speak of the nature or impact of their work upon what is today the active field of cognitive development.

5 Weekly colloquia were places where one displayed one's cleverness. The first question was always asked by a senior faculty member, always standing up from the front row, facing the audience. After all, the speaker was only the vehicle; the important folks were the ones in the audience. A long first question, with a twinkle in the eye, displaying wit, erudition, and insight. Who else dared match that question? One of us (D.A.N.) remembers one occasion where a young Center member poked him toward the end of the talk and whispered, "I can't think of a question; can you think of one for me?" As for the answers to the questions – irrelevant.

6 The writing of this chapter has caused us to recognize yet another powerful influence of the Center upon each of our lives: as a role model for our own development, both as research scientists and as proponents of similar research centers. Thus, Norman has built up a similar, although more limited, enterprise jointly with Dave Rumelhart at the Institute for Cognitive Science at the University of California, San Diego. Levelt has done a similar thing on a somewhat larger scale at the Max-Planck-Institut für Psycholinguistik, Nijmegen, The Netherlands. Students, postdoctoral fellows, visiting scientists. Provide good facilities. Set up a climate for the holding of frequent seminars and discussions. Take away the administrative burden from the younger workers. And leave people alone.

References

Deese, J. (1969). Behavior and fact. *American Psychologist, 24,* 515–22.

Miller, G. A. (1964). *Mathematics and Psychology.* New York: Wiley.

Miller, G. A. (1962). *Psychology, the Science of Mental Life.* New York: Harper & Row.

Miller, G. A., Bregman, A. S., & Norman, D. A. (1965). The computer as a general-purpose device for the control of psychological experiments. In B. Waxman & R. W. Stach (Eds.), *Computers in Biomedical Research.* New York: Academic Press.

Osgood, C. (968). Towards a wedding of insufficiencies. In T. R. Dixon & D. L. Horton (Eds.), *Verbal Behavior and General Behavior Theory.* Englewood Cliffs, N.J.: Prentice-Hall.

PART III Psycholinguistics

George had been interested in language since his undergraduate days at the University of Alabama. As a result, many of the members of the Center for Cognitive Studies that he and Bruner invited were interested in the psychology of language. The list of psycholinguists that either spent time at or were trained at the Center is large and impressive. Three of these, Thomas Bever, Eric Wanner, and Jacques Mehler, write about psycholinguistics at the Center, the issues that intrigued them then, and how these issues have been transformed since the heyday of the Center. Morris Halle is a close friend of George's who tutored George in the complexities of linguistics. Halle's chapter traces the changing concept of the phoneme.

9   The psychological reality of grammar: a student's-eye view of cognitive science

Thomas G. Bever

> Never mind about the why:
> figure out the how, and the why will take care of itself.
> Lord Peter Wimsey

Introduction

This is a cautionary historical tale about the scientific study of what we know, what we do, and how we acquire what we know and do. There are two opposed paradigms in psychological science that deal with these interrelated topics: The behaviorist *prescribes* possible adult structures in terms of a theory of what can be learned; the rationalist *explores* adult structures in order to find out what a developmental theory must explain. The essential moral of the recent history of cognitive science is that it is more productive to explore mental life than prescribe it.

The classical period

Experimental cognitive psychology was born the first time at the end of the nineteenth century. The pervasive bureaucratic work in psychology by Wundt (1874) and the thoughtful organization by James (1890) demonstrated that experiments on mental life both can be done and are interesting. Language was an obviously appropriate object of this kind of psychological study. Wundt (1911), in particular, gave great attention to summarizing a century of research on the natural units and structure of language; (see especially, Humboldt, 1835; Chomsky, 1966). He reported a striking conclusion: The natural unit of linguistic knowledge is the *intuition* that a sequence is a sentence. He reasoned as follows:

All of the cited articles coauthored by me were substantially written when I was an associate in George A. Miller's laboratory, first at Harvard University and then at Rockefeller University. That is no accident.

112

> We cannot define sentences as sequences of words because there are single-word sentences (e.g., "Leave").
>
> We cannot define sentences as word uses that have meaningful relations because there are meaningful relations within certain word sequences that, nevertheless, are not sentences (e.g., "the days of the week").

Hence, the sentence must be defined as a sequence that native speakers of a language intuitively believe to convey a complete proposition in a linguistically acceptable form.

At the outset, this framed the problem of linguistic description as a problem of linguistic knowledge – to describe what speakers of a language know when they know a language. Wundt's formal analyses of this knowledge summarized a tradition of continental research on local and exotic languages. Most important was the assignment of purely abstract syntactic structures to sentences, independent of their meaning. Among these structural features were several levels of representation, which expressed grammatical relations between words and phrases. At a surface level, a set of hierarchically embedded frames symbolized the relative unity of word sequences grouped into phrases. For example, in sentence (1), "the" is clearly more related within a unit to "Rubicon" than to "crossing"; similarly, in sentence (2), "was" is closer to "crossed" than to "Rubicon." The surface level also defines a set of surface grammatical relations between the phrases: In sentence (1), "Caesar" is the grammatical subject, namely, the phrase that determines the morphological agreement with the verb. In sentence (2), the corresponding grammatical subject is "The Rubicon." In sentence (3), it is the entire act, "Crossing the Rubicon."

(1) Caesar was crossing the Rubicon.
(2) The Rubicon was crossed by Caesar.
(3) Crossing the Rubicon was what Caesar did.

It was obvious that the propositional relations between the phrases could not be captured by the surface grammatical relations. As Wundt noted, "Caesar" is the acting one in each of these cases. The propositional relations between phrases must be represented by a separate level, the "inner form" of the sentence. At this level, sentences (1) to (3) share the same relations between "Caesar" (agent), "cross" (action), and "Rubicon" (object). The different actual sequences at the surface grammatical level were related to the propositional level by processes of transformation *(umwandlung)*; these processes reorder surface phrases in surface patterns allowed by the particular language. The propositional relations were not purely semantic, but were the formal expression of relations between semantic units of meaning (Blumenthal, 1970; 1975).

The continental model of language was rich and made many claims about the capacity of humans to manipulate abstract entities. But, alas, the theory never became an object of experimental importance. The reasons are, no doubt, politically and scientifically complex. One sufficient fact is that Wundt classified the study of language as a branch of social psychology, and hence, for him, not a subject fit for experimental investigation. His vast structural catalog of language is more an anthropological survey rather than a scientific scrutiny of the mind. The linguistic model and its richness became lost to scientific psychology.

But the model was not lost to everbody interested in language. It was popularized in the infant field of linguistics by a young professor of German, Leonard Bloomfield. Bloomfield's (1914) enthusiastic exegesis of Wundt's multileveled model might have installed it as the basis for the newly emerging science of language. However, in all social sciences at the time, there was a growing preoccupation with behaviorist injunctions against unobservable entities and relations. Clearly, the notions "intuition" and "inner grammatical level" were not acceptable in the operationalist framework. Bloomfield capitulated to such restrictions as enthusiastically as he had earlier espoused the Wundtian model. His foundational book, *Language* (1933), presents a totally operationalist framework for linguistic theory. In that book, the sentence is hardly mentioned, while meaning is given an amusing (and brief) treatment in terms of the association of stimuli and responses. The interdict had fallen.

The dark ages

Behaviorism is a seductive doctrine that has dominated psychological theories of learning for the majority of this century. It is seductive because it *simultaneously* purports to answer three questions:

> What do we learn?
> How do we learn?
> Why do we learn?

According to behaviorism, the reason that we learn is that the environment provides pleasure when we do – that is, it reinforces our activity. Selective reinforcement accounts for the way we learn; it associates environmentally successful pairs of behaviors and situations as permanently learned units. Accordingly, what we learn must be expressed in terms of definable pairs of behaviors and situations. These principles provide a chain of inference from the motive to learn back to the structure of what is learned, a chain that has fettered generations of psychologists. The functional importance of reinforcement justifies the scientific investigation of isolated sources of pleasure and displeasure. The focus on behavior/situation pairs licenses investigation of the learning of meaningless associations between situations and behaviors. The requirement that learned associations are between definable entities transfers to the operationalist requirement that theoretical terms must be inductively reducible to observable entities.

By the late 1950s, sophisticated elaborations of these principles had crystallized, most notably in the proposal by Hull (1943) that they could account for hierarchically organized chains of behavior. Even when transferred to descriptions of language behavior (Osgood, Suci, & Tannenbaum, 1957), the basic behaviorist doctrine about the structure of what was learned remained: It must offer recognizable links between isolatable situations and behaviors (Fodor, 1966; Bever, 1968). The implications of this doctrine for theories of language were severe. Consider how these procedures affected theories of the relationship between two levels of description, words and phrases. Following Bloomfield's conversion, linguists had adopted the behaviorist restrictions on how to pursue the analysis of language structure. They imposed on themselves a set of *discovery* procedures that would guarantee the scientific acceptability of linguistics and the learnability of the resultant linguistic descriptions. Language was to be described in a hierarchy of levels of learned units such that the units at each level can be expressed as a grouping of units at an intuitively lower level. The lowest level in any such hierarchy was necessarily composed of physically definable units. For example, sentences (4)–(7) could all be resolved to a basic sequence of the same kinds of phrases, a noun phrase, a verb, and an adjective phrase.

(4) Harry was eager.
(5) The boy was eager.
(6) The tall boy was eager to leave.
(7) He was something.

The behaviorist principles demanded that phrases not be free-floating, abstract objects: Each must be reducible back to a single word that could serve as a lexical substitute for the entire phrase, as in sentence (7). In this way, "phrases" were rendered theoretically as units that could be resolved as "words." At the same time, the description gave an account of the fact that words within phrases seem to be more closely related to each other than across phrases. Finally, it seemed possible to hope for a description of all possible types of phrases, since longer ones seemed to resolve into combinations of shorter ones, which in turn could resolve to single words.

This behaviorist implementation of linguistics may seem harmless enough, but it had a particular result: The theoretical notion of the *sentence* could not be described by linguistic theory. This is true for three empirical reasons: First, the number of sentences seemed unfathomably large; second, in a single sentence, there are often relations between words in different phrases; there are grammatical relations between phrases, which cannot be described as superficial facts about the phrases themselves. In addition, as Wundt had noted, it is methodologically impossible to define sentences operationally. To deal with such phenomena as these, linguistic theory would have required levels of representation and theoretical entities that could not be resolved by reduction to independently observable units. Most behaviorist linguists were sufficiently aware of these problems to leave the description of the sentence alone; the reducible phrase was the pinnacle of behaviorist linguistics.

One unconventional linguist attempted to apply the operationalist descriptive principles to sentences. From the operationalist standpoint, the sentence is a component of a complete discourse in the same sense that a phrase is a component of a sentence. Harris (1957, 1958) capitalized on this perspective: He developed a descriptive scheme in which sentences (and clauses) that can occur in the same discourse frame are reduced to canonical sentence forms. This scheme depends on the fact that sentences occur in structural families: For example, sentences (1)–(3) are part of a larger set of constructions, as follows:

> Caesar crossed the Rubicon.
> It is the Rubicon that Caesar crossed.
> What Caesar did was cross the Rubicon.
> The Rubicon is what Caesar crossed.
> . . . that Caesar crossed the Rubicon . . .
> . . . Caesar's crossing the Rubicon . . .
> . . . the Rubicon's being crossed by Caesar . . .
> . . . the crossing of the Rubicon by Caesar . . .

Harris noted that all of these variants can often co-occur in the same discourse environment – that is, all of them can be substituted for the blank in the following discourse frame (ignoring changes needed to accommodate the clausal variants):

> Caesar marched north.
> Then _____ .
> This surprised the local inhabitants.

The notion of co-occurrence was intended to be the same as that describing the substitutability of phrases in discourse-based sentence frames. The difference is that unlike phrases, sentences cannot be reduced to canonical words ("it," "did"). Rather, Harris suggested that they be reduced to a *standard canonical sentence* form, the "kernel" of each structural sentence family. Kernel sentences are the simple declarative construction; for example, co-occurrence "transformations" express the relation between the kernel sentence and its variants. The kernel and the passive sentence (2) are related by the co-occurrence transformation, as follows:

"NP_1, V + ed by NP_2 '$\longleftrightarrow$' NP_2 was V ed by NP_1"

There are several important points to retain about this theory. First, the co-occurrence transformations can only relate specific observable sentences. (Harris actually apologized for using abstract terms of the previous kind, but argued that this was only a descriptively temporary notion, not a true violation of operationalist purity; see Katz & Bever, 1975.) Second, the relative priority of the kernel sentence form had an intuitive appeal but still did not unambiguously meet the requirement that it be both observable and operationally definable. Finally, it was inordinately difficult to make the program work in detail. In retrospect, one can view co-occurrence transformational grammar as an insightful attempt to describe sentence structure within a taxonomic paradigm. The failures of the attempt were illuminating and set the scene for the later developments in linguistic theory, to which I return after reviewing progress in psychology of the day.

The middle ages

For several decades, psychological research on language proceeded largely without explicit benefit of linguistic analysis. The beginnings were modest: the study of the processing of unrelated word sequences to discover how universal laws of learning apply to human beings. This deceptively simple paradigm, "verbal learning," became the focus of an enormous amount of research (many hundreds of articles, with several journals devoted to little else – see Underwood & Schulz, 1960; Cofer, 1961; Cofer & Musgrave, 1963, for representative reviews). Enormous effort was devoted to exploring the formation of associations between adjacent and remote words in strings, the influence of different kinds of practice, of different kinds of reinforcement, of subjects' age, mental capacity, and so on. These studies might appear to be about language as well as learning because they used words as stimuli. But they were about words only coincidentally; words were merely handy units that humans could learn to string together in unrelated ways (much later, it became clear that even this was an illusion, but that is another story; Anderson & Bower, 1973). The focus was on learning, motivation, and memory, not language. Of course, one could have viewed this as propaedeutic to an understanding of how words are processed when they are organized in whole sentences. Unfortunately, this promise was never realized. As we shall shortly see, words in whole sentences are processed differently from words in random sequences.

Just as wholes are the natural enemies of parts, gestalt psychology is the natural enemy of associationist behaviorism. Crucial demonstrations had long been available that percepts have higher-order structures that cannot be accounted for by merely associating the parts. Linguistic structures would seem to have been prime candidates for gestalt investigations: Sentences are wholes that bind together and transcend words and phrases as their parts (Lashley, 1951; Mandler & Mandler, 1964). Such obviously true observation rarely stops associationists from going about their business, and had absolutely no impact on the prediction that the study of verbal learning would lead to an understanding of language (Skinner, 1957). The failure of the gestalt demonstrations to undercut associationistic accounts of language was due in part to the inability of gestalt psychology to develop a generative theory of possible gestalten; in any domain, most "principles" of how gestalten are formed seemed true but inexplicable. Furthermore, gestalt psychologists themselves had little interest in language, since to them it seemed obvious that language was both abstract and learned, and therefore not the proper object of their investigation (Koffka, 1935). Once again, a methodological preconception barred a potentially fruitful approach to language.

Until the 1950s, linguists and psychologists worked apart, though sharing the fundamental theoretical restrictions of behaviorism. An early burst of psycholinguistics occurred when the two groups discovered that they could mate each others' theories: learning theory was allegedly capable of describing the acquisition of "behavioral hierarchies" of just the type that linguists had found to be the ultimate grammatical aspect of language, namely, words-in-phrases (Osgood & Sebeok, 1954). The first mating between psychology and linguistics was intense but sterile. The reason was that the two disciplines were mutually compatible just because they shared the same behaviorist preconceptions: The psychologist was willing to postulate of the language learner only the inductive capacity to learn what the linguist had already restricted himself to describe. Yet the shared descriptive restrictions robbed linguistic theory – and psychology – of the sentence. The project of the first psycholinguistics – to show how linguistic structures followed from psychological laws of learning – was successful, brilliantly – and pyrrhically.

There was a separate stream of research that emerged during the same period – the study of how language behavior is organized in adults, independent of any theoretical preconceptions about learning (Miller, 1951a, 1951b). It was unarguable that at some point in the understanding of the sounds of spoken language, listeners arrive at an abstract conceptual analysis of its meaning and structure, but it was still arguable that the meaning conveys the structure and not the reverse. Miller and Selfridge (1950) demonstrated the behavioral relevance of sentence structure, in particular, by showing that memory for the word sequences improves as they approach the statistical regularities of English. This suggested that language behavior involves a transfer of the physical signal into a linguistic world that can access regularities of structure and meaning. The perceptual question was formulated in terms of a search for *the* units of speech perception in which the acoustic-to-linguistic transfer takes place from an acoustic to a linguistic representation.

A standard experimental method to investigate this question was based on an everyday fact: Spoken language is extremely resistant to acoustic interference. Imagine yourself next to a large waterfall: Even though the noise is tremendous, you are able to understand somebody talking to you, so long as the conversation is in your language. The question is, why? Clearly, you are using your knowledge of the language to aid your perception. But which aspect of your linguistic knowledge do you access first? A straightforward hypothesis is that you have memorized the *words* of your language. In this view, the unit of transfer from acoustic to linguistic information in speech perception is the word: A listener first maps the acoustic signal onto separate words and then computes the meaning from them.

The proposal that the unit of speech perception is the word may seem daunting, since there are so many of them. But one thing we know: People do learn thousands of words in their language. Since the number of effectively necessary words is finite (though large), it is possible to imagine that they are the learned basis for speech perception. A laboratory-controlled variant of the speech-by-waterfall experience offered a technique to test the word hypothesis (Miller, Heise, & Lichten, 1951; Miller & Isard, 1963). Suppose we adjust the loudness of a noise source relative to recordings of the words in sentence (8) so that each word is recognized correctly 50 percent of the time when the words are heard alone. If it is the word level at which the acoustic information is mapped onto linguistic representations, then a sentence composed by stringing together the same words should be perceived 25 percent of the time. This follows from the hypothesis that the acoustic shape of each word is mapped independently onto a linguistic representation. The actual facts are striking: When strung together into a sentence, the word sequence is often recognized much more than 50 percent of the time. Most important is the intuitive fact that the words seem acoustically clearer *as you hear them* when they are in a sentence.

(8)   Horses, eat

The outcome of a series of such studies was the demonstration that it is at least the *sentence* that is the unit of speech perception. Even sentences that do not make semantic sense enhance perception of the words in them.

This finding created two problems that still dominate investigations of language: How do we use our knowledge of sentences in behavior? What do we know when we know the sentences of our language? The first issue is a direct example of the problem of integrating abstract knowledge with concrete behavior. For decades, psychologists had assumed that beliefs cannot affect perception except in very limited cases. This belief was consistent with the behaviorist strictures on what we can learn: If beliefs can influence perception, then what the child learns cannot be limited to what is in the world to be perceived. The apparent influence of abstract sentence structure on acoustic decisions [and other kinds of sensory judgments (Miller, Bruner, & Postman, 1954)] suggested that perceptual activity involves the *simultaneous* integration of abstract and concrete levels of representation.

There are two views how this integration occurs: Abstract levels of knowledge can directly influence concrete levels ("top-down processing") or can interact only after lower-level representations are formed ("bottom-up processing"). Since it was first discovered, this issue has been vigorously pursued in language perception, because language offers well-defined, distinct levels of linguistic structure. The pendulum of scientific fashion has swung back and forth, with current investigators in favor of a bottom-up theory of perception (Forster, 1979; Fodor, 1983; Pylyshyn, 1984). This issue may never be entirely resolved. The clear experimental demonstration of the behavioral importance of sentence level discredited behaviorist restrictions on theories of language comprehension. More enduringly, the issue has been the engine for decades of empirical and theoretical research.

Another matter was raised by the acoustic clarity of sentences: How can something as varied as the sentence be the unit of transfer from acoustic to linguistic representations? Unlike the number of words, there is no meaningful upper bound to the number of sentences; hence, when we listen, we cannot transfer information from acoustic to linguistic structure sentence by sentence. Clearly, we must know a system of rules for describing the sentences in our language, and we must apply that categorical knowledge actively during speech behaviors such as comprehension.

This conclusion from experiments on adult behavior presented an unanticipated challenge to the behaviorist doctrine about learning. The sentence level of knowledge plays an active role in perception, yet that level cannot be described or acquired according to behaviorist principles. By ignoring the problem of learning altogether and focusing on adult behavior, it was discovered that adults use representations that cannot be learned by induction: People actively use categorical rules in ongoing behavior. This seemed typical of many behaviors once some thought was given to the question (Miller, Galanter, & Pribram, 1960). Behaviorism was surely doomed as a theory of language, but the final fall awaited a viable theory of what kind of knowledge generates the sentences of a language.

What *is* a sentence? Harris had attempted to include the sentence level within an operationalist framework, but his success was limited by the discovery procedures. In the late 1950s Chomsky (1957a) offered a new kind of grammar as a formal answer to this question: A sentence is what the grammar describes as a sentence. The motivations and details of this new theory were similar in many respect to those summarized by Wundt (though without awareness of this similarity at the time) (Chomsky, 1957b). The configuration of the syntactic model that described sentence structure was also similar to that of much earlier times and included a reformulated notion of transformation. But the new transformational grammar had novel formal devices, as well as a completely new goal for grammatical description. The grammar was generative: It described sentence structures of a language as a natural part of human knowledge. The new approach flatly rejected operationalist discovery procedures and allowed abstract terms and rules that were not reducible to observable entities. This represents in linguistics the same kind of shift away from behaviorist principles of learning that was occurring within psychology. Chomsky was also diligent in pointing out the general failures of behaviorist accounts of language (Chomsky, 1959). The goal of linguistic analysis was to describe an adult's linguistic knowledge, not language behavior: The staple facts that reflect that knowledge are intuitions about the acceptability of sentences in one's language. Hence, masses of data relevant to linguistic analysis are easy to collect; one merely consults a native speaker on how he feels about a language sequence. By assigning sentence status to only those sequences that are intuitively acceptable, the grammar constitutes a theory of the speaker's underlying linguistic knowledge.

The most important feature of the new syntactic model was that several levels of representation are included in the description of every sentence. Obviously, only one of these levels is directly observable. This level, the surface structure, corresponds roughly to the kind of phrase structure Wundt described for surface grammatical relations, as well as that arrived at by behaviorist linguists. Every sentence at this level was paired with an underlying "kernel" structure, which presented the propositional relations for each verb in a canonical form.

A set of transformations specified the possible pairs of deep and surface phrase structures. Unlike co-occurrence transformations, these transformations operate unidirectionally. Each transformation applies a successive deformation of the input tree – for example, changing a structure that will end up as an active into one that will end up as a passive:

tree 1 $====================$⟩ tree 2

Certain transformations combined kernel trees into complex sentences like sentences (9) and (10) (⟨⟩ represents a position into which a complement sentence is to be inserted):

(9) John defied Bill to go.
(10) John desired Bill to go.

The way in which different kernel sentences are combined reveals interesting differences in the deep-structure organization of sentences that are superficially similar. For example, in the complex sentences with

John past defy Bill ⟨⟩ $==$⟩ John past defy Bill to go
Bill go

John past desire ⟨⟩ $==$⟩ John past desire Bill to go
Bill go

"desire" and "defy" appear to have superficially identical structures. But they have different corresponding structural variations, which attests to their underlying distinctness. For example, the complement sentence can be passivized as a whole unit with "desire" but not with "defy." Contrast your intuitions about the acceptability of the following two sequences:

(11) For Bill to go was desired by John.
(12) For Bill to go was defied by John (unacceptable).

The fact that the complement sentence can act as a whole unit in passive constructions demonstrated that at the deep structure level the entire complement sentence is a direct object of verbs like "desire," whereas only the following noun phrase is the direct object of verbs like "defy."

Similar kinds of reasons demonstrated the difference at the underlying structure level of other superficially identical sentence structures:

(13) John was eager to please.
(14) John was easy to please.

John past BE eager $\langle\rangle$
John please someone $= =\rangle$ John was eager to please

It past BE easy $\langle\rangle$
Someone please John $= =\rangle$ John was easy to please

Thus, knowing the syntax of a language consisted of knowing a set of phrase structure rules that generate the underlying kernel structures and the transformations that deform and combine those underlying structures into sentences. The kernel structures were not representations of meaning of sentences but of their underlying syntactic configuration. The meaning of a sentence was a function of semantic operations on underlying structure representation (Katz & Postal, 1964; Chomsky, 1965); the sound was produced by operations on the surface representation.

Linguists made a firm point of insisting that, at most, a grammar was a model of "competence" – what the speaker knows. This was distinguished from "performance" – how the speaker implements his knowledge. But, despite this distinction, the syntactic model had great appeal as a model of the processes we carry out when we talk and listen. It offered a precise answer to the question of what we know when they know the sentences in their language: We know the different coherent levels of representation and the linguistic *rules* that interrelate those levels. It was tempting to postulate that the theory of what we know is a theory of what we do, thus answering two questions simultaneously:

What do we know when we know a language?
What do we do when we use what we know?

The first answers were couched in terms of the linguistic model and a direct assumption about how the model was linked to behavioral systems. We know two systems of syntactic rules and the levels of representation that they describe; phrase/structure rules define underlying kernel structures, and transformations derive surface phrase structures from the kernels. This knowledge is linked to behavior in such a way that every syntactic operation corresponds to a psychological process. The hypothesis linking language behavior and knowledge was that they are identical.

The way to test the direct linking hypothesis was to demonstrate the "psychological reality" in ongoing behavior of linguistic structures. Surface phrase structures were taken to be noncontroversial because they were allegedly definable within the behaviorist framework. (In fact, they probably are not; Bever, 1968b; Bever, Foder, & Weksel, 1968.) But the claim that *deep* structures were psychologically "real" was a direct challenge to behaviorism: Deep structures were obviously abstract in the sense that they are not actual sentences, but rather the "inner form" to which Wundt referred. Note that even the simplest kernel structure ("he (past leave)") is not an actual sentence. A set of morphological transformations always applies to even the simplest sentences (e.g., changing "he past leave" to "he left"). The further claim that transformations were real mental processes was an additional challenge, both because the rules are themselves abstract and because they define intermediate levels of phrase structure representations as they do their transformational work.

The first step was to define a structural paradigm that would generate a family of studies of the psychological validity of the grammar as a mental model. Three optional transformations defined eight sentence types in a three-dimensional cube (Miller, 1962b). Sentences can be either active or passive, declarative or interrogative, positive or negative. In linguistic theory of the day, each of these dimensions corresponded to transformation. Accordingly, in testing the behavioral implications of the formal relations between these sentences as arrayed on the transformational cube, one could test the psychological relevance of the grammatical model.

The initial results were breathtaking. The amount of time it takes to produce a sentence, given another variant of it, is a function of the distance between them on the transformational cube (Miller & McKean, 1964); transformational distance between sentences also predicts confusability between them in memory (Mehler, 1963; Clifton, Kurcz, & Jenkins, 1965; Clifton & Odom, 1966). Furthermore, the ease of memorizing the sentences was predicted by the number of transformations that have applied to them: Simple declaratives are easier than passives, which are easier than passive questions, and so on (Mehler, 1963). Finally, such transformationally complex sentence forms as passives were more resistant to acoustic distortion (Compton, 1967), took longer to comprehend than corresponding actives (McMahon, 1963; Gough, 1965, 1966), and put a greater load on immediate memory (Savin & Perchonock, 1965).

It is hard to convey how exciting these developments were. It appeared that there was to be a continuing direct connection between linguistic and psychological research: Linguistic analysis would support structural analyses, which would directly become hypotheses for investigation in language behavior. Abstract models of linguistic structure and performance could give clear direction and critical importance to empirical research (Chomsky & Miller, 1963; Miller & Chomsky, 1963). The hypothesized link between the structure of knowledge and the processes of behavior was wildly successful. The golden age had arrived.

The enlightenment

It soon became clear that either the linking hypothesis was wrong or the grammar was wrong, or both. The support for the psychological relevance of transformations had been based only on those three that defined the transformational "cube." But the overall program implied a broad empirical hypothesis about the relation between all rules in a grammar and sentence processing: the so-called derivational theory of complexity. (The complexity of processing a sentence corresponds to the number of transformations in its description.)

It had long been known that the derivational hypothesis was wrong for many constructions. As a predictive principle, it was both too strong and too weak (Fodor & Garrett, 1967; Bever, 1970). It was too weak because it failed to predict the obvious complexity of numerous kinds of sentences.

(15) Center embedding: *the oyster the oyster the oyster split split split.* (Contrast to the structurally identical, but easier, *the reporter everyone I met trusts predicted the coup.*)

(16) Object relative clauses without relative pronouns: *the horse raced past the barn fell.* (Contrast to the structurally identical, but easier, *the horse ridden past the barn fell.*)

It was too strong because it incorrectly predicted that various sentence constructions with more transformations are harder to understand than corresponding sentences with fewer transformations:

(17) Heavy noun phrase (NP) shift: *We showed the long-awaited and astoundingly beautiful pictures of the Himalayan trip to Mary.* is transformationally less complex than the easier *We showed Mary the long-awaited and breathtakingly beautiful pictures of the Himalayan trip.*

(18) Extraposition: *That Bill left early with Mary surprised Hank.* is transformationally less complex than the easier *It surprised Hank that Bill left early with Mary.*

These direct demonstrations of the inadequacy of the derivational theory of complexity were backed up by several experiments that examined the implications for perceptual difficulty of transformations other than those that defined the transformational cube. For example, the transformation that optionally moves a particle/preposition to the position following the verb was well motivated as starting with the *Verb + particle NP* deep structure and then being transformed to the *Verb-NP-prt* sequence, as shown subsequently. This order of structures is indicated by the fact that verbs are lexically associated with some particle/prepositions and not others (e.g., we have "call up" and "call NP over" but not "call NP under"). If such verbal sequences are entered as complex lexical items and *then* transformed, we can capture these lexical regularities.

John called up Mary $==\rangle$ John called Mary up
verb prt NP   verb NP prt

Despite this clear motivation for treating the *Verb-prt-NP* variant as less complex transformationally, such sentences turned out to be processed more slowly than the corresponding transformed versions (Bever & Mehler, 1967). Other studies of specific transformations also failed to show that perceptual difficulty corresponds to the number of transformations (Bever, Fodor, Garrett, & Mehler, 1966; Jenkins, Fodor, & Saporta, 1965; Fodor & Garrett, 1967).

Such failures were baffling in light of the initial success of the structures arranged on the transformation cube. The failures motivated reconsideration of the theoretical interpretation of the three-dimensional model. This further consideration revealed that if the grammatical theory were taken literally, it would not have motivated many of the original predictions. First, the linguistically provided route from one construction to another is not along the surface of the three-dimensional cube; rather, it must involve returning to the underlying kernel structure and then reemerging to the target structure. For example, the grammatically defined pathway from the negative-passive to the active construction is not provided by undoing the negative and then the passive; rather, it is provided by undoing the morphologically necessary transformations, the passive transformation, and then the negative transformation, to recover the kernel structure: then that structure must have the morphological transformations reapplied to it to produce the declarative sentence. Each time two sentences are related, it must be by way of a return to the inner kernel structure and a new path out to the target sentence structure. This strict interpretation of the grammar had the consequence that confusions between two complex sentences adjacent on the transformation cube (e.g., between the negative passive and the passive question) would be far less likely than between two simpler structures (the negative and the question). Yet, this was not confirmed. Sentences were confusible as a function of their adjacency on the *surface* of the sentence cube. This fact had to be reinterpreted in light of the lack of motivation due to a strict implementation of the grammar. One possibility was that their language cube was a real but temporary representation that subjects themselves constructed to deal with the temporarily repetitive experimental problem set for them: The repeated presentation of a small number of sentence types stimulated their arrangement on a cube (Bever, 1970a). This offered an explanation of why small variations in response technique could change the evidence for the transformational cube. For example, the frequency of decisions that a sentence is appearing for the first time is low if a transformational variant of it appeared recently (Clifton & Odom, 1966). The amount of interference, however, appears to be a function of the similarity of the two sentences at the underlying structure level: For example, active and passive constructions mutually interact more than active and negative constructions. This is explained by the fact that the "negative" is marked in the deep structure, as well as occasioning a transformational rule (Katz & Postal, 1964; Chomsky, 1965).

It was also necessary to understand why the relative difficulties of comprehension and perception were predicted by the transformational distance from the kernel structure on the cube. First, two of the transformations actually changed the meaning of the sentence: question and negation. It is not surprising, upon reflection, that such sentences might be relatively hard to process precisely because of their semantic complexity (i.e., the negative has the same propositional structure as the declarative, with an additional semantic operator). The importance of semantic analysis was emphasized by the finding that passive constructions are relatively complex *only* when they are semantically reversible (Sobin, 1966; Walker, Gough, & Wall, 1968; e.g., "Vercingetorix was crossed by Caesar" is more difficult than its corresponding active construction, but "The Rubicon was crossed by Caesar" is not).

The conclusion of such demonstrations, and of further theoretical analysis, was that there is no direct evidence for grammatical transformations in speech behaviors. The behavioral relevance of grammatical levels of representation fared better. Surface phrase structure can be construed as making the behavioral claim that the members of a phrase have a stronger bond to each other than to the members of other phrases. This was directly tested by Levelt (1970). He demonstrated that surface phrase structure can be derived by hierarchical clustering analyses of subjects' reports of "relatedness" among the word pairs of a sentence (see Chapters 4 and 8 of this volume). Accordingly, words are better prompts for other words in the same surface phrase than in different phrases (Johnson, 1965; Suci, Ammon, & Gamlin, 1967; Stewart & Gough, 1967).

Other kinds of studies demonstrated that surface phrase structure is imposed on sentences as we perceive them (Mehler & Carey, 1967; Mehler, Bever, & Carey, 1970). The surface structure pattern was dramatically revealed in the perceived location of nonspeech sounds that interrupt a sentence. Such sounds characteristically are reported as having occurred in a phrase break, especially between clauses, rather than in their actual location (Fodor & Bever, 1965; Garrett, 1966). This effect is not due to guessing biases (Garrett, 1965; Holmes,

1970; Seitz, 1972; Bever & Hurtig, 1974) or to variation in word sequence probability (Bever, Lackner, & Stolz, 1969). Carefully designed materials also showed that this effect is not due to local intonational cues; for example, the italicized sequence in sentences (20) and (21) is common to both syntactic organizations (Garrett, Bever, & Fodor, 1966). Yet, the perceived location of the nonspeech sound objectively at the slash is determined by the syntactically driven clause boundary (marked by the # for each structural version). As the authors of this particular study put it, the use of surface phrase structure to organize speech during perception is "active." This was a convincing demonstration of what was foreshadowed by the studies of the comprehension of speech-in-noise: Grammatical knowledge is actively deployed in a way that clarifies the speech signal.

(20)   In her *hope of marrying An/na was impractical*
                                      #
(21)   Harry's hope of *marrying An/na was impractical*
                                      #

The most tendentious hypothesis in generative grammar was that every sentence has a deep structure representation, which is abstract. This hypothesis was the subject of greatest debate in linguistic circles because it was the most striking challenge to behaviorist principles. On the one hand, deep structure is not directly observable in the surface sequence; on the other, it is not definable in semantic terms. Rather, it is a formal structure that mediates between surface form and meaning. Several psychologists proposed that deep syntactic structure was, in fact, the "code" in which sentences are organized and retained (Mehler, 1963; Miller, 1962b). The "coding hypothesis" was just formulated in terms of a "schema plus correction" model for memory based on Bartlett (1932). Sentences are retained in the simple declarative form, plus transformationally motivated "tags" that express the actual construction of the sentence (passive, negative, etc.) (Mehler, 1963; Miller, 1962a). This theory was originally based on a literal interpretation of the language cube in which the kernel structure was taken to be the simple declarative sentence. There was further support for the interpretation that the coding hypothesis applied to abstract underlying structures as defined in syntactic theory. *Ceteris paribus,* perceived relatedness between words is greater when they are in the same deep structure phrase [Levelt, 1970; e.g., "John" and "eager" would be perceived to be more closely related than "John" in sentence (13) and "easy" in sentence (14)]. Words are better prompts for other words in the same deep structure phrase than in other phrases (Walker, Gough, & Wall, 1968; Davidson, 1969). In fact, a word is a better prompt for recall of the entire sentence if it is represented several times in the deep structure representation [e.g., "John" would be a better prompt in sentence (13) than in sentence (14), since only in sentence (13) is it the subject of two deep structure predicates; Blumenthal, 1967; Blumenthal & Boakes, 1967; Wanner, 1968].

The nonspeech interruption studies offered evidence that the deep structure is actively computed during speech perception. The perceived location of nonspeech sounds is influenced by the "clause" structure at the *deep* structure level of representation, as shown in sentences (22) and (23) (Bever, Lackner, & Kirk, 1969). See the preceding discussion of sentences (4) and (5). The slash indicates the objective location on the nonspeech sound, and the # indicates the relatively dominant perceived location of the sound.

(22)   The general defied the t/roops to fight
                              #
(23)   The general desired the t/roops to fight
                              #

Thus, the levels of representation proposed by transformational grammar were vindicated as active participants in sentence perception; even the deep structure level of representation is actively computed as part of comprehension. But it seemed clear that the grammatical rules that defined these levels of representation did not systematically correspond to psychological operations. In that case, how are grammatical levels of representation elicited during speech processing?

One possibility is that the representation-forming processes of perception are entirely distinct from grammatical operations (Fodor & Garrett, 1966; Fodor, Bever, & Garrett, 1974). In one version of this view, listeners acquire an extragrammatical set of *perceptual strategies* that map surface structures onto deep structures (Bever, 1968a, 1970a). These strategies are not grammatical rules but state relations between levels of representations based on salient features at the surface level. The most powerful of these strategies (in English) is that the surface sequence "NP-verb-NP" corresponds to "agent verb object." That strategy gives a nontransformational explanation for the one fact that unambiguously had supported the hypothesis that transformations correspond to psychological operations: Passives are harder than actives. This is explained by the fact that passives violate the NP-verb-NP strategy. Similarly, the strategy explains the salience of NP-verb-NP structures as exemplified in sentence (16). It also explains the preference for the transformed version of sentences with particle/prepositions, and the transformed version places the object directly after the verb.

Research on sentence comprehension in children confirmed the behavioral independence of such perceptual strategies. During their third year, children rely heavily on this strategy for comprehension, although there is no concomitant change in their linguistic knowledge (Bever, Mehler, Valian & Epstein, 1969; Bever, 1970; Maratsos, 1972; DeVilliers & DeVilliers, 1972; Slobin & Bever, 1980). The relation between grammatical rules and the processes of speech production seemed similarly remote: Both intuition and speech errors suggest that speaking involves mapping underlying structures onto surface structures (Fodor, Bever, & Garrett, 1974; Garrett, 1975). But the mapping mechanisms themselves are not grammatical rules: Speakers appear to talk by inserting words into syntactically defined frames (Garrett, 1975; Bever, Carroll, & Hurtig, 1975).

Distinguishing grammatical rules from psychological strategies stimulated investigation of how the latter interact with other psychological processes, such as attention, perception, and memory. There are capacity limits that require immediate memory to be cleared periodically for new input (Miller, 1957; Miller, Galanter, & Pribram, 1960). The perceptual strategies can clear immediate memory by recoding surface sequences on deep structure propositions; this motivated the hypothesis that the proposition is the unit of recoding during speech perception (Bever, 1970a; Bever, Kirk, & Lackner, 1969; Fodor, Bever, & Garrett, 1974). This proposal gives special status to the end of each proposition, since it is there that definitive recoding can take place. In fact, just at the end of clauses, reaction times to clicks are slow (Abrams & Bever, 1969), detection of clicks is poor (Bever, Hurtig, & Handel, 1974), tones are hard to discriminate (Holmes & Forster, 1972), and evoked potentials are suppressed (Seitz, 1973), whereas the relative magnitude of orienting responses to shock suggest greatest preoccupation at that point (Bever et al. 1969). The loss of attention capacity was ostensibly due to the mental load associated with the final stage of recoding the sentence into a deep representation (Abrams & Bever, 1969; Bever, Garrett, & Hurtig, 1973). At first, it was argued that the surface clause was the relevant unit that defined the scope of the perceptual strategies (Fodor & Bever, 1965); then the deep structure "sentence" (Bever, Lackner, & Kirk, 1969). Finally, it became clear that the relevant unit as a psychological object was in part defined as a "functionally complete" proposition (Carroll, 1964; Carroll & Tanenhaus, 1975).

The decade of research on speech processing between 1965 and 1975 offered a complete account of the relation between linguistic theory and behavioral systems: Grammar defines the levels of representation, but ordinary behavior depends on statistically valid strategies. Grammatical rules may find behavioral instantiation, but only as a backup system slowly brought into play on the rare cases when the behavioral strategies fail (Bever, 1972).

The moral of this experience is clear. We made progress by separating the question of what people understand and say from how they understand and say it. The straightforward attempt to use the grammatical model directly as a processing model failed. The question of what humans know about language is not only distinct from how children learn it, it is distinct from how adults use it. In retrospect, this should not have been a surprising result. It is a philosophical truism that there is a difference between knowing *that* X and knowing *how to* X – knowing that a sound sequence is an arpeggio on a French horn is quite different from playing one. Musical knowledge may inform both performers and listeners about the structure inherent in their shared experience, but the knowledge does not describe the actual experiential processes. The same distinction is true of linguistic knowledge.

Further consideration also suggests a straightforward functional reason why grammars are not models of specific kinds of language behaviors: There are too many classes of language behavior, each with its own neurological and physical constraints. In particular, humans ordinarily both talk and comprehend; the constraints on the ear are obviously different from those on the mouth. A grammar represents exactly those aspects of language that are true, no matter how the language is used. The representation of such knowledge must be abstracted away from any particular system of use.

The most positive result of this exercise was the demonstration of the importance of abstract levels of linguistic representation during language behavior. It definitively rejected a behaviorist model of language learning, which cannot account for the incorporation of such abstract structures. It also offered the hope of a new kind of gestalt psychology, one in which the relevant gestalten would be given a theoretical foundation; the grammar can be called on to define the "good figures" of language (Neisser, 1967). The golden age was tarnished, but there was a solid prospect for a period of normal science in which abstract mental structures could be taken as the object of serious inquiry.

Modern times

Behaviorism springs eternal. New theories in both linguistics and experimental psychology proposed arguments against the notion of a syntactic deep structure. Generative semanticists in linguistics grappled with the problem of the relationship between deep structure and semantic representations. Their argument was that if a shared deep structure represents the relation between an active and a passive construction, a shared deep structure can underlie both an active and a causative structure (e.g., expressing the structural relation between "John killed Bill" and "John caused Bill to die"); or it can underlie an active and a superficially remote construction ("I'm telling you, that what happened was that the thing that John caused Bill to do was changed from being alive to being not alive"). Generative semanticists also noted technical problems with the transformational syntactic model that focused on its relation to semantic structure. They eventually proposed that the semantic representation of a sentence *is* its deep structure (Lakoff, 1971a; Lakoff & Ross, 1976; McCawley, 1968; Postal, 1967). In this view, there was no intermediate, purely syntactic configuration that represented the inner grammatical structures. Rather, they were viewed as an arbitrary subset of the semantic representation (Lakoff, 1972a). The entire semantic representation itself served as the input to the transformations, which derived surface phrase structures from it.

This theory had great appeal and caused considerable controversy among syntacticians. It appeared to simplify linguistic description, and to do so without recourse to a purely formal level of syntactic representation, but this position was not tenable: Semantic representations themselves either must be stated in a normal form or must comprise all conceptual knowledge. Either way, the generative semantics program collapses. If the semantic representation is in a canonical, propositional, or some other normal form, the model still includes an intermediate formal level of representation that mediates structurally between thoughts and the outer form of language (as in McCawley, 1976). If semantic representations are purely conceptual, they must include all possible human knowledge (Lakoff, 1971a, 1972a, 1973). This conclusion was a *reductio ad totam,* since it is impossible to define grammatical rules for all possible knowledge (Katz & Bever, 1975). For this and other reasons generative semantics was largely abandoned as a grammatical project (see Katz & Bever, 1975; Newmeyer, 1980, for general discussions).

The wars in linguistics highlighted another problem: Linguistic theory changes like quicksilver. Psychologists think they have their hands on it, but it slips through. The rapid development of linguistic theory is one of the reasons it is such an influential discipline in behavioral science. It is also one of the reasons that merging linguistics and experimental psychology is difficult. It takes a month to develop a new syntactic analysis of a phenomenon; it takes a year to develop an experimental investigation of it. All too often, the psychologist is in the position of completing an arduous series of empirical studies, only to discover that the linguistic theory underlying them is no longer operative. During the 1970s, syntactic theory received particularly great attention in linguistics; the transformational model evolved and alternative models emerged. The rejection of the early transformational grammar as a literal model of processing had discouraged psychologists from attending to linguistic theory. The sudden multiplicity of syntactic theories confirmed the psychologists' suspicion that linguists were hopelessly fickle.

For all that, psychologists were not to be left out of attempts to develop a behaviorist revival of language. The salient target was the deep structure coding hypothesis, which gives priority to deep syntactic structure as the code for remembered sentences. The obvious alternative hypothesis is that people actually remember sentences in terms of semantic schemata. Many experimental demonstrations of the syntactic coding hypothesis seemed interpretable as degenerate cases of semantic rather than syntactic coding; for example, "John" in sentence (13) is not only the subject of two deep structure sentences, it is also the agent of two propositional "ideas." There were also positive demonstrations of the importance of nonsyntactic representations. Sentences in a story are misrecalled or gratuitously imputed to the story in a way consistent with the story line (Bransford & Franks, 1971, 1972) – a story originally with sentences about a robbery, shots, and dying may be incorrectly recalled as having included a sentence about killing. Such results, and the apparent disarray in linguistic theory, encouraged many to assume that linguistics-based psychology of language was an adventure of the past. In fact, some took this discouraging thought to its behaviorist conclusion: Syntax is not real; only probabilistic language behavior exists. What appears to be evidence of syntax is the gratuitous by-product of perceptual processes (Clark & Haviland, 1974), speech behavior learning strategies (Bates, 1977; Bates & MacWhinney, 1982), or an overimaginative and flawed linguistic methodology (Schank, 1973, 1975).

Nonetheless, the same crucial empirical problem remained, both for linguistics and for psychology: Sentences have behaviorally relevant inner forms, phrase-grouped representations that are neither conceptual nor superficial. Independently of how they are behaviorally integrated with conceptual world knowledge, these structures play a role in the formal description of linguistic knowledge, aspects of sentence comprehension, and the concrete analysis of language learning. One can see some clear trends in the evolution of syntactic theory that may lead to a renewed collaboration between psychology and linguistics. The overwhelming shift has been away from restrictions expressed in transformations to verb-based structural restrictions. Three syntactic models have emerged in this direction (see Sells, 1985, and Tanenhaus, 1986, for a review of current linguistic and psycholinguistic issues, respectively).

(1) Government and binding theory: The original transformational model, with the following changes from the original:

Increase in the importance of lexical information in determining sentence structure.
Reduction in the variety of transformations to one movement rule.
Introduction of explicit "filters" that constrain the distinct levels of representation and relations between the levels of representation.

In the original transformational model, the transformations themselves specified the relation between the deep and the surface level; a derivation is possible only if there are particular transformations that construct it. In the current variant, there is only one transformational rule, essentially a universal movement rule that randomly changes the deep tree; constraints on possible trees then filter out potentially ungrammatical structures (Chomsky, 1981, 1985).

(2) Lexical functional grammar: A separate model (which may be a notational variant of the preceding model) treats most transformational variations as specified within the lexicon itself (Bresnan & Kaplan, 1983).
(3) Finally, a recently introduced variant of phrase structure proposes to describe sentence structure. Unlike earlier models of phrase structure, this model in-

cludes an enriched repertoire of the kinds of abstract constituent nodes that are intended to overcome the empirical inadequacy of earlier phrase structure systems (Gazdar, Klein, Pullum, & Sag, 1985).

Each of these three syntactic models has its champions as a model of speech behavior: Crain and Fodor (1985) for generalized phase structure grammar; Bresnan and Kaplan (1983) for lexical functional grammar; Frazier (1985) and Freedman and Forster (1985) for government and binding theory. The common argument is that the only thing wrong with the previous attempts to take the syntactic theory as a psychological model was that the syntactic theory itself was wrong. Yet the old difficulties persist; consistent linking assumptions between the formal model and the behaving person are hard to state. A consistent theory of direct implementation of grammatical knowledge in behavior continues to elude us. (See Bever, 1987, for a discussion of current attempts to formulate direct linguistic linking assumptions.)

Back Again?

Several recent developments in cognitive psychology and the study of language suggest a certain recycling of previous approaches. First, concomitant with the increasing emphasis on lexically driven grammatical analyses, a large body of research in the last decade has been devoted to "lexical access," the recognition, immediate processing and recall of single words in various contexts, including sentences (see Simpson, 1981; Seidenberg & Tanenhaus 1986; and Tanenhaus, Carlson, & Seidenberg, 1985, for reviews). Sentence-level syntax offered few structures for a psychologist to study after establishing the behavioral relevance of abstract levels of representation. A language has a small number of constructions that can act as crucial cases, for example, paired constructions like sentences (13) and (14) or (22) and (23), which are identical in their surface representation but different at the underlying level; or paired constructions like sentences (24) and (25), which share a substantial acoustic segment, with distinct surface phrase structures.

But a language has a large number of words. It will take a long time to run out of things to study about them. And it appears that such work will always be relevant; surely, whatever we find out today about processing words will be relevant to a future integrated theory of language behavior. Unfortunately, scientific history tells us that this is not necessarily so; the only people who we can be absolutely sure will profit from our scientific work, brilliant or parochial, are the future historians of science. Otherwise, we would today be profiting from the decades of research on verbal learning. Today's studies seem to offer more hope;

they typically (but not always) involve the relation among words in sentences. They sometimes focus on the relation between lexical levels and other levels of processing. Such studies offer an unequivocal answer to the question of how much of sentence processing is controlled by categorical information in words. But many lexically focused studies are done entirely without the benefit of a more general theory of language behavior; the word has returned, and it is not always good.

This raises a separate but intellectually coordinated development, now in its first blush of high fashion in cognitive psychology: "connectionist" models of complex behavior (Feldman, 1986; McClelland & Rumelhart, 1986). Connectionism is a descriptive term for a class of theories based on associative connections between elements. There are few constraints on how abstract the units themselves can be or how many clusters they are arranged in. In this sense, connectionism is associationism without behaviorism. How the modern technological version will fare remains to be seen. Practitioners of the art take the laudable stance that the theories should be precise enough to be testable. But "testability" is easily conflated with "modeled," and much energy is given to instantiating specific proposals in computer programs. This is intriguing and guarantees a theory's local consistency, but by no means guarantees its correctness. Superficially, successful computational models can be the undoing of the science they purport to aid. The ability of a model to deal with a large but manageable number of isolated facts has little to do with having a correct theory. In fact, factual success can unnaturally prolong the life of an incorrect theory. As the unknown wag says, if Ptolemy had had a computer, we would still believe that we are the center of the universe.

One of the things we know about words is that a language has a manageably small number of them. Hence, studies of lexical processes and connectionist models go well together. Such associative models can even simulate the effect of morphological combination rules (Rumelhart et al., 1986). This success tempts one to speculate that the consequences of such linguistic rules are represented in an associative network without any actual representation of the rules themselves: That is, the system *is* the rule (see Rumelhart & McClelland, 1968, chap. 18; Feldman, 1986). This is a conflation of competence and performance opposite to the conflation of transformational grammar and a performance model, discussed previously. Twenty-five years ago, psycholinguists claimed that the grammar is the performance system; now the corresponding connectionist claim would be that the performance system is the grammar. The grammarian's claim was wrong because categorical grammatical knowledge cannot explain the continua of actual behavior. The connectionist claim may turn out to be wrong for the corresponding reason: Contingent probabilities cannot explain categorical knowledge. Of course, given enough associative connections between explicit and internal elements, any rule-governed behavior can be approximated. Such models are the equivalent of the sculptor's plaster of paris: Given them an articulate structure and they will shape themselves to it. Associative simulations do not explain morphological structure in lexical morpheme combinations; they only conform to it as an automatic consequence of simulating a description of the combinations. If there is anything we know about sentences, it is that a language has an *un*manageably large number of them. This contrast was one of the strong motivations for embarking on the study of the acquisition and deployment of rules in behavior rather than memorized connections and automatic elicitations (Miller, Galanter, and Pribram, 1960). No doubt connections and elicitations exist and dominate much measurable behavior in an adult. The perennial puzzle is how to prestructure associations so that they systematically *impose* rulelike organization on what they learn. The specific challenges for an associative theory of language learning remain: What is the nature of the categorical information encoded in words, sentences, and rules? How is such categorical information learned and represented? Last (but not least), how does it come to be used and translated into contingent connections? (See Lachter & Bever, 1988.)

There is a recent development in one interpretation of grammar that appears to reunite the study of syntax with a theory of language acquisition. The child acquires the rich internal structure of his or her language from scanty data (Chomsky, 1965), a fact that implies that language structure must be deeply constrained to accord with the child's specific language capacity. This underlies the recent development of so-called learnability theory – an attempt to construct a model of language acquisition that explains specific linguistic rules and constraints on the grounds that they make language learnable (Wexler & Culicover, 1980; Osheron, Stob, & Weinstein, 1982; Pinker, 1984).

Such functionalist proposals are innocuous as a selectional model of learning. But if they are taken to constrain the form of possible linguistic theories, we will have come full circle to the methodological position on linguistic analysis that characterized behaviorism. To be sure, current syntactic models are not constrained by either behaviorist or associative descriptive principles. But we must be warned by our own history: Theories of learning are not good prospects as theories of knowledge.

Conclusion: the mystery of structure

This has been a tale about the merits of being methodologically flexible and answering only one question at a time. Progress was made in understanding how language behavior works by divorcing it from the question of how it is learned. Further progress depended on making a distinction between the models of linguistic knowledge and language behavior. Despite all of this progress, however, we are left with an essential empirical puzzle, the answer to which will involve solutions to most of the issues raised in this chapter:

How does syntactic structure improve the acuity of the ear?

Note

I have received comments from many linguists and psychologists on an earlier version of this chapter. Generally, psychologists find it an accurate picture of the intellectual period; linguists tend to think that it overlooks much of what was happening within linguistics at the time. The typical comment is: "But linguists were not confused about that matter (e.g., the derivational theory of complexity), so why report the psychologists' confusion over it?" I am not convinced that most linguists were – and are – not just as confused as most psychologists on most matters. However, such responses prompt me to add an explanatory caveat: This chapter is intended to give an account of how the world looked to psychologists and psycholinguists at the forefront of the field during the years of 1955–75. A parallel history of developments within linguistics would be of parallel interest – especially with respect to how linguists viewed language behavior. For example, during the period covered in this chapter, almost all linguists disdained research on the role of syntactic and semantic structures in language processing. This situation has changed somewhat in the last decade, though not always with a clarifying effect, as mentioned at the end of the chapter.

References

Abrams, K., & Bever, T. G. (1969). Syntactic structure modifies attention during speech perception and recognition. *Quarterly Journal of Experimental Psychology, 21,* 280–90.

Anderson, J. R., & Bower, G. H. (1973). *Human Associative Memory.* Washington, D.C.: V. H. Winston.

Bartlett, F. C. (1932). *Remembering.* Cambridge: Cambridge University Press.

Bates, E. (1977). Comments on the paper by Culicover and Wexler. In P. Culicover, T. Wascow, & A. Akamagian (Eds.), *Formal Syntax.* New York: Academic Press.

Bates, E., & MacWhinney, B. (1982). Functionalist approaches to grammar. In E. Wanner & L. Gleitman (Eds.), *Language Acquisition: The State of the Art.* New York: Cambridge University Press.

Berry, R. (1970). A critical review of noise location during simultaneously presented setences. Ph.D. dissertation, University of Illinois.

Bever, T. G. (1968a). A survey of some recent work in psycholinguistics. In W. J. Plath (Ed.), *Specification and utilization of a Transformational Grammar: Scientific Report Number Three.* Yorktown Heights, N.Y.: Thomas J. Watson Research Center, International Business Machines Corporation.

Bever, T. G. (1968b). Associations to stimulus–response theories of language. In T. R. Dixon & D. L. Horton (Eds.), *Verbal Behavior and General Behavior Theory.* Englewood Cliffs, N.J.: Prentice-Hall, pp. 478–94.

Bever, T. G. (1970a). The cognitive basis for linguistic structures. In J. R. Hayes (Ed.), *Cognition and the Development of Language.* New York: Wiley.

Bever, T. G. (1970b). The integrated study of language. In J. Morton (Ed.), *Biological and Social Perspectives in Language.* Logos Press, pp. 158–206.

Bever, T. G. (1972). The limits of intuition. *Foundations of Language, 8,* 411–12.

Bever, T. G. (1973). Serial position and response biases do not account for the effect of syntactic structure on the location of brief noises during sentences. *Journal of Psycholinguistic Research, 2,* 287–8.

Bever, T. G. (1974). The ascent of the specious of there's a lot we don't know about mirrors. In David Cohen (Ed.), *Explaining Linguistic Phenomena.* Washington, D.C. Hemisphere, pp. 173–200.

Bever, T. G. (1987). Three paradigms for the study of language and cognition. In M. Macken et al. (Eds.), *Proceedings of the SCLI Workshop on Language and Context.*

Bever, T. G., Carroll, J. M., & Hurtig, R. (1976). Analogy of ungrammatical sequences that are utterable and comprehensible are the origins of new grammars in language acquisition and linguistic evolution. In T. G. Bever et al. (Eds.) *An Integrated Theory of Linguistic Ability.* New York: Crowell, pp. 149–82.

Bever, T. G., Fodor, J. A., Garrett, M. F., & Mehler, J. (1966). Transformational operations and stimulus complexity. Unpublished paper, MIT.

Bever, T. G., Fodor, J. A., & Weksel, W. (1965). Is linguistics empirical? *Psychological Review, 72,* 493–500.

Bever, T. G., Fodor, J. A., and Weksel, W. (1968). A formal limitation of associationism. In T. R. Dixon & D. L.Horton (Eds.), *Verbal Learning and General Behavior Theory,* Englewood Cliffs, N.J.: Prentice-Hall.

Bever, T. G., Garrett, M. F., & Hurtig, R. (1973). Ambiguity increases complexity of perceptually incomplete clauses. *Memory and Cognition, 1,* 279–81.

Bever, T. G., & Hurtig, R. (1975). Detection of a nonlinguistic stimulus is poorest at the end of a clause. *Journal of Psycholinguistic Research, 4,* 1–7.

Bever, T. G., Hurtig, R., Handel, A. (1976). Analytic tasks stimulate right-ear processing in listening to speech. *Neuropsychologia, 14,* 174–81.

Bever, T. G., Kirk, R., & Lackner, J. (1969). An autonomic reflection of syntactic structure. *Neuropsychologia, 7,* 23–8.

Bever, T. G., Lackner, J. R., & Kirk, R. (1969). The underlying structures of sentences are the primary units of immediate speech processing. *Perception and Psychophysics, 5,* 225–31.

Bever, T. G., Lackner, J. R., & Stolz, W. (1969). Transitional probability is not a general mechanism for the segmentation of speech. *Journal of Experimental Psychology, 79,* 387–94.

Bever, T. G., & Mehler, J. (1967). The coding hypothesis and short-term memory, *AF Technical Report.* Cambridge, Mass.: Harvard Center for Cognitive Studies.

Bever, T. G., Mehler, J., Valian, V., Epstein, J., & Morrissey, H. (1969). Linguistic capacity of young children. (Unpublished.) Referred to in J. Fodor, T. G. Bever, & M. F. Garrett (Eds.), *The Psychology of Language.* New York: McGraw-Hill, p. 502.

Bloomfield, L. (1914). *The Study of Language.* New York: Henry Holt.

Bloomfield, L. (1933). Prompted recall of sentences. *Journal of Verbal Learning and Verbal Behavior, 6,* 203–6.

Blumenthal, A. L., (1970). *Language and Psychology.* New York: Wiley.

Blumenthal, A. L. (1975). A reappraisal of Wilhelm Wundt. *American Psychologist, 30,* 1081–8.

Blumenthal, A. L., & Boakes, R. (1967). Prompted recall of sentences, a further study. *Journal of Verbal Learning and Verbal Behavior, 6,* 674–6.

Bransford, J. D., Barclay, J., & Franks, J. J. (1972). Sentence memory: Constructive vs. interpretive approach. *Cognitive Psychology, 3,* 193–209.

Bransford, J. D., & Franks, J. J. (1971). The abstraction of linguistic ideas. *Cognitive Psychology, 2,* 331–50.

Bransford, J. D., & Johnson, M. K. (1972). Contextual prerequisites for understanding: Some investigations for comprehension and recall. *Journal of Verbal Learning and Verbal Behavior, 11,* 717–26.

Bresnan, J. (1978). A realistic transformational grammar. In M. Halle, J. Bresnan, & G. Miller (Eds.), *Linguistic Theory and Psychological Reality.* Cambridge, Mass.: MIT Press.

Bresnan, J., & Kaplan, R. (1983). Grammars as the mental representation of language. In J. Bresnan (Ed.), *The Mental Representation of Language.* Cambridge, Mass.: MIT Press.

Carey, P. W., Mehler, J., & Bever, T. G. (1970). Judging the veracity of ambiguous sentences. *Journal of Verbal Learning and Verbal Behavior, 9,* 243–354.

Carroll, J. (1967). *Language and Thought.* Englewood Cliffs, N.J.: Prentice-Hall.

Chomsky, N. (1957b). *Syntactic Structures.* The Hague: Mouton.

Chomsky, N. (1959). Review of "Verbal Behavior." *Language, 30,* 26–58.

Chomsky, N. (1965). *Aspects of the Theory of Syntax.* Cambridge, Mass.: MIT Press.

Chomsky, N. (1966). *Cartesian Linguistics.* New York: Harper & Row.

Chomsky, N. (1967). The formal nature of language. In E. Lennenberg (Ed.), *Biological Foundations of Language,* New York: Wiley, 397–442.

Chomsky, N. (1975). *Logical Structure of Linguistic Theory.* New York: Plenum.

Chomsky, N. (1981). *Lectures on Government and Binding.* Dordrecht, Holland: Foris.

Chomsky, N. (1985). *Knowledge of Language.* New York: Praeger.

Chomsky, N. & Miller, G. A. (1958). Finite state languages. *Information and Control, 1,* 91–112.

Chomsky, N. & Miller, G. A. (1963). Introduction to the formal analysis of natural languages. In D. Luce, R. Bush, & E. Galanter (Eds.), *Handbook of Mathematical Psychology.* New York: Wiley.

Clark, H. H. (1965). Some structural properties of simple active and passive sentences. *Journal of Verbal Learning and Verbal Behavior, 4,* 365–370.

Clark, H. H., & Haviland, S. E. (1974). Psychological processes in linguistic explanation. In D. Cohen (Ed.), *Explaining Linguistic Phenomena.* Washington, D.C.: Hemisphere.

Clifton, C., Kurcz, I., & Jenkins, J. J. (1965). Grammatical relations as determinants of sentence similarity. *Journal of Verbal Learning and Verbal Behavior, 4,* 112–117.

Clifton, C., & Odom, P. (1966). Similarity relations among certain English sentence constructions. *Psychological Monographs, 80,* (Whole No. 613).

Cofer, C. N. (Ed.) (1961). *Verbal Learning and Verbal Behavior.* New York: McGraw-Hill.

Cofer, C. N. & Musgrave, B. S. (Eds.). (1963). *Verbal Behavior and Learning: Problems and Processes.* New York: McGraw-Hill.

Compton, A. J. (1967). Aural perception of different syntactic structures and length. *Language and Speech, 10,* 81–87.

Crain, S., & Fodor, J. D. (1985a). How can grammars help the parser? In D. Dowty, L. Kartunnen, & A. M. Zwicky, (Eds.). *Natural language parsing: Psychology, computational and theoretical perspectives.* London: Cambridge University Press.

Crain, S. & Fodor, J. D. (1985b). Rules and contraints in sentence processing. *Proceedings of the 15th New England Linguistic Society, 15,* Amherst, Mass.: New England Linguistic Society.

Davidson, R. E. (1969). Transitional errors and deep structure differences. *Psychonomic Science, 14,* 293.

DeVilliers, P. A., & DeVilliers, J. G. (1972). Early judgments of semantic and syntactic acceptability by children. *Journal of Psycholinguistic Research, 1,* 299–310.

Epstein, W. (1961). The influence of syntactical structure on learning. *American Journal of Psychology, 74,* 80–5.

Feldman, J. A. (1986). *Neural Representation of Conceptual Knowledge.* Cognitive Science Technical Report, Rochester, N.Y.: University of Rochester.

Fodor, J. A. (1965). Could meaning be an rm? *Journal of Verbal Learning and Verbal Behavior, 4,* 73–81.

Fodor, J. A. (1983). *The Modularity of Mind.* Boston: MIT Press.

Fodor, J. A., & Bever T. G. (1965). The psychological reality of linguistic segments. *Journal of Verbal Learning and Verbal Behavior, 4,* 414–20.

Fodor, J. A., Bever, T. G., & Garrett, M. R. (1974). *The Psychology of Language: An Introduction to Psycholinguistics and Generative Grammar.* New York: McGraw-Hill.

Fodor, J. A., & Garrett, M. F. (1967). Some syntactic determinants of sentential complexity. *Perception and Psychophysics, 2,* 289–96.

Forster, K. (1979). Levels of processing and the structure of the language processor. In W. E. Cooper & E. C. T. Walker (Eds.), *Sentence Processing: Psycholinguistic Studies Presented to Merrill Garrett*. Hillsdale, N.J.: Erlbaum, pp. 27–85.

Frazier, L. (1985). Modularity and the representational hypothesis. *Proceedings of the 15th Northeast Linguistics Society, 15*. Amherst, Mass.: New England Linguistic Society.

Frazier, L. (1986). The mapping between grammar and processor. In I. Gopnick & M. Gopnick (Eds.), *From Models to Modules: Studies in Cognitive Science from the McGill Workshops*. Norwood, N.J.: Ablex Press.

Freedman, S. E., & Forster, K. I. (1985). The psychological status of overgenerated sentences. *Cognition, 19*, 101–32.

Garrett, M. F. (1965). Syntactic structures and judgments of auditory events. Ph.D. dissertation, University of Illinois.

Garrett, M. F. (1975). The analysis of sentence production. In G. H. Bower (Ed.), *The Psychology of Learning and Motivation*. New York: Academic Press, pp. 133–77.

Garrett, M. F., Bever, T. G., & Fodor, J. A. (1966). The active use of grammar in speech perception. *Perception and Psychophysics, 1*, 30–2.

Gazdar, G., Klein, E., Pullum, G., & Sag, I. (1985). *Generalized Phrase Structure Grammar*. Cambridge, Mass.: Harvard University Press.

Gough, P. B. (1965). Grammatical transformations and speed of understanding. *Journal of Verbal Learning and Verbal Behavior, 4*, 107–11.

Gough, P. B. (1966). The verification of sentences. The effects of delay of evidence and sentence length. *Journal of Verbal Learning and Verbal Behavior, 5*, 492–6.

Harris, Z. (1957). Co-occurrence and transformation in linguistic structure. *Language, 33*, 283–340.

Harris, Z. (1958). Linguistic transformations for informational retrieval. Washington, D.C.: *Proceedings of the International Conference on Scientific Information, 2*, NAS-WRC.

Holmes, V. M., & Forster, K. I. (1970). Detection of extraneous signals during sentence recognition. *Perception and Psychophysics, 7*, 297–301.

Hull, C. L. (1943). *Principles of Behavior*. New York: Appleton-Century-Crofts.

Humboldt, W. V. (1835/1903). *Ueber die Verschiedenheit des menschlichen Sprachbaues und ihren Einfluss auf die geistige Entwicklung des Menschengeschlechts*. In *Gessamelte Schriften*, Vol. 7. Berlin: Koeniglich Preussische Akademie der Wissenschaften.

James, W. (1890). *Principles of Psychology*. New York: Henry Holt.

Jenkins, J. J., Fodor, J. A., & Saporta, S. (1965). An introduction to psycholinguistic theory. Unpublished.

Johnson, N. F. (1965). The psychological reality of phrase structure rules. *Journal of Verbal Learning and Verbal Behavior, 4*, 469–75.

Katz, J. J., & Bever, T. G. (1975). The fall and rise of empiricism. In T. G. Bever, J. Katz, & D. T. Langendoen (Eds.), *An Integrated Theory of Linguistic Ability*. New York: T. Y. Crowell.

Katz, J. J. & Postal, P. M. (1964). *An Integrated Theory of Linguistic Descriptions*. Cambridge, Mass.: MIT Press.

Koffka, K. (1935). *Principle of Gestalt Psychology*. New York: Harcourt, Brace & World.

Koplin, J. H., & Davis, J. (1966). Grammatical transformataions and recognition memory of sentences. *Psychonomic Science, 6*, 257–8.

Lachter, J., & Bever, T. G. (1988). The relation between linguistic structure and theories of learning – A constructive critique of some connectionist learning models. *Cognition*.

Lakoff, G. (1971a). On generative semantics. In D. Steinberg & L. Jakobovits (Eds.), *Semantics*. Cambridge: Cambridge University Press, pp. 232–96.

Lakoff, G. (1971b). Presupposition and relative well-formedness. In D. Steinberg & L. Jakobovits (Eds.), *Semantics*. Cambridge: Cambridge University Press, pp. 329–40.

Lakoff, G. (1972a). The arbitrary basis of transformational grammar. *Language, 48*, 76–85.

Lakoff, G. (1972b). Hedges: A study in meaning criteria and the logic of fuzzy concepts. *Papers from the Eighth Regional Meeting of the Chicago Linguistic Society*, 182–228.

Lakoff, G. (1973). Fuzzy grammar and the performance/competence terminology game. *Papers from the Ninth Regional Meeting of the Chicago Linguistic Society*, 271–91.

Lakoff, G., & Ross, J. (1976). Is deep structure necessary? In J. McCawley (Ed.), *Syntax and Semantics*, Vol. 7. New York: Academic Press, pp. 159–64.

Lashley, K. S. (1951). The problem of serial order in behavior. In L. A. Jeffress (Ed.), *Cerebral Mechanisms in Behavior: The Hixon Symposium*. New York: Wiley.

Levelt, W. J. M. (1970). A scaling approach to the study of syntactic relations. In G. B. Flores d'Arcais & W. J. M. Levelt (Eds.), *Advances in Psycholinquistics*. New York: American Elsevier, pp.

Licklider, J. C. R., & Miller, G. A. (1951). The perception of speech. In S. S. Stevens (Ed.), *Handbook of Experimental Psychology*. New York: Wiley, pp. 1040–74.

Mackay, D. G., & Bever, T. G. (1967). In search of ambiguity. *Perception and Psychophysics, 2,* 193–200.

Mandler, G., & Mandler, J. (1964). Serial position effects in sentences. *Journal of Verbal Learning and Verbal Behavior, 3,* 195–202.

Maratsos, M. (1974). Children who get worse at understanding the passive: A replication of Bever. *Journal of Psycholinguistic Research, 3,* 65–74.

McCawley, J. (1968a). The role of semantics in grammar. In E. Bach & R. Harms (Eds.), *Universals in Linguistic Theory*. New York: Holt, Rinehart and Winston, pp. 127–70.

McCawley, J. (1968b). Lexical insertion in a transformational grammar without deep structure. *Papers from the Fourth Regional Meeting of the Chicago Linguistic Society,* 71–80. Reprinted in McCawley (1976), pp. 155–66.

McCawley, J. (1976). *Grammar and Meaning*. New York: Academic Press.

McClelland, J. L., & Rumelhart, D. E. (1986). Distributed memory and the representation of general and specific information. *Journal of Experimental Psychology: General, 114,* 159–88.

McMahon, L. (1963). Grammatical analysis as part of understanding a sentence. Ph.D. dissertation, Harvard University.

Mehler, J. (1963). Some effects of grammatical transformations on the recall of English sentences. *Journal of Verbal Learning and Verbal Behavior, 2,* 346–51.

Mehler, J., Bever, T. G. & Carey, P. (1967). What we look at when we read. *Perception and Psychophysics, 2,* 213–18.

Mehler, J., & Carey, P. (1967). Role of surface and base structure in the perception of sentences. *Journal of Verbal Learning and Verbal Behavior, 6,* 335–8.

Miller, G. A. (1951a). Speech and language. In S. S. Stevens (Ed.), *Handbook of Experimental Psychology*. New York: Wiley, pp. 769–810.

Miller, G. A. (1951b). *Language and Communication*. New York: McGraw-Hill.

Miller, G. A. (1954). Psycholinguistics. In G. Lindzey (Ed.), *Handbook of Social Psychology*. Cambridge, Mass.: Addison-Wesley, pp. 693–708.

Miller, G. A. (1956). The magical number seven, plus or minus two: Some limits on our capacity for processing information. *Psychological Review, 63,* 81–97.

Miller, G. A. (1962a). Decision units in the perception of speech. *IRE Transactions on Information Theory, 2,* IT-8.

Miller, G. A. (1962b). Some psychological studies of grammar. *American Psychologist, 7,* 748–62. (Presidential address to the Eastern Psychological Association, April 1962.)

Miller, G. A. (1963). Comments on Professor Postman's paper. In C. N. Cofer & B. Musgrave (Eds.), *Verbal Behavior and Learning*. New York: McGraw-Hill, pp. 321–29.

Miller, G. A., Bruner, J. S., & Postman, L. (1954). Familiarity of letter sequences and tachistoscopic identification. *Journal of General Psychology, 50,* 129–39.

Miller, G. A., & Chomsky, N. (1963). Finitary models of language users. In D. Luce, R. Bush, & E. Galanter (Eds.), *Handbook of Mathematical Psychology*. New York: Wiley.

Miller, G. A., Galanter, E., & Pribram, K. (1960). *Plans and the Structure of Behavior*. New York: Holt.

Miller, G. A., Heise, G. A., & Lichten, W. (1951). The intelligibility of speech as a function of the context of the test materials. *Journal of Experimental Psychology, 41*, 329–35.

Miller, G. A., & Isard, S. (1963). Some perceptual consequences of linguistic rules. *Journal of Verbal Learning and Verbal Behavior, 2*, 217–28.

Miller, G. A., & McKean, K. O. (1964). Chronometric study of some relations between sentences. *The Quarterly Journal of Experimental Psychology, 16*, 297–308.

Miller, G. A., & Nicely, P. E. (1955). An analysis of perceptual confusions among some English consonants. *Journal of Acoustical Society of America, 27*, 338–52.

Miller, G. A., & Selfridge, J. A. (1950). Verbal context and the recall of meaningful material. *American Journal of Psychology, 63*, 176–85.

Neisser, U. (1967). *Cognitive Psychology*. New York: Appleton-Century-Crofts.

Newmeyer, F. (1980). *Linguistic Theory in America*. New York: Academic Press.

Osgood, C. E., & Sebeok, T. A., (Eds.). (1954). *Psycholinguistics: A Survey of Theory and Research Problems*. Supplement to the *International Journal of American Linguistics, 20* (4). Reprinted by Indiana University Press, 1969.

Osgood, C., Suci, G., & Tannenbaum, P. (1957). *The Measurement of Meaning*. Urbana: University of Illinois Press.

Osheron, D. N., Stob, M., & Weinstein, S. (1982). Learning strategies. *Information and Control, 53*, 32–51.

Pinker, S. (1984). *Language Learnability and Language Development*. Cambridge, Mass.: Harvard University Press.

Postal, P. (1967). Linguistic anarchy notes. In. J. McCawley (Ed.), *Syntax and Semantics*, Vol. 7. New York: Academic Press, pp. 201–26.

Pylyshyn, A. (1984). *Computation and Cognition*. Boston: MIT Press.

Rumelhart, D. E., & McClelland J. L. (1986). On learning the past tenses of English verbs. In J. L. McClelland, D. E. Rumelhart, and the PDP Research Group (Eds.), *Parallel Distributed Processing: Explorations of the Microstructure of Cognition*. Cambridge, Mass.: MIT Press.

Savin, H. & Perchonock, E. (1965). Grammatical structure and the immediate recall of English sentences. *Journal of Verbal Learning and Verbal Behavior, 4*, 348–59.

Schank, R. C. (1973). Identification of conceptualizations underlying natural language. In R. C. Schank & K. M. Colby (Eds.), *Computer Models of Thought and Language*. San Francisco: Freeman, pp. 187–247.

Schank, R. C. (1976). The role of memory in language processing. In C. N. Cofer (Ed.), *The Structure of Human Memory*. San Francisco: Freeman, pp. 162–89.

Seidenberg, M. S., & Tanenhaus, M. K. (1986). Modularity and lexical access. In I. Gopnick & M. Gopnick (Eds.), *From Models to Modules: Studies in Cognitive Science from the McGill Workshops*. Norwood, N.J.: Ablex, pp. 117–34.

Seitz, M. (1972). AER and the perception of speech. Ph.D. dissertation, University of Washington.

Sells, P. (1985). *Lectures on Contemporary Syntactic Theories*. Palo Alto, Calif.: CSLI Publications.

Simpson, G. B. (1981). Meaning, dominance and semantic context in the processing of lexical ambiguity. *Journal of Verbal Learning and Verbal Behavior, 20*, 120–36.

Skinner, B. F. (1957). *Verbal Behavior*. New York: Appleton-Century-Crofts.

Slobin, D. I. (1966). Grammatical transformations and sentence comprehension in childhood and adulthood. *Journal of Verbal Learning and Verbal Behavior, 5*, 219–27.

Slobin, D., & Bever, T. G. (1980). Children use canonical sentence schemas in sentence perception. *Cognition, 12,* 229–65.

Stewart, C., & Gough, P. (1967). Constituent search in immediate memory for sentences. *Proceedings of the Midwestern Psychology Association.*

Suci, G. Ammon, P., & Gamlin, P. (1967). The validity of the probe-latency technique for assessing structure in language. *Language and Speech, 10,* 69–80.

Tanenhaus, M. K. (in press). Psycholinguistics: an overview. In F. Newmeyer (Eds.), *Linguistics: The Cambridge Survey.* Volume 3, Biological and Psychological Perspectives. Cambridge, Mass.: MIT Press.

Tanenhaus, M. K. & Carroll, J. M. (1975). Functional clause hierarchy . . . and Nouniness. In R. Grossman, J. San, & T. Vance (Eds.), *Papers from the Parasessian on Functionalism.* Chicago: Chicago Linguistics Society.

Tanenhaus, M. K., Carlson, G. N., & Seidenberg, M. S. (1985). Do listeners compute linguistic representations? In D. R. Dowty, L. Karttunen, & A. M. Zwicky (Eds.), *Natural Language Parsing,* New York: Cambridge University Press, pp. 359–408.

Tanenhaus, M. K., Carroll, J. M., & Bever, T. G. (1976). Sentence-picture verification models as theories of sentence comprehension: A critique of Carpenter and Just. *Psychological Review, 83,* 310–17.

Underwood, B., & Schultz, R. (1960). *Meaningfulness and Verbal Learning.* Philadelphia: Lippincott.

Walker, E., Gough, P., & Wall, R. (1968). Grammatical relations and the search of sentences in immediate memory. *Proceedings of the Midwestern Psychological Association.*

Wanner, E. (1968). On remembering, forgetting, and understanding sentences: A study of the deep structure hypothesis. Ph.D. dissertation, Harvard University.

Wexler, K., & Culicover, P. (1980). *Formal Principles in Language Acquisition.* Cambridge, Mass.: MIT Press.

Wingfield, A., & Klein, J. F. (1971). Syntactic structure and acoustic pattern in speech perception. *Perception and Psychophysics, 9,* 23–5.

Wundt, W. (1874). *Grundzuge der psyiologischen Psychologie.* Leipzig: Engelmann.

Wundt, W. (1911). *Volkerpsychologie & Erster Band: Die Sprache.* Leipzig: Englemann.

10 Psychology and linguistics in the sixties

Eric Wanner

Although psychology and linguistics have a long and honorable history of co-operative efforts to explain the acquisition and use of language (see Blumenthal, 1970), in the 1960s these efforts took on a particularly focused character that is generally considered the origin of modern psycholinguistics. Perhaps a dozen linguists, psychologists, and philosophers were principally involved in this movement, but for me the center has always seemed to lie in the collaboration between Noam Chomsky and George Miller, the main tangible results of which were the chapters they co-authored for the *Handbook of Mathematical Psychology* in 1963.

I was a first-year graduate student in social psychology at Harvard then, and language was only one of far too many items on my intellectual agenda. But during our first fall in Cambridge, my wife happened, quite by chance, to land a job at MIT as secretary to Morris Halle and Noam Chomsky. She began to smuggle out preprints for me, and pretty soon I was hooked. By far the hardest but most riveting legacy of her larceny was the set of three *Handbook* chapters. I studied them as though they were holy writ, at a rate of about five pages a day. It was difficult going for someone with little background in mathematics and linguistics, but if you read enough of the references to understand what Chomsky and Miller were talking about, what you got was an essential education in psycholinguistics. Everything was there: an introduction to stochastic models, generative grammar, automata theory, and the Chomsky hierarchy of languages, a general characterization of language performance models, and a sketch for a theory of complex behavior. Even now, these chapters seem to me the clearest foundational statement of the field; certainly much subsequent work in psycholinguistics has cycled around the issues first developed there.

What excited me most about the *Handbook* chapters was the idea (then several years old but still new to me) that just as linguistic knowledge could be described as a set of rules from which all and only admissible sentences could be generated, so too could a performance system be modeled as an automaton of a definite, specifiable kind. (An *automaton*, I learned by reading the references, is an ab-

143

stract mathematical representation of a computational device, discrete mathematics' means of studying the powers and limitations of computing systems.) An automaton, if guided by the right rules, could process all possible English sentences. Importantly, automata of different powers were needed for different rule systems. In the *Handbook* chapters, Chomsky and Miller carefully articulated the relation between possible systems of linguistic rules and the kind of automaton needed to realize these rules in a production model.

For those of us who were new to the struggles of behaviorism, the *Handbook* chapters underlined an important result derivable from this formalism: that the class of automata needed to model the kind of linguistic rules posited by standard learning theory was demonstrably inadequate to process natural language. This result seemed then, as it does now, a very powerful antibehaviorist argument, one dependent on well-grounded empirical assumptions and straightforward logic that needed no polemics to make it convincing.

But what also excited me as a young student was the fact that not all of Miller and Chomsky's arguments were equally airtight. There was, after all, a little work left to be done. It was one thing to show that natural language was neither a regular language processable by a finite-state automaton nor a context-free language processable by a push-down store automaton, but it was much more difficult to show just which of the many imaginable unrestricted rewrite systems would provide a psychologically appropriate account of linguistic knowledge. Chomsky, of course, favored transformational grammars, but his preference seemed to me to be based much more on aesthetic criteria concerning the nature of scientific laws than on psychological criteria about what should count as linguistic knowledge. Transformational grammars have the virtue of expressing certain apparently natural generalizations by means of single rules, whereas an earlier candidate grammar, context-sensitive phrase structure, requires a number of rules to achieve the same results. Chomsky favored grammars that captured these "linguistically significant generalizations" (Chomsky, 1965, p. 42) but the question that immediately struck many psychologists was whether linguistically significant generalizations were also psychologically significant.

Two approaches to that psychological question seemed open. One tack was to look at the natural course of language acquisition to see whether children readily arrive at the generalizations stated in transformational grammar (e.g., Klima and Bellugi, 1966). The other was to formulate and test models of adult linguistic performance that incorporate a transformational grammar as a subcomponent. If transformational grammar describes the language user's tacit syntactic knowledge (or competence), then an empirically successful performance model of sentence processing should be derivable by showing how the rules of the grammar are actually put to use in sentence production or perception.

In the third of their *Handbook* chapters, Miller and Chomsky sketched a model of sentence perception that became the prototype for all subsequent performance models. Their model had two components: a preprocessor with a limited short-term memory that "take[s] a sentence as input and give[s] us as output a relatively superficial analysis of it (perhaps the derived phrase marker . . .)" and a secondary component that "utilize[s] the full resources of the transformational grammar to provide a structural description, consisting of a set of P-markers and a transformational history, in which deeper grammatical relations and other structural information are represented" (p. 480). According to Miller and Chomsky, the output of such a model "[is] the complete structural description assigned to the input sentence by the grammar that it stores" (loc. cit).

This sketch, brief as it was, provided the essential rationale underlying much of the empirical work undertaken by psycholinguists for the remainder of the decade. These were the experiments that, in the unhappy label hung on them by the textbooks (e.g., Fodor, Bever, & Garrett, 1974), attempted to determine the psychological "reality" of the grammatical structures and rules specified by a transformational grammar. Miller and Chomsky made the case for this research program with typical circumspection: "The psychological plausibility of a transformational model of the language user would be strengthened, of course, if it could be shown that our performance on tasks requiring an appreciation of the structure of transformed sentences is a function of the nature, number, and complexity of the grammatical transformations involved" (op. cit., p. 481). On the strength of this modest statement, a small research industry was born.

The "reality" experiments

No one, of course, was philosophically naive enough to suppose that the psychological reality of transformational grammar could ever ultimately be determined. Reality is not a matter that science can decide. But it is possible to determine the range of coverage of some explanatory concept, and I think this is the right way to look back at the "reality" experiments. Transformational grammar in 1963 had been tested externally against certain kinds of data (acceptability judgments) and tested internally according to certain theoretical criteria (the ability to capture linguistically significant generalizations). The question that the reality experiments sought to answer was whether the empirical coverage of transformational grammar could be extended to other kinds of behavioral phenomena by formulating a successful transformationally based model of performance data (such as memory errors and reaction times).

If successful, this line of work would have had two important consequences. First, for generative linguistics, it would have given real substance to Chomsky's (1957) claim that linguistic knowledge, or competence, is distinct and logically separable from linguistic performance, the application of the knowledge. Uncoupled from a performance model, testability of a model of grammatical competence remains quite elusive, since any unsuccessful prediction can be attributed to unspecified performance factors. However, if a grammar could be successfully embedded in a family of performance models (for sentence production, perception, linguistic judgment, and the like), then the competence model's testable predictions might be more unambiguously determined. Second, for psycholinguistics, successful reality tests would have meant that grammars based exclusively upon linguistic criteria could be plugged directly into performance models. In this way, successful reality experiments would have shown that linguistically significant generalizations were psychologically significant, and the laborious work required to develop an independent psychological characterization of linguistic knowledge might have been avoided. Although it is now fashionable to regard the reality experiments as somehow naive, the issues at stake were by no means trivial. If the structures and rules of transformational grammar had turned out to be psychologically real, the progress of the field would have been enormously accelerated. Unfortunately, the story did not turn out quite so simply.

Three hypotheses, all derivable from Miller and Chomsky's incorporation model, received the lion's share of experimental attention. Two of these concerned the reality of grammatical structure and one concerned the reality of the transformations themselves. These hypotheses vary both in the strength of their connection to the transformational performance model and in the amount of empirical support that they received. Unfortunately for the transformational model, the variation along these two dimensions turned out to be negatively correlated: The more closely connected to the transformational model, the weaker the empirical support.

The phrase structure hypothesis:

According to this hypothesis, the language user naturally (although tacitly and unconsciously) groups words into phrases while processing a sentence. This hypothesis is the weakest of the reality hypotheses because evidence in its favor does not require us to conclude for a transformation-based performance model. Such phrase grouping might be evidence of the kind of preliminary analysis that Miller and Chomsky envisioned in the sentence perception model *or* it might be the final analysis of a syntactic system that, unlike a transformational analysis, assigns only one phrase marker to the sentence. The defect of this hypothesis is thus its lack of theoretical leverage; its virtue, however, is an overwhelming amount of support.

On my count, there were at least sixteen studies between 1961 and 1972 that independently verify the phrase structure hypothesis. By the standards of experimental psychology, this is a massive convergence of evidence – smacking somewhat of overkill. It was as if psychologists, who had been brought up to believe in strictly associative accounts of list learning, could not get over the fact that grouping words into phrases made them easier to learn. The hypothesis turned out to be true whether grouping was induced by the physical spacing of words (Anglin & Miller, 1968), by the placement of function words (Epstein, 1961), or by the ordinary process of comprehending sentences (Suci, 1967). Moreover, the mnemonic trace for memorized sentences gave strong evidence of having phrasal structure. Errors in recall turned out to be greater across phrase boundaries than within phrases (Johnson, 1965), and two probe words could be more quickly judged to be present or absent from a previously memorized sentence if they were both within the same phrase (Stewart & Gough, 1967).

These results, and others, served spectacularly well to break the grip of associative learning theory, which recognized only bonds between immediately neighboring items in time or space. But they did little to help decide whether a transformational grammar was employed during linguistic performance. Even the justly famous click experiments, beginning with Fodor and Bever (1965), which strongly suggested (but never quite proved) that constituents are computed on the fly during comprehension, didn't concern the transformational question. That required another sort of test entirely.

The deep structure hypothesis:

The 1965 version of transformational grammar, most completely set forth in Chomsky's *Aspects of the Theory of Syntax,* distinguishes between the surface structure and deep structure of a sentence. The deep structure of a sentence represents its basic grammatical relations (logical subject, logical object, etc.). It serves as the input to the transformation cycle, and it is at the level of deep structure that lexical interpretation occurs. Transformations convert deep structure into surface structure, the grammatic form of the actual sentence. Thus, the two sentences "John hit the ball" and "The ball was hit by John" have similar deep structure, with "John" being the logical subject and "ball" the logical object, even though, in the surface structure, the grammatical arrangement of words in the two sentences differs.

In the mid-1960s, deep structure was an exciting idea. It provided a formal justification for the intuitively appealing notion that sentences have an underlying logical form that differs from the surface arrangement of words and phrases. This idea goes back at least as far as the seventeenth-century Port-Royale grammars of French philosophers, and it was used by the inventors of modern logic to get around the nasty problems of ambiguity and paraphrase. Transformational grammar significantly improved upon these earlier ideas by giving deep structure an explicit definition, by supplying formal machinery (via the transformational cycle) to relate deep and surface structure, and by providing a way of bringing evidence to bear on questions about the form of deep structure. This evidence was obtained by determining whether deep structure could be configured so as to both represent basic grammatical relations and provide input to the transformational rules in a way that would allow their optimal application.

For psychologists, deep structure suggested a solution to the ancient problem of memory for prose. It has been known ever since the pioneering work of Binet and Henri (1894) that subjects who listen to a story or to a set of sentences will, unless they make special efforts at memorization, recall the meaning of these sentences much more accurately than they will recall the exact form. This fact might be explained quite nicely by a model that incorporates a transformational grammar. On this hypothesis, the listener tacitly applies the grammar to each incoming sentence to obtain its deep structure and then retains only deep structure in memory. When asked to recall, the listener applies transformations to the remembered deep structures to synthesize a paraphrase of the original.

To test this idea, it was necessary to see whether the memory trace left by a sentence bears any resemblance to its deep structure phrase marker. This is a difficult assessment, so it may not be surprising that no more than a handful of studies addressed the question. The experimental effects tend to be small, and their interpretation is not easy. One example may make the point.

In 1967, Arthur Blumenthal published two interesting experiments that used prompted recall to assess the mnemonic reality of deep structure. In Blumenthal's paradigm, subjects commit a list of sentences to memory and then attempt to recall them with the aid of one prompt word from each sentence. Since the accuracy of prompted recall is ordinarily better than free recall, prompt effectiveness can be measured by assessing the improvements in prompted versus free recall. In perhaps the most interesting of his experiments (Blumenthal & Boakes, 1967), Blumenthal used sentences based upon Chomsky's famous demonstration sentences:

(1) John is eager to please.
(2) John is easy to please.

Although these two sentences have similar surface structures, they have different deep structures. "John" is the logical subject of the two predicates ("be eager" and "please") in sentence (1) but is the logical object of only one predicate ("please") in sentence (2). If the ease with which the sentences can be recalled depends on their deep structure representation, then "John" should be a more effective prompt for sentence (1) than for sentence (2) for two reasons. First, "John" is multiply represented in sentence (1) and not in sentence (2), and it is plausible that the more often an item is represented in memory, the better chance it has of prompting the sentence. Second, "John" is the subject of the so-called matrix predicate ("be eager") in sentence (1) but not in sentence

(2), and it is also plausible that the subject of the main predicate of a sentence would be a more effective cue than the object of the predicate of a subordinate clause. This line of reasoning turned out to be supported by the facts; "John" is a more effective prompt for sentence (1) than for sentence (2).

Blumenthal's result is interesting and hardly intuitive. But does it show that deep structure is mnemonically real? The answer, I think, depends upon how carefully we define our tests of deep structure. Subsequent work of mine (Wanner, 1974) showed that the effectiveness of a prompt word is due not to its location in the deep phrase marker but to the number of times it appears in deep structure. Thus, the correct generalization of Blumenthal's result is simply that the more underlying propositions a prompt word is involved in, the more effective the prompt is. Does this generalization implicate deep structure? At first, I thought that it did (Wanner, 1974), but since then I have had doubts (Wanner, 1977). After all, propositional representation must be common to all semantic representations that decompose complex sentences into underlying propositions, each with a single predicate (Anderson & Bower, 1973). To show that prompt effectiveness is a function of propositional involvement therefore entails only that sentence memory involves decomposition into propositions. To provide positive evidence for the deep structure hypothesis, we need to test one aspect of the deep structure phrase marker that is *unique* to that representational form. For reasons I will come to, I strongly doubt that such evidence will ever be forthcoming.

The transformational hypothesis:

Of course, the most direct way to test the psychological reality of transformational grammar is to determine whether transformations are in any way involved in sentence processing. This game soon became known as the "derivational theory of complexity (DTC)." According to the DTC, the difficulty of producing or perceiving or remembering any sentence should be a direct function of the number (and possibly the complexity) of transformations in its derivational history.

At first, the DTC appeared to be spectacularly true. Lee McMahan (1963) and Dan Slobin (1966) both found, for instance, that the time required to judge a sentence true or false increases with the number of transformations used to derive it. Jacques Mehler (1963), George Miller (with K. A. McKean, 1964), and Harris Savin (with E. Perchonock, 1965) all found evidence that sentences are more difficult to remember verbatim the more transformations there are in their derivational history. Or so it seemed. But on closer inspection, much of this early evidence for the transformational hypothesis gave way.

The principal problem concerned the nature of the transformations used to test the DTC. For historical reasons that are difficult to disentangle, these tests were confined to the so-called major optional singulary transformations in Chomsky's 1957 version of the grammar: passive, negative, and question. The problem with these rules, of course, is that they introduce correlated changes in meaning (negative and question) or sentence length (passive and negative) into any sentence whose derivation involves them. Thus memory and comprehension time effects that first appeared to result from derivational complexity turned out to depend upon much more mundane facts about sentence length and meaning. To take just one example, Savin and Perchonock (1965) developed a truly elegant test of the "size" of the memory trace for a sentence by asking subjects to memorize a sentence together with a list of words and then measuring the numbers of words correctly recalled after verbatim recall of the sentence. This handsomely Archimedean method for measuring trace size showed apparently linear increases with the number of transformations in the derivational history of the memorized sentences. But, unfortunately for the DTC, efforts to replicate these effects failed using transformations such as particle movement, which change neither length nor meaning (Bever, Fodor, Garrett, & Mehler, 1966, reported in Fodor, Bever, & Garrett, 1974). Not surprisingly perhaps, the measured trace size for "John called Bill up" does not exceed the size of "John called up Bill" even though one more transformation is required to derive the former sentence.

Beyond reality

These results, and others like them, led to the virtual abandonment of the DTC by the late 1960s. Within psychology at large there were rumors, some finding print, that the adventure into transformational grammar had reached a dead end. But within psycholinguistics proper the range of responses was much more varied and interesting.

The most influential of these was what I have called elsewhere the "weak reality" hypothesis (Wanner, 1977). Surveying the pattern of partial success and partial failure achieved by the three reality hypotheses, Fodor, Bever, and Garrett (1974) offered the generalization that the structural descriptions generated by the grammar were psychologically significant, but not the rules used to generate those descriptions. This proposal seems a direct induction from the results that we have reviewed, but it has a flaw. Recall that the architecture of deep structure is in part determined in order to permit the general operation of the transformational rules. If the transformational rules are psychologically unreal, why should those aspects of deep structure that are motivated by the nature of the transformations be real? Such an accident of nature would seem monumentally improbable.

It is possible, of course, that only nontransformationally motivated aspects of deep structure are psychologically relevant. But if so, then the claim for the psychological reality of deep structure begins to collapse because it is precisely the transformationally motivated aspects of deep structure that separate it from other semantic representations. If transformationally motivated aspects are psychologically insignificant (and a review of the literature suggests that they are), then there is no unique evidence for deep structure. Listeners appear to recover underlying propositions when they understand a sentence, and these propositions undoubtedly contain information about the basic grammatical relations of the input sentence, but they do not recover deep structure per se.

This logic, or something like it, seems to have won a silent argument with the field. After 1975, there is very little mention of deep structure recovering during linguistic performance – either via transformations or in any other way. Instead, attention turned to proposals about how the basic grammatical relations might be determined directly from the surface structure phrase marker. Leading candidates have included Fodor, Bever, and Garrett's (1974) "heuristic" strategies, the augmented transition network parser (Kaplan, 1973; Wanner & Maratsos, 1978), the "sausage machine" parser (Fodor & Fraser, 1978), and, most recently, a processing model based upon lexical functional grammar (Ford, Bresnan, & Kaplan, 1982). Some of these moves abandon the idea that a performance model literally incorporates a grammar; others retain incorporation as a principle but employ a nontransformational grammar. Which, if any, will work is an open question. But it is important to remember that the results of the reality experiments – even, and perhaps most especially, where they departed from the expectations of the first generation of experimenters – set the terms on which this question must now be answered.

References

Anderson, J. R., & Bower, G. H. (1973). *Human Associative Memory*. Washington: Winston and Sons.

Anglin, J. M., & Miller, G. A. (1968). The role of phrase structure in the recall of meaningful verbal material. *Psychonomic Science, 10,* 343–4.

Bever, T. G., Fodor, J. A., Garrett, M. F., & Mehler, J. (1966). Transformational operations and stimulus complexity. Unpublished paper, MIT.

Binet, A., and Henri, V. (1894). La Memoire des mots. *L'Annal Psychologuique, 1,* 1–59.

Blumenthal, A. L. (1967). Prompted recall of sentences. *Journal of Verbal Learning and Verbal Behavior, 6,* 203–6.

Blumenthal, A. L. (1970). *Language and Psychology*. New York: Wiley.

Blumenthal, A. L. & Boakes, R. (1967). Prompted recall of sentences. *Journal of Verbal Learning and Verbal Behavior, 6,* 674–6.

Chomsky, N. (1967). *Syntactic Structures*. The Hague: Mouton.

Chomsky, N. (1963). Formal properties of grammar. In R. D. Luce, R. Bush, & E. Galanter (Eds.), *Handbook of Mathematical Psychology*, Vol. 2. New York: Wiley, pp. 323–418.

Chomsky, N. & Miller, G. A. (1963). Introduction to the formal analysis of natural languages. In R. D. Luce, R. Bush, & E. Galanter (Eds.), *Handbook of Mathematical Psychology*, Vol. 2. New York: Wiley, pp. 269–322.

Chomsky, N. (1965). *Aspects of the Theory of Syntax*. Cambridge, Mass.: MIT Press.

Epstein, W. (1961). The influence of syntactical structure on learning. *American Journal of Psychology, 74*, 80–5.

Fodor, J. & Bever, T. (1965). The psychological reality of linguistic segments, *Journal of Verbal Learning and Verbal Behavior, 4*, 414–20.

Fodor, J., Bever, T., & Garrett, M. (1974). *The Psychology of Language*. New York: McGraw-Hill.

Ford, M., Bresnan, J., & Kaplan, R. M. (1982). A competence-based theory of syntactic closure. In J. Bresnan (Ed.), *The Mental Representation of Grammatical Relations*. Cambridge, Mass.: MIT Press, pp. 727–97.

Frazier, L., & Fodor, J. (1978). The sausage machine: A new two-stage parsing model. *Cognition, 6*, 291–325.

Johnson, N. F. (1965). The psychological reality of phrase structure rules. *Journal of Verbal Learning and Verbal Behavior, 4*, 469–75.

Kaplan, R. (1973). A general syntactic processor. In R. Rustin (Ed.), *Natural Language Processing*. Englewood Cliffs, N.J.: Prentice-Hall, pp. 193–242.

Klima, E. S., & Bellugi, U. (1966). Syntactic regularities in the speech of children. In T. I. Lyons & R. J. Wales (Eds.), *Psycholinguistics Papers*. Edinburgh: Edinburgh University Press, pp.

McMahon, L. (1963). Grammatical analysis as part of understanding a sentence. Unpublished Ph.D. dissertation, Harvard University.

Mehler, J. (1963). Some effects of grammatical transformations on recall of English sentences. *Journal of Verbal Learning and Verbal Behavior, 2*, 346–51.

Miller, G. A., & Chomsky, N. (1963). Finitary models of language users. In R. D. Luce, R. Bush, & E. Galanter (Eds.), *Handbook of Mathematical Psychology*, Vol. 2. New York: Wiley, pp. 419–92.

Miller, G. A., & McKean, K. A. (1964). A chronometric study of some relations between sentences. *Quarterly Journal of Experimental Psychology, 16*, 297–308.

Savin, H., & Perchonock, E. (1965). Grammatical structure and the immediate recall of English sentences. *Journal of Verbal Learning and Verbal Behavior, 4*, 348–53.

Slobin, D. J. (1966). Grammatical transformations and sentence comprehension in childhood and adulthood. *Journal of Verbal Learning and Verbal Behavior, 5*, 219–27.

Stewart, C., & Gough, P. (1967). Constituent search in immediate memory for sentences. *Proceedings of the Midwestern Psychological Association*.

Suci, G. (1967). The validity of pause as an index of units in language. *Journal of Verbal Learning and Verbal Behavior, 6*, 26–32.

Wanner, E. (1974). *On Remembering, Forgetting, and Understanding Sentences*. The Hague: Mouton.

Wanner, E. (1977). Review of *The Psychology of Language* by J. A. Fodor, T. G. Bever, and M. F. Garrett. *Journal of Psycholinguistic Research, 3*, 261–70.

11   Language use and linguistic diversity

Jacques Mehler

What was the single most influential contribution of George Miller to the Center for Cognitive Studies in the first half of the 1960s? Surely, it was to found psycholinguistics as the study of language processing. Books on the psychology of language had been published generally with little or no concern for processing. Consider the intellectual environment that preceded Miller's work. At Harvard, as almost everywhere else, behaviorism was dominant. Behaviorists argued that the study of language was very simple. Words encoded in the acoustic wave triggered a response in an organism, and that was it. Operant conditioning supposedly explained how behavior was actually linked to the physics of signals. Behaviorism viewed stimuli and responses, in conjunction with a mechanism to link one to the other – namely, association through conditioning – as sufficient to explain behavior. Observable behavior was the only accepted information on the basis of which psychology was to be built. Organisms were viewed as basically identical to one another. Perhaps the difference between human and rat was in the number of units available to make associations, but certainly not in terms of qualitative distinctions.

George Miller and the Center for Cognitive Studies changed all that. In collaboration with Noam Chomsky, Miller opened psycholinguistics to universal grammatical structures. Miller argued that much of behavior was determined by the formal structures underlying the domain to which processes applied. Thus, subjects' performance in memorizing strings of symbols could be predicted in terms of an automaton capable of generating all sequences. Likewise, Miller predicted that with natural language it would be the grammatical structure rather than the conditions under which this or that sentence had been heard before that would predict behavior.

I would like to thank the following organizations for their financial support during the writing of this chapter: CNRS (ATP Aspects Cognitifs et Neurobiologiques du Langage), the Ministere de l'Industrie et de la Recherche (Decision No. 84C1390), and CNET (Convention 837 BD 2800790). I would also like to express my gratitude to Anne Cutler for her comments and invaluable assistance and to William Hirst for his patience and helpful suggestions.

153

At the same time, Eric Lenneberg was teaching other investigators at the Center that biological constraints were essential in allowing us to explain how language comes about and how it can be lost. Lenneberg and Chomsky were arguing that biological determinants, innate dispositions, explain why humans acquire language, whereas other vertebrates do not. Miller was to incorporate biological constraints and innateness into much of his later theorizing.

The net result of the environment that Miller created at the Center for Cognitive Studies was to allow him to redefine the aim of psycholinguistics. Indeed, for Miller, psycholinguistics was to describe processing in detail. It was no longer enough to talk loosely about stimuli and responses, as behaviorists were doing. Psycholinguists had to provide an information processing account of perception, a model of encoding and recoding, and explain how sentences were comprehended. Psycholinguists were urged to abstain from making any claims if they could not explain how a process took place. In particular, Miller did not accept many of the overoptimistic claims frequently made during those days (e.g., that chimps could learn language). George used to joke about this and comment that it was like teaching them to fly: "Have they learned to fly?", he would ask the animal psychologist in charge of the training, who would reply, "Well, actually not, but boy, can they jump."

All of this provided us with the best possible environment in which to be graduate students in psychology. Indeed, we lived in an atmosphere that only graduate students tend to create. We were convinced that we were right, not only in our ideas but also in our conceptions. We contended that we were living on the brink of a major breakthrough. Little did it matter that we were often out of touch with other studies of language processing being carried out elsewhere. Sometimes I had trouble understanding why George did not share our optimism. Be that as it may, the Center was certainly one of the most exciting places in the world during those days.

However, there was one sense in which I always felt a little different from my fellow graduate students and teachers. Miller and most colleagues focused their attention on English. I, on the other hand, was switching frantically from bad Spanish and German to even worse English and Italian, and finally settling for broken French. And, like Lenneberg, I was not always able to share the linguists' intuitions. Were sentences like "Some teddybears fight each other more often than not" or "She pass under the stars" grammatical or not? How could I know? I learned from Eric to worry about foreign accents, language learning, critical periods, and the like. The spirit of the time didn't include much interest in the study of comparative psycholinguistics. But, even if it had, there was little that could have been done about that in Cambridge, Massachusetts. However, I returned to France in 1967, and Europe was to offer me many languages within short distances. Furthermore, what I had learned for English had to be evaluated for French. In the process of adapting to Europe, I did not give up my own theoretical preferences. Indeed, I was convinced that language arises because we are built to sustain it. I was also convinced that competence is the same in all of us, even if the *us* are the French.

In this chapter, I summarize three lines of research in which, together with other investigators, I attempted to address this very basic issue. First, I review research in collaboration with Lecours and Parente on the effect of literacy on brain and language performance; then I review work carried out with Cutler, Norris, and Segui on specific language effects on speech processing. Finally, I present data that show that the effects of the linguistic environment are felt even after only a few hours of life.

Stabilization of language processing

In the following pages, I discuss briefly some of the investigations referred to previously. In part, data help to clarify many theoretical issues, and in part, they illustrate the virtues of the experimental method in cognitive science.

Brain functions and environmental pressures

Brains have a species-specific tendency to organize themselves in ways that are adaptive to the organism as a whole. Although in most humans the left hemisphere is dominant for language comprehension and production, some humans, presumably with different genetic programs, display right dominance for language. Early brain damage may result in a dominance different from the one genetically programmed. The influence of the environment in determining the effectiveness and eventually the amount of cerebral dominance has not yet, barring some exceptions, been explored. Bellugi and her collaborators (Bellugi, Poizner, & Klima, 1983; Poizner, Klima, & Bellugi, 1986; Poizner, Kaplan, Bellugi & Padden, 1984) have shown that cortical representation of language is similar in deaf and hearing populations. Sasanuma (1975) claims that the scripts used to represent speech in Japanese determine different cortical representations for the writing ability of Kana and Kanji. Much more research will be needed to understand the relation between brain processes and language processing.

In collaboration with Lecours and Parente, we have compared language performance in literate and illiterate subjects with or without brain damage. Prior to our own research, literate and illiterate populations had been compared using dichotic listening tests and had also been compared after brain damage. Damasio, Damasio, Castro-Caldas, and Hamsher (1979), using a dichotic test on words with different initial consonants, found a right ear advantage (REA) in literates but a left ear advantage (LEA) in illiterates. In contrast, Tzavaras, Kaprinis, and Gatzoyas (1981), using digits, found a REA in both populations. These discrepant results may arise from the materials employed, from different methodologies, or from differences in subject populations. The ages of the subjects differed as well. Obviously, such results cannot settle patterns of ear advantage in literate as compared to illiterate populations.

Aphasiological investigations of adult illiterate patients have been the object of a number of case studies (Lecours, Mehler, & Parente, 1987a, 1987b). However, systematic studies on the effects of brain injury in these two populations have been rare. Cameron, Currier, and Haerer (1971) and Damasio, Castro-Caldas, Grosso, and Ferro (1976) are probably the main exceptions. Cameron et al. found that transitory aphasia was more frequently observed in literates than in illiterates; this led them to conclude that language is less well represented in the dominant hemisphere of illiterates than in that of literates. They speculated that language is more ambilaterally represented in illiterates.

Damasio et al. studied a sample of literate and illiterate focal brain-damaged patients. Fifty-five percent of the literate and 54 percent of the illiterate patients presented aphasic symptoms. Furthermore, no differences were found on the token test between the left brain-damaged illiterates compared to a matched group of literate patients. These authors concluded that brain specialization for language does not depend on literacy. The discrepancy between the results in these two sets of studies prompted Lecours, Mehler, and Parente to compare literate and illiterate populations suffering from similar lesions.

The bulk of our field work was carried out mainly in Brazil, where a total of 157 illiterate and 139 literate subjects of an average age of sixty years were interviewed and tested. The literate subjects had had, on the average, over eight years of schooling, whereas the illiterates had never attended school and were totally incapable of reading or writing even their own names.

We used a directed interview and a test (a translation of the Montreal M1-Alpha test). Globally, our results can be summarized as follows. By and large, as Damasio et al. had found, left cerebral dominance for language is characteristic of right-handed adults regardless of their literacy status. In literates and illiterates, as the classical view suggests, language comprehension and production mechanisms are mediated by the left hemisphere. However, our results also suggest that naming requires more ambilateral involvement in illiterates than in literates. Given that naming is a major item in assessment of linguistic functioning, this result can explain Cameron et al.'s conclusions.

The results of the directed interview also indicate that the left brain-damaged patients have comparable problems with language regardless of their literacy status. However, subjective scores by speech therapists who interviewed the patients show that more right hemisphere illiterate patients have language-related problems than right hemisphere literate patients. However, on the more objective M1-Alpha scores, we found that on almost all items, right brain-damaged patients have scores similar to those of control subjects matched for age, socioeconomic factors, and sex.

The one exception was the naming scores of right-lesion illiterates, which were significantly lower than those of control subjects.

On the basis of these results, we concluded that left hemisphere dominance is characteristic of all populations, irrespective of literacy status. Even so, some tasks may require greater reliance by illiterates on the subsidiary hemisphere. Thus, biologically determined tendencies cannot be countered by sociocultural pressures. Nonetheless, since the resources for different tasks change, depending on subjects' familiarity with them, strategies that require reliance on different cortical tissue ensue. The differences between populations for naming may thus only reflect changes in processing strategies, and not changes in the cortical representation of linguistic function.

The interpretation of our results might also be valid for Bever and Chiarello's (1974) results for music. They found that musical literacy induces a change in dominance, as assessed by a dichotic listening task. Some recent results by Peretz, Morais, and Bertelson (1987) have confirmed those reports. However, clinical data by Basso (personal communication) indicate that a right-handed professional musician after a cerebrovascular accident (which destroyed most of his left hemisphere cortex) retained his musical ability but lost his capacity for language. If there is a shift in dominance through literacy, then, at the very least, previous (right hemisphere) capabilities are not destroyed. Here again, however, clinical data on cerebrovascular patients uncover problems arising from the loss of specialized structures, whereas dichotic listening tests, sensitive to attentional and strategic resources, uncover modifications in the management of test-taking aptitudes.

The resistance of cortical structures to sociocultural pressures meshes well with post-Lamarckian teachings in biology. Behavior, however, is affected by sociocultural factors. This is where cognitive psychologists come into the picture. They must ask themselves at what level environmental effects modify functional architecture. Speech perception is an optimal domain for exploring this issue. Miller, as well as Lenneberg, speculated about the *raison d'etre* of foreign accents. Why is it difficult to learn a language without a foreign accent after a certain age? We can ask ourselves if there are similar problems with perception. During the early days at the Center for Cognitive Studies, we were concerned about these issues. However, I have come to deal with them only recently, and for two reasons. First, in the late 1960s, I met Segui, whose interests were quite close to mine, and later Cutler and Norris. They were all instrumental in getting this research program off the ground. Second, the multilingual environment in Europe is very conducive to this kind of work.

Speech processing units across languages

Fodor (1983) argues that input systems convert the output of sensors into a format fit for the central processor. Indeed, the inferences of the input analyzers convert representations of proximal stimuli into representations related to the distribution of objects in the world. Fodor states that "Input systems constitute a family of modules: domain-specific computational systems characterized by informational encapsulation, high-speed, restricted access, neural specificity and the rest" (p. 101).

Much of the information available to such systems is innately specified. Indeed, "the neural mechanisms subserving input analysis develop according to specific, endogenously determined patterns under the impact of releasers" (Fodor, 1983, p. 100). These claims deserve proper empirical assessment.

Segui and I, in collaboration with Cutler and Norris, have explored the units used in speech perception and the effect that the first language may have in determining them. I believe that this issue bears directly upon Fodor's input systems and their environmental releasers.

Cutler, Mehler, Norris, and Segui (1986) have used a syllable monitoring technique to elicit fast responses from subjects. Subjects hear lists of words and are instructed to monitor for a given word-initial target. Mehler, Dommergues, Frauenfelder, and Segui (1981) had found that a target is detected faster when it coincides precisely with the first syllable rather than when it is larger or smaller than the first syllable in the target-bearing item. Thus the target "pa" was detected faster in "palace," where it is the first syllable, than in "palmier," where it is smaller than the first syllable, whereas the target "pal" is detected faster in "palmier," where it is the first syllable, than in "palace," where it is larger than the first syllable.

Mehler et al. argued from this result that syllabification plays an important role in processing – in fact, that syllables are the basic processing units in speech perception and lexical access. However, we initially failed to question the universality of this unit. Mehler et al.'s experiment was conducted in French. Linguists demonstrate that languages have very different syllabic structures. Although all languages have syllables, some (e.g., Japanese) have mostly consonant-vowel (CV) syllables, whereas others (e.g., English) tolerate syllables as simple as V and as complex as CCCVCCC (e.g., "sprints"). Likewise, languages differ in the distinctiveness of their syllabic boundaries. On the one hand, some languages, like English, have ambisyllabic consonants, that is, consonants that can belong to either of two syllables. In many stress languages, intervocalic consonants before unstressed vowels are often ambisyllabic. On the other hand, languages like French have much less ambisyllabicity. Thus, French and English differ in the distinctiveness with which they mark the boundary of first syllables. Furthermore, English has lexical stress, whereas French is a purely oxytonic language without lexical stress. Therefore, the questions we should have asked concerned the functional validity of syllables for native speakers of both languages. We knew that French speakers rely consistently on syllabification, but we needed to ascertain whether English speakers also syllabify. We found that English subjects listening to English words that incorporate either CV[C]/—or CVC/—onset syllables detected a target in ambisyllabic items more rapidly, irrespective of target type, than in CVC/—items. Thus, in "palace" the targets "pa" and "pal" were detected extremely rapidly, and in "palpitate" the target "pa" was detected less rapidly than "pal."

To evaluate in greater detail the procedures underlying behavior, we tested English subjects on the French tape and French subjects on the English tape. All subjects were monolinguals. The French tape contains only items that are easy to syllabify, but English speakers showed no tendency to syllabify, even on items that had elicited such behavior in French. French speakers syllabify the English language words. The interaction is significant, although it is mostly due to CVC items rather than to the unfamiliar ambisyllabic ones.

These results suggest that French and English speakers differ in regard to syllabification. French speakers syllabify familiar as well as unfamiliar items, whereas English speakers fail to syllabify regardless of the status of items. This difference may be due to several causes. English subjects are slower than the French by over 100 milliseconds when both monitor their own language. This observation is compatible with the conjecture that both populations syllabify, but only when responses are fast. Slow responses triggered from a different buffer mask the effects of syllabification. In other words, English-speaking subjects might be slower because they need more information to determine whether the first segmented syllable carries stress or not. It would be useless to identify CONtact as conTACT or vice versa. French has no lexical stress, and such information is irrelevant to its processing. Of course, another possibility is that speech segments differ for English and French native speakers.

At this time, unpublished results from Bradley, Sanchez-Casas, and Garcia Albea show that the behavior of native speakers of Spanish closely resembles that of native French speakers; both populations syllabify. Since Spanish is a language with lexical stress, the preceding explanations become unlikely for explaining the difference between French and English speakers.

In brief, at this time, syllabification must be viewed as just one of several options to use in coping with speech. Possibly, during acquisition, subjects may have to adjust their speech perception system to extract the properties of speech relevant to processing in their native language. Our results suggest that the initial state is set to reflect the phonological properties of the mother tongue. Thereafter, even when listening to a foreign language, subjects still use procedures elaborated for their native language.

According to Fodor's thesis that language is an input–output system par excellence, speech perception should be mediated by a specialized module. This module uses its own data base to guide its decisions. In the preceding experiments, we have demonstrated that this data base is compiled during first-language learning. It must be remembered that according to the thesis defended in the *Modularity of Mind,* only central processes have access to all of the knowledge of the organism. Modules are encapsulated, fast, mandatory, and sensitive to knowledge provided by their proprietary data base. This difference between central and input faculties deserves ontogenetic investigation. How does the speech module adapt to the constraints of native language learning? How does it extract the properties that will optimize its functioning? Is this process compatible with the encapsulated nature of modules, or should we imagine that modules start as Quinean, to become modular after some years of functioning? Unfortunately, the data that might allow us to answer these questions do not yet exist. Hopefully, in the coming years, relevant research will become available. In the meantime, I would like to throw some new light on the capacity for speech processing in very young infants from studies that have been carried out in France, the United States, and Canada.

Languages in infancy

A number of very good reviews of the infant's ability to discriminate speech sounds can be found in Eimas (1982), in Aslin, Pisoni, and Jusczyk (1983), and in several of the chapters in Mehler and Fox (1984). In substance, by one or two months of age, infants discriminate most, if not all, of the phonetic contrasts discriminated by adults. Eimas (1975) has shown that infants can even discriminate contrasts that their parents can no longer make. Trehub (1976) has found similar results. In a series of recent experiments, Werker and Tees (1984a, 1984b) confirmed this early ability and also showed that, by the end of the first year, infants start ignoring contrasts that they discriminated earlier. In brief, the very young infant reacts to contrasts irrespective of his or her linguistic background. By the end of the first year, the infant reacts distinctively to the contrasts used in the native language. It is difficult, at this time, to understand how the infant achieves this ability. It is also unclear whether the newborn baby has the same competence as the one- or two-month-old infant, though results from my laboratory in Paris suggest that this is the case. Thus we can conjecture that the ability to distinguish all potential speech contrasts is part of the initial state. This faculty, impressive as it is, does not exhaust the list of abilities that tune the newborn baby to language. Indeed, infants recognize speakers (Mills & Meluish, 1974; Mehler, Barriere, & Jassik-Gerschenfeld, 1976; DeCasper & Fifer, 1980) and, like adults, they stream signals (Demany, 1982). But again, we have almost no idea of how the infant accomplishes these tasks. However, the ability itself indicates that the infant pays selective attention to a source and organizes several concomitant sounds into structures that correspond to those of the adult.

These abilities provide little or no insight into how the infant copes with his or her linguistic environment on the basis of partial and often erroneous information. Currently, a considerable effort is being made to understand the formal properties of systems for language acquisition (Osherson, Stob, & Weinstein, 1986; Wexler & Culicover, 1980). Hopefully, studies on learnability will uncover systems that stabilize in behaviors resulting in the acquisition of natural language. However, in parallel with such studies, empirical investigations of the newborn can also provide the boundary conditions of the initial state system that allow it to acquire language.

In collaboration with Lambertz, Jusczyk, and Amiel, we have explored the infant's ability to recognize a language – for instance, the mother's language – irrespective of the utterance and of the speaker. A French-Russian bilingual female speaker, with equal competence in both languages, recorded the same story twice, once in French and once in Russian. Her recordings were then edited into sequences averaging 15 seconds each, selected so as not to disturb the integrity of the prosody. Four-day-old infants born in Paris to French-speaking parents were then tested with a variant of the nonnutritive sucking technique developed by Siqueland and Delucia (1969). Two groups of babies were presented first with Russian and two other groups with French, and their sucking rates were measured. It was found that the infants sucked at higher rates when listening to French than to Russian. A group of infants born in Paris to parents who spoke a foreign language were also tested. These infants had almost no experience with French, the language in which they were tested. Their sucking rate corresponded to that of French babies listening to Russian. These results, see Figure 11.1, show that the four-day-old infant reacts differently to French and to Russian.

If we turn our attention back to the French infants in the four groups described earlier, when these infants reached the preestablished criterion, one of the groups that started with Russian and one that started with French were switched to the other language. The infants in the other two groups, namely, the control groups, continued listening to the same language after they attained the criterion. The experimental and control groups starting with French did not differ from each

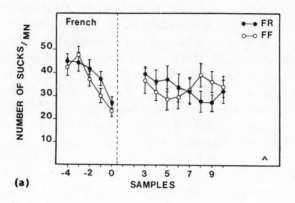

(a)

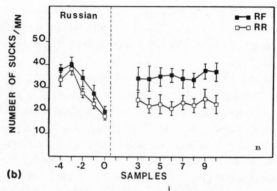

(b)

Figure 11.1   Results for infants hearing either French or Russian during the first phase
of the experiment. (a) Results for the two groups (FF: 10 subjects and FR: 10 subjects)
who, after achieving criterion for entering the second phase, switched to Russian for the
FR group and continued to hear French for the FF. (b) Comparable results for infants who
heard Russian during the first phase.

other after achieving the criterion. In contrast, the groups starting with Russian
differed significantly from each other after reaching the criterion. These results
are shown in Figure 11.2.

We conjectured that two factors account for these results. One is preference.
As shown earlier, French, the familiar and preferred language, elicits greater
sucking activity during the first phase, and the sucking is sustained for longer
intervals. This explains the finding that the French control group continued to
suck at a high rate after reaching the criterion. The other factor is related to
novelty, namely, an increase in sucking rate whenever a change is discriminated.

With these two factors, we can interpret our results. The two groups starting

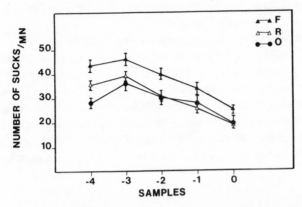

Figure 11.2 Display of the change in sucking rate for the last five samples during the first phase of the experiment. Group F (20 infants) had significantly higher sucking rates than group R (20 infants). Group 0 included 10 infants of foreign language–speaking parents.

with Russian behaved differently after the switch because, whereas the control group decreased its sucking rate, given that it continued listening to an unfamiliar language (i.e., Russian), the experimental group, discriminating a change, had a tendency to increase its own sucking rate. However, this tendency was increased because the change was from a nonpreferred to a preferred language, namely, French. In contrast, the groups starting with French looked similar after the switch. The control group, as already mentioned, sustained high sucking rates in the presence of the preferred language, whereas the experimental group had two tendencies that canceled each other out. One was to increase the sucking rate because a change in language had been noticed; the other was to decrease the sucking rate because the change was from a preferred to a nonpreferred language.

This experiment suggests that infants as young as four days old can discriminate between Russian and French, languages that differ considerably. No data are yet available to ascertain whether infants can discriminate between languages that are more like each other. Regardless of the answer to this question, our results suggest that infants extract dynamic parameters from the signal. (Indeed, two groups of subjects failed to react differentially to Russian and French when the sequences were played backward. This control rules out some parameters that could have accounted for the results, as for instance, systematic differences in the height of F_0.)

Even at four days, therefore, infants extract information from the environment to characterize the preferred language, presumably the language that has become reinforcing because it is the one used by the mother. On average, a four-day-old infant has been fed more than twenty-four times, providing ample opportunity for familiarity with its mother's language.

Our results partially answer the question asked previously, namely, when and what kind of information determines the nature of the proprietary data base that guides the speech perception module? Indeed, though we cannot say much about the nature of this information, we can say that it is effective from the first moments of life on. It remains to be seen whether this information is acquired through general knowledge structures or by parameters that are specified within the module. The ontogenetic path for the acquisition of the data base will determine whether the notion of a module does or does not play a critical role in development.

Conclusion

From the evidence of the three lines of research discussed, it appears that the brain's structure remains unchanged regardless of the linguistic environment, provided only that language is made available. The linguistic environment, however, changes the nature of the processes involved in speech perception. The four-day-old infant is already changed by the effects of the environment.

The fundamental concerns of George Miller and the Center for Cognitive Studies in the early 1960s irreversibly changed the way psychology is conceived and research is carried out. Processing has become the concern of most psycholinguists. As a result of the investigations that Miller's approach stimulated, the relationship of behavior to brain structures is understood somewhat better, and so are the biological determinants of language. Finally, the path to language acquisition is being actively explored with success. All of these were the concerns that George Miller argued were important. A quarter of a century later, his intuitions have been borne out.

Consider the quote from Voltaire's *Micromégas*:

L'âme est un esprit pur qui a reçu dans le ventre de sa mère toutes les idées metaphysiques, et qui, en sortant de là, est obligée d'aller a l'école, et d'apprendre tout de nouveau ce qu'elle a si bien su et qu'elle ne saura plus.[1]

Voltaire's ironic approach to nativist theories of language acquisition was justified. However, psycholinguistic research, for which the intellectual climate at the Center laid the groundwork, has provided a solid empirical basis upon which intellectually respectable nativist theorizing can now proceed.

However, it would be misleading to conclude this tribute to George and the environment that was provided for us at the Center by mentioning only intellectual events. The exceptional atmosphere that existed in the 1960s at the Center was also created by people and events. The people were the ones already mentioned, as well as Chris Alexander, Ursula Bellugi, Tom Bever, Tom Bower, Al

Bregman, Bill Huggins, Paul Kolers, David McNeill, Don Norman, Harris Savin, Molly Potter, and many others. The events were varied. For instance, many of us participated in a musical creation: "Passagio" by Luciano Berio. It was of outstanding psycholinguistic significance in that its inaugural performance starred Ursula Bellugi, Rick Cromer, Ed Klima, Susan Berio, Marilu Kuiper, and others who would become famous psycholinguists. Berio later composed "Psycholinguistic Clinic," an episode of his well-known A-RONE that was also very successful, even though we were not used as performers.

The exceptional climate at the Center for Cognitive Studies promoted work and creativity that was to influence the field. Many attempts have been made to imitate the Center. However, even when successful, they have failed to match the exceptional climate that George and his colleagues created. Partly this was because it was then that George was shaping the field and because the intuitions about the direction in which to go were right: Try to use psychology, linguistics, and biology in your work.

Notes

1 In my own translation, Voltaire states: "The mind is a pure substance that has received all metaphysical ideas in the mother's womb, and yet after birth it has to go to school to learn all it once knew so well but no longer knows."

References

Aslin, R. N., Pisoni, D. B., & Jusczyk, P. W. (1983). Auditory development and speech perception in infancy. In M. Haith & J. Campos (Eds), *Carmichael's Handbook of Child Psychology: Infant Development*. New York: Wiley.

Bellugi, U., Poizner, H., & Klima, E. S. (1983). Brain organization for languages: Clues from sign aphasia. *Human Neurobiology, 2,* 155–70.

Bever, T. G., & Chiarello, R. (1974). Cerebral dominance in musicians and non-musicians. *Science, 185,* 537–9.

Cameron, R. F., Currier, R. D., & Haerer, A. F. (1971). Aphasia and illiteracy. *British Journal of Disorders of Communication, 6,* 161–3.

Cutler, A., Mehler, J., Norris, D., & Segui, J. (1986). The syllable's differing role in segmentation of French and English. *Journal of Memory and Language, 25,* 385–400.

Cutler, A., Mehler, J., Norris, D., & Segui, J. (1987). Phoneme identification and the lexicon. *Cognitive Psychology, 19,* 141–77.

Damasio, A. R., Castro-Caldas, A., Grosso, J. T., & Ferro, J. M. (1976). Brain specialization for language does not depend on literacy. *Archives of Neurology, 33,* 300–1.

Damasio, H., Damasio, A. R., Castro-Caldas, A., & Hamsher, K. S. (1979). Reversal of ear advantage for phonetically similar words in illiterates. *Journal of Clinical Neuropsychology, 1,* 331–8.

DeCasper, A. J., & Fifer, W. P. (1980). Of human bonding: Newborns prefer their mother's voices, *Science, 208,* 1174–6.

Demany, L. (1982) Auditory Stream Segregation in Infancy. *Infant Behavior and Development, 5,* 261–76.

Eimas, P. D. (1975). Auditory and phonetic coding of the cues for speech *Discrimination of the (r—1) distinction* by young infants, *Perception and Psychophysics, 18,* 341–7.

Eimas, P. D. (1982). Speech perception: A view of the initial state and perceptual mechanisms. In J. Mehler, S. Franck, M. Garrett, & E. Walker (Eds.), *Perspectives in Mental Representation: Experimental and Theoretical Studies of Cognitive Processes and Capacities.* Hillsdale, N.J.: Erlbaum.

Fodor, J. A. (1983). *The Modularity of Mind.* Cambridge, Mass.: MIT Press.

Lecours, A. R., Mehler, J., & Parente, M. A. (1987a). Illiteracy and brain damage: 1. Aphasia testing in culturally contrasted populations. *Neuropsychologia, 25,* 1B, 231–45.

Lecours, A. R., Mehler, J., & Parente, M. A. (1987b). Illiteracy and brain damage: 2. Manifestations of unilateral neglect in testing "auditory comprehension" with iconographic materials, *Brain and Cognition* (in press).

Mehler, J., Barrière, M., & Jassik-Gerschenfeld. (1976). Reconnaissance de la voix maternelle par le nourrisson. *La Recherche, 7,* 786–8.

Mehler, J., Dommergues, J. Y., Frauenfelder, U., & Segui, J. (1981). The syllable's role in speech segmentation. *Journal of Verbal learning and Verbal Behavior 20,* 298–305.

Mehler, J., & Fox R. (Eds.) (1984) *Neonate Cognition: Beyond the Buzzing, Blooming Confusion,* Hillsdale, N.J.: Erlbaum.

Mehler, J., Lambertz, G., and Jusczyk, P. W. (1986). Discrimination de sa langue maternelle par le nouveau-ne de quatre jours. *C.R. de l'Academie de Sciences de Paris, 303,* 637–40.

Mills, M., & Meluish, E. (1974). Recognition of mother's voice in early infancy. *Nature, 252,* 123–4.

Osherson, D. N., Stob, M., & Weinstein, S. (1986). *Systems That Learn.* Cambridge, Mass.: MIT Press.

Peretz, I., Morais, J., & Bertelson, P. (1987). Shifting ear differences in melody recognition through strategy inducement. *Brain and Cognition* (in press).

Poizner, H., Kaplan, E., Bellugi, U., & Padden, C. A. (1984). Visual-spatial processing in deaf brain-damaged signers. *Brain and Cognition, 3,* 281–306.

Poizner, H., Klima, E., & Bellugi, U. (1986). *What the Hands Reveal About the Brain.* Cambridge, Mass.: MIT Press.

Sasanuma, S. (1975). Kana and Kanji processing in Japanese aphasics. *Brain and Language, 2,* 369.

Siqueland, E. R., & Delucia, C. A. (1969). Visual reinforcement of non-nutritive sucking in human infants. *Science, 165,* 1144–6.

Trehub, S. E. (1976). The discrimination of foreign speech contrasts by infants and adults. *Child Development, 47,* 466–72.

Tzavaras, A., Kaprinis G., & Gatzoyas, A. (1981). Literacy and hemispheric specialization for language: Digit dichotic listening in illiterates. *Neuropsychologia, 19,* 565–70.

Werker, J. F., & Tees, R. C. (1984a). Phonemic and phonetic factors in adult cross-language speech perception. *Journal of the Acoustical Society of America, 75,* 1866–78.

Werker, J. F., & Tees, R. C. (1984b). Cross-language speech perception: Evidence for perceptual reorganization during the first year of life. *Infant Behavior and Development, 7,* 49–63.

Wexler, K., & Culicover, P. (1980). *Formal Principles of Language Acquisition.* Cambridge, Mass.: MIT Press.

12   The immanent form of phonemes

Morris Halle

The role of linguistic knowledge in phonetics

Perhaps the most intriguing aspect of language is its dual nature. On the one hand, an utterance is an acoustical signal produced by readily observable gymnastics of the human vocal tract: the lips, tongue, soft palate, larynx, and so on, that is, the anatomical structures that make up the upper end of our digestive and respiratory tracts. On the other hand, an utterance always involves knowledge of a special kind, for it is only by virtue of this knowledge that the physical signal that strikes our ears has meaning. For the person who does not know English, the sounds made by someone speaking English are just that – meaningless noises. Moreover, such a person would not only fail to understand an English utterance; he would also experience great difficulty if he were asked to reproduce a segment of spoken English. For example, a person who does not know English is unlikely to be able to reproduce the eight-word sequence "the noun phrase that I am now uttering," and will, of course, have no idea of the meaning of this phrase. By contrast, a speaker of English would understand the meaning of the phrase and would find little difficulty in repeating the eight words that make up "the noun phrase that I am now uttering." Knowledge of language thus affects aspects of linguistic behavior that at first appear to be quite mechanical, such as the ability to reproduce a short phrase.

The study of the production and perception of spoken utterances has been the province of the science of phonetics. Among the questions phonetics has been trying to answer are, not surprisingly, questions concerning the neurophysiological organization of the speaking process. Phoneticians want to understand precisely what sort of gymnastics a fluent speaker of English engages in in producing an English utterance and how this gymnastics differs from as well as resembles the gymnastics engaged in by speakers of Japanese, Javanese, Arabic, or Kwakiutl. Phoneticians also want to know how this vocal tract gymnastics is

This work was supported in part by the Center for Cognitive Science, MIT.

167

anatomically structured and controlled. Although the speaking process has been subject to serious physiological inquiry for almost a century and a half, our understanding of this aspect of language is still rather rudimentary: We know much less about how we speak than about how cockroaches walk, fish swim, or monkeys reach for objects in their visual field. Some will no doubt attribute this disparity in our knowledge to the fact that we are limited in the type of experimentation to which we can subject humans. It seems to me, however, that a much more serious impediment to progress has been the failure of phoneticians to take adequate advantage of a large body of information that is accessible to study, namely, the linguistic knowledge that – as previously noted – is intimately involved in the production of every utterance.

In what follows, I attempt to illustrate how some aspects of this knowledge have been utilized to draw inferences about the way in which the gymnastics of the speaking process is controlled. I present evidence and arguments for a specific organization of the speaking process, and I spell out specific implications that this organization appears to have for the motor physiology of speaking.

Phonological representations are three-dimensional

I assume that naive speakers are correct in their belief that every utterance is a sequence of words and that every word is a sequence of speech sounds. Moreover, I assume that speech sounds or phonemes are complexes of binary distinctive features of the sort discussed in Jakobson, Fant, and Halle (1952) and illustrated in (1).

	p	b	m	k	g	ŋ	
							(1)
labial	+	+	+	−	−	−	
dorsal	−	−	−	+	+	+	
nasal	−	−	+	−	−	+	
voiced	−	+	+	−	+	+	

It was suggested by Jakobson that speech sounds are complexes of such distinctive features and nothing else. To Jakobson the formula meant that, for the speaker, speech sounds are not unanalyzable entities, as might be suggested by the letters of the alphabet with which speech sounds are represented in writing; rather, each speech sound is a complex of properties such as those represented in (1). As evidence for the validity of this proposition, I cited in Halle (1978) the fact – brought to my attention by Lise Menn – that English speakers have no difficulty forming plurals of foreign nouns ending in phonemes that do not exist in English. That English speakers form the plural of the German names Bach with /s/ in "boots," rather than with /z/ as in "cows" or with /Iz/ as in "bushes," can be explained only if it is assumed that the rule for forming English plurals is formulated in terms of features rather than phonemes and that English speakers are able to analyze phonemes into their features. If the English plural rule had been stated in terms of phonemes, it could not have included a phoneme that is not part of the language, and if speakers could not analyze phonemes into their component features, there would be no explanation for their ability to form the plural of words that are not part of their language and that contain sounds that are not English. In sum, there is reason to assume that words are represented in the speaker's memory in the form of feature matrices of the kind illustrated in (1).

Research of the last decade has shown that this is only a partial picture of the actual situation. For example, all languages utilize variations in the fundamental pitch of the voice to give melodic shape to their utterances. Thus, in English, utterances are pronounced with quite different melodies (pitch curves) when they are used as a response to a neutral question than when they are intended to convey surprise, dismay, or other emotions. It has been established that pitch curves represent sequences of discrete tones. Like tone sequences in a song, the tone sequences encountered in spoken language frequently can be spread over an arbitrary number of syllables. Thus, the melody appropriate for asking a question in English remains essentially unchanged, without regard to the number of syllables over which it must be spread. This means, in effect, that as in the musical score of a song, we are dealing with two parallel sequences of discrete entities: tones and speech sounds or "phonemes," as illustrated in (2), which has been adapted from Pierrehumbert (1980).

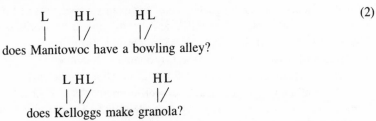

We note that in (2) not every phoneme is linked to a tone, nor is a single tone linked to a phoneme. It is well known that in the usual case tones are linked only to vowels, and that in English only certain vowels in a phrase are supplied with a tone, as shown in (2). As a result of work by Goldsmith (1979), Williams (1976), Liberman (1975), McCarthy (1979), Pulleyblank (1986), Levin (1985), and others, we have learned a great deal about the formal apparatus that is required to deal with this type of information. An important result of this work has been a change in the nature of the relation between the phonemes and the tones. Rather than link the tones to the phonemes directly, as was done in (2), it was found necessary to establish a somewhat more indirect relationship between the

two sets of segment sequences that are now connected by being linked to a
sequence of timing slots, as illustrated in (3).

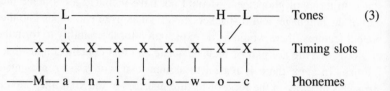

We have in (3) three parallel lines of units: the tones, the timing slots, and the
phonemes. It is an elementary fact of solid geometry that two parallel lines define
a plane. It is, therefore, possible to think of (3) as consisting of two half-planes
that intersect in the line constituted by the timing slots. The phonemes represented by complexes of distinctive features, as in (1), are contained in the bottom
half-plane of (3), and the tones represented by a different set of distinctive features are represented in the top half-plane. The obvious question suggested by a
representation such as (3) is whether there are additional half-planes above and
beyond the two given in (3) and what function such half-planes might perform.

Perhaps the most striking result obtained by utilizing the three-dimensional
format just sketched has been John McCarthy's treatment of the discontinuous
morphemes of the Semitic languages, an old conundrum of linguistic theory. We
now briefly discuss the problem and present McCarthy's solution.

Every language has constraints on what strings of phonemes constitute well-
formed sequences in that language. Thus, for example, speakers of English will
usually agree that "blick," "snill," and "trun" might be words of English,
whereas "lbick," "nsill," and "rtun" might not. It has been discovered that
the domain over which sequential well-formedness is defined in all languages is
the *syllable*. Languages, of course, differ as to what types of syllables they allow, but in all languages a sequence of well-formed syllables constitutes a well-
formed word or utterance. Work by Steriade (1982), Levin (1985), and others
has shown that syllables have internal constituent structure of the sort illustrated
in (4).

The syllable is thus a complex of nested binary constituents. It is composed of the rime, which may or must be preceded by one or more timing slots linked to consonants. The rime itself is composed of the nucleus, which must or may be followed by one or more timing slots linked to consonants. Finally, the nucleus may or may not be branching; it must, however, dominate a timing slot linked to a vowel or phoneme of high sonority. Different phonemes or phoneme sequences are admitted in different positions in the syllable. For example, in English /ž/, as in "rouge," is admissible in the rime but not in the onset, whereas tones in English are admitted in the nucleus but not elsewhere. These restrictions can readily be expressed if the syllable structure is represented on a separate half-plane that intersects the half-planes of (3) – that is, the half-planes carrying information about the phonemes and the tones – in the line of timing slots.

The structure of the syllable in classical Arabic, as well as of many other Semitic dialects, is of the fairly simple variety given in (5).

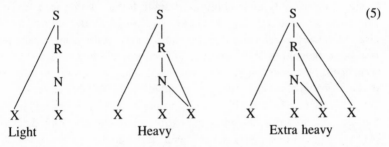

(5)

Heavy syllables have either a branching rime or nucleus, whereas in an extra-heavy syllable an extra consonant is added to a heavy syllable.

Arabic shares an interesting property with all Semitic languages, as well as with a number of non-Semitic languages such as the American Indian language Yokuts (Archangeli, 1984). In these languages the syllabification of a word is determined not by the phonemes that happen to compose the word, but rather by its morphological structure. To illustrate, I cite in (6) some forms from McCarthy (1982a) epitomizing the formation of the so-called broken plurals of Arabic.

			(6)
jundab	janaadib	"locust"	
sultaan	salaatiin	"sultan"	
duktar	dakaatir	"doctor"	
safarjal	safaarij	"quince"	
maktab	makaatib	"office"	
miktaah	mafaatiih	"key"	
nuwar	nawaawir	"white flower"	
9andaliib	9annaadil	"nightingale"	

The first thing to observe about these examples is that whereas the singular forms are either bi- or trisyllabic, the plural forms are uniformly trisyllabic. Moreover, the structure of the syllables in the plural is fixed. The first syllable is light, the second syllable is heavy, and the third syllable, which always ends with a consonant, has a vowel that is identical in length with that of the second syllable in the singular. This is a typical instance of what is meant by morphology-driven syllabification; that is, syllable structure that is imposed not by the phoneme composition of the word, but by the fact that the word belongs to a particular grammatical category, the plural in the case under discussion.

Nor is syllable structure all that is determined by the fact that the form is a plural noun. Note that the vowel pattern in all plural forms is the same: /i/ in the last syllable, /a/ in the first two syllables. The vowel pattern of the plural is thus totally unrelated to that of the singular: It is determined not by the noun that is pluralized, but rather by the fact of pluralization. This leaves only the consonants to signal the identity of the pluralized noun: to tell us that we are speaking of "doctors" or "sultans" rather than of "nightingales" or "quince"; everything else in the word is determined by the morphology of the word, by the fact that it is a noun belonging to a particular inflectional class. The distribution of the consonants, moreover, is severely restricted: They occur only in those positions in the word where consonants are admitted by the syllable structure, and there are precisely four such positions in every plural form. If the word has more than four consonants in the singular, the extra consonants are omitted, as shown in (6) by the nouns meaning "quince" and "nightingale."

We illustrate in (7) the three-dimensional template of the Semitic broken plural forms.

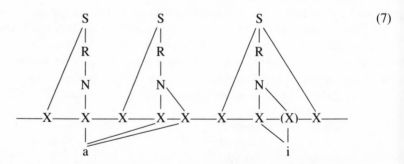

(7)

The question that is posed by the template is clearly that of the way the consonants of the base noun are to be inserted. Since we have already established the need for three half-planes – one to represent syllable structure, another to represent the tones, and a third to represent the phonemes – our first move would be to represent the consonants on the same plane as the vowels. It can, however, be readily seen that this would make it impossible for us to link the consonants to the appropriate timing slots without crossing the lines linking the vowels to their timing slots. The crossing of linking lines, however, must be prohibited if one wishes to preserve the logical coherence of the representation (Sagey 1986). In light of these considerations, it has been proposed that the consonants – that is, the phonemes of the base noun – should be represented on a separate plane intersecting the line of timing slots. Moreover, it was proposed by McCarthy that in all cases the phonemes of the base noun are linked to the slots of the template by the general convention (8).

> Link unlinked phonemes to empty timing slots from left to (8)
> right and one for one subject to the constraint that the linking
> results always in well-formed syllables.

In the case of the broken plurals, this means that only the consonant phonemes of the base noun can be linked, since, as already noted, all timing slots that may be occupied by vowels are prelinked in the template (7). We illustrate this procedure in (9) with the derivation of the plural for the noun meaning "quince." Underlining indicates that a timing slot is prelinked in (9).

$$s \quad a \quad f \quad a \quad\quad r \quad\quad j \quad a \quad l \qquad\qquad (9)$$
$$| \quad\quad | \quad\quad\quad\quad | \quad\quad |$$
$$X \quad \underline{X} \quad X \quad \underline{X} \quad \underline{X} \quad X \quad \underline{X} \quad X$$

What is especially significant here is the case in which phonemes cannot be linked, either because their linking would create an ill-formed syllable or, as in the case of all vowels and the last consonant of the stem, because there are no more empty timing slots to which they might link, they do not appear in the phonetic realization of the form. Put differently, the vowels of the base noun cannot be linked because all timing slots that admit vowels are prelinked in the template (7), whereas the last consonant of the base noun cannot be linked because all timing slots where consonants are admissible have already been preempted, and these phonemes are omitted in the output because only phonemes that are linked to timing slots can be pronounced.

There is good corroborative evidence for the "psychological reality" of this three-dimensional phonological representation. Perhaps the most convincing evidence known to me is the ability of children to learn various "secret" languages that consist of the insertion of extraphonetic material into the original word. For example, consider a secret language in which the word "Latin" is recoded as "lapatipin." Given the formalism developed here, the recoded word appears as in (10).

$$
\begin{array}{ccccc}
l & a & t & i & n \\
| & \diagup\diagdown & | & \diagup\diagdown & | \\
-\text{X}-\text{X}-\text{X}-\text{X}-\text{X}-\text{X}-\text{X}-\text{X}-\text{X}- \\
| \qquad\qquad | \\
p \qquad\qquad p
\end{array}
\tag{10}
$$

Formally, this type of language requires the following rule: In every syllable, insert before the rime a copy of the rime vowel followed by the consonant /p/. Much more complicated secret languages have been studied by McCarthy (1982b) and Yip (1982). It is quite difficult to imagine an alternative account of this type of language deformation without making use of essential aspects of the three-dimensional representations that have been described here. The fact that naive speakers can readily master the distortions exemplified here suggests rather strongly that they have access to representations of this type or their equivalent.

The immanent structure of phonemes

A common phonological process is "feature assimilation," a process whereby a given value of a feature is spread from one phoneme to one or more adjacent phonemes. For example, the rule of implementing the *s*-suffix of the English plural discussed in the section "The role of linguistic knowledge in phonetics" must include a subpart specifying that if the stem ends with a [−voiced] sound, and the suffix is actualized as ([−voiced]) [s], whereas in all other contexts the morpheme appears as ([+voiced]) [z], for we pronounce [s] in "books," "boots," "loops," "coughs," and "sixths," but [z] in "roads," "groves," "cans," "ways," and so on. It has therefore been assumed that the basic plural suffix is the voiced /z/. After a voiceless obstruent this suffix becomes the voiceless /s/. In the three-dimensional notation developed in the preceding section, this fact can be formalized by spreading the feature [−voiced] from the stem segment to that of the suffix while simultaneously delinking its [+voiced] feature. We illustrate this in (11).

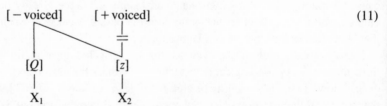

$$\tag{11}$$

where Q and z stand for the feature complexes, excluding voicing, associated with the last stem consonant and the suffix, respectively; X_1 and X_2 for the two timing slots; the dotted arrow for the spreading of the feature [voiced] from X_1 to X_2; and the = sign for the delinking of [+voiced] from X_2.

Many languages distinguish short and long vowels and/or short and long consonants. (The latter are frequently referred to as "geminate" consonants.) In the three-dimensional notation previously developed, such "long" phonemes are naturally represented by linking two consecutive timing slots to every feature in a given feature complex, as illustrated in (12).

(12)

This type of notation implies, on the one hand, that adjacent timing slots may share any number of features in common, and, on the other hand, that the complexity of shared features increases in direct proportion to their number. When actual assimilation processes are examined, it is readily seen that both implications are incorrect. The markedness of sequences with shared features that are the result of assimilation processes is quite unrelated to their number. There do not seem to be severe restrictions on the sharing of a single feature or of *all* features in a complex. By contrast, the sharing of feature subsets composed of two or more features, yet less than the entire complex, is subject to extremely heavy constraints; a few such multiple assimilations appear to be quite common, but the large majority are never encountered. For example, the sharing of the two features [anterior] and [distributed] is not uncommon, whereas the simultaneous assimilation of the feature pair [nasal] and [round] is unattested to.

These restrictions have been the subject of a number of recent studies (Mascaro, 1983; Mohanan, 1983; Clements, 1985; Sagey, 1986). The chief result of these investigations has been to attribute internal structure to the feature complexes. Specifically, features subsets that are readily assimilated are grouped together into hierarchically superordinate classes; some of the classes, in turn, are grouped together in still higher hyperclasses, which, as proposed by Mohanan, are grouped under a single ROOT node. In (13) I have illustrated this hierarchization of the feature complex, modifying somewhat the proposal made in Sagey (1986).[1]

In (13) the set of terminal features represented in the column on the left is organized into a hierarchy of superordinate classes represented by the labeled nodes in the tree shown to the right of the terminal features. If, following Mohanan (1983), assimilation processes are restricted to single nodes in the tree structure (13) (including those of the terminal features), almost all of the attested and none of the unattested, assimilatory processes are accounted for. In other words, given Mohanan's restriction, we expect single features to be assimilated. We also expect sharing of each of the feature subsets dominated by the different

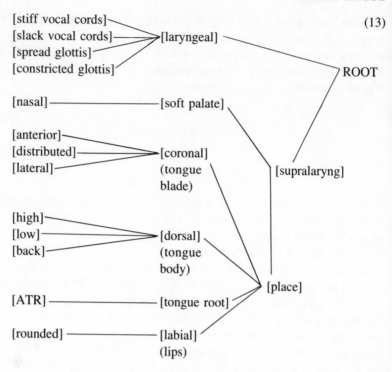

(13)

class nodes. Thus, our model leads us to expect assimilation of the four terminal features dominated by the class node [laryngeal] or of the nine terminal features dominated by the class node [place], but not to expect the simultaneous assimilation of [nasal] and [round], since these two features are not dominated by a single class node.

We illustrate this situation with an example discussed by Clements (1985). In the American Indian language Klamath, the phonological alternations shown in (14) have been found.

$$nl{\rightarrow}ll \quad nL{\rightarrow}lh \quad nl'{\rightarrow}l?$$
$$lL{\rightarrow}lh \quad ll'{\rightarrow}l?$$

where $L = [l]$ with $[+ \text{spread glottis}]$
$l' = [l]$ with $[+ \text{constricted glottis}]$

(14)

These alternations are the result of two rules. The first rule turns a nasal into a lateral before a following lateral;[2] it spreads to the former all but the laryngeal features of the latter. The subsequent rule removes from the second consonant in the sequence all but its laryngeal features. In (15) I present the first of these two processes in the tree hierarchy notation previously developed.

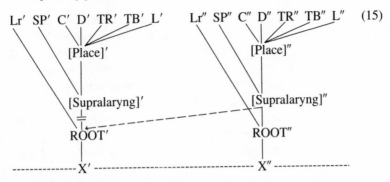

In (15) each timing slot X is linked to a feature complex, as before. The complex, however, is no longer without internal structure, but rather is organized in the manner shown in (13) and (15). Formally, each feature tree is represented in a plane that is orthogonal to the line of timing slots. Because of limitations on my capabilities for graphic representation, I have omitted all terminal features that are dominated by the class nodes at the top of (15); the reader can, I hope, imagine the additional branching lines extending above the topmost nodes.

As noted by Clements, the proposed modifications affect rather markedly the form of phonological representations. Whereas up to this point phonological representations could be envisaged as consisting of a number of half-planes intersecting in a single line on which the timing slots are represented, in representations such as (15) the half-plane on which features were represented is split into a family of half-planes intersecting in lines running parallel to the central line of timing slots. Specifically, in (15) at the ROOT node, the half-plane containing the timing slots and the ROOT nodes is split into two half-planes, one containing the consecutive [Laryngeal] nodes and the other the consecutive [Supralaryngeal] nodes. A further split into two half-planes occurs at the [Supralaryngeal] node and at every other nonterminal node. Because of the already mentioned limitations on my graphic capabilities, these further half-planes are not illustrated graphically.

The Klamath process that we have characterized in (15) is one in which the first phoneme in the sequence assimilates from the second all but the terminal features dominated by the class node Lr″ ([Laryngeal]″). We implement this by connecting the node ROOT′ to the [Supralaryng]″ node while simultaneously disconnecting the ROOT′ node from the [Supralaryng]′ node. The result is two timing slots that agree in their supralaryngeal features but differ in their laryngeal features. The second rule previously mentioned applies to the representation in (15) and cuts the link between ROOT″ and [Supralaryngeal]″, so that at the end ROOT′ is linked to the terminal features dominated by Lr′ and [Supralaryng]″, whereas ROOT″ is linked to Lr′ but not to any supralaryngeal features.

One consequence of the Klamath rules thus is to generate a timing slot (phoneme) specified for the laryngeal features but unspecified for any of the other features. At first, it might seem that such defective timing slots should be ruled out by a condition governing the well-formedness of phonological representation. When we examine the sounds that are represented by these "defective" timing slots, we discover that a good case can be made for their defectiveness. The sounds represented by the defective timing slots are the glides [h] and [?]. These sounds are produced by particular configurations in the larynx: The [h] requires that the vocal cords be spread, whereas to produce a glottal stop ([?]) the vocal cords must be constricted. The only other requirement for the production of these sounds is that there should be no constrictions in the vocal tract narrow enough to impede the flow of the expiratory air stream. If we can assume that such an unconstricted state is characteristic of the vocal tract in its "neutral" position and that, in the absence of specific instructions to the contrary, the vocal tract automatically goes into this neutral position, then glides like [h] and [?] are correctly characterized by specifying laryngeal features only and omitting specifications for all other features. As remarked by Clements, the possibility of omitting specifications of classes of features – of the sort just illustrated – is one of the arguments in favor of the hierarchical tree structure previously sketched: The structure permits us to express in a simple manner specific properties of speech sounds that could not be expressed except by ad hoc stipulations in earlier frameworks.

The hierarchical tree structure in (13) was proposed in order to facilitate the statement of phonological rules of various kinds. It should, therefore, come as a gratifying surprise that the hierarchical tree in (13) has a direct interpretation in terms of vocal tract anatomy, a fact that was also observed by Clements. In other words, the organization that we were led to impose on the basis of purely grammatical considerations turned out to be one that is directly interpretable in terms of the functional anatomy of the vocal tract.

It is obvious that the six class nodes immediately dominating the terminal features in (13) represent each of the six articulators that control the shape of the vocal tract: the larynx, the soft palate, the tongue blade, the tongue body, the tongue root, and the lips. Phoneticians have always been aware of the obvious fact that speech is the result of changes in the shape of the vocal tract and that the only way in which vocal tract shape can be changed is by changing the positioning of its movable parts, that is, of articulators such as the larynx, the soft palate, the lips, and the tongue. In spite of this, articulators play only a secondary role in all major phonetic frameworks such as that of the International Phonetic Association or that of Jakobson et al. (1952). It is one of the obvious advantages of the framework in (13) that it explicitly recognizes this fundamental aspect of the speech production process. It should also be remarked that this recognition was not imposed a priori on the framework, but emerged as a consequence of the attempt to group features in a manner that was optimal for purposes of characterizing certain abstract phonological processes. Thus, we have two independent lines of evidence – one stemming from a study of the rules of phonology and the other from a study of the process of speaking – converging on a single result: the need for explicit recognition of the role of the articulators.

An obvious articulatory difference between features that has not been taken explicit account of in previous frameworks is that between features such as [nasal], [high], [round], or [stiff vocal cords], which can be executed only by a particular articulator, and features like [continuant] or [consonantal], which may be implemented by a number of different articulators. The framework in (13) includes features of the former kind, but none of the latter. Clearly, it is necessary to indicate how features such as [continuant] and [consonantal] are dealt with in the theoretical framework under discussion. I follow here the treatment proposed in Sagey (1986).

Sagey shows that it is not possible to represent the feature [continuant] on the Place node because in many languages place of articulation is assimilated without simultaneous assimilation of the feature [continuant]. For example, in Sanskrit words, the final /s/ optionally assimilates in place of articulation to the following obstruent but retains its [+ continuant] character regardless of whether the following obstruent is [+ cont] or [− cont]. For similar reasons, it is impossible to represent the feature [continuant] on any of the nodes hierarchically subordinate to Place. Sagey concludes, therefore, that [continuant] must be represented in (13) on a node that is superordinate to Place, and we follow Sagey in representing the feature on the ROOT node, the topmost node in the hierarchy.

The feature [continuant] is universally restricted to [+ consonantal] phonemes. In many, perhaps even most, languages the [continuant] feature that controls the degree of closure in the vocal tract is implemented by a single articulator. Thus, in English we have labial, coronal, and dorsal (= velar) consonants, that is, consonants where the [continuant] feature is executed by the lips, tongue blade, tongue body, or tongue root, respectively. The problem, therefore, is how to link the [continuant] feature represented on the ROOT node to the articulator that actually executes the feature. Sagey's proposal is to supplement the notation by introducing a special pointer that indicates the articulator in question. We illustrate this in (16).

It was noted previously that each of the seven class nodes dominating the different groups of terminal features in (13) represents a specific articulator. There is (as yet) no direct anatomical interpretation for the three remaining nodes in (13), that is, for the nodes labeled "Place," "Supralaryng," and "ROOT." These may be thought of as higher-level controls in the neurological organization of the vocal tract. Implicit in (13), then, is the empirical hypothesis that in the

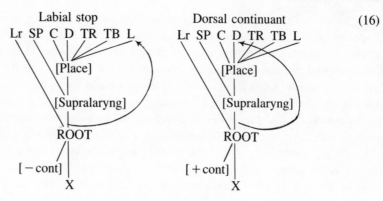

production of speech the tongue and lips together are controlled by a single center, the one labeled "Place." Analogous hypotheses are implied by the nodes Supralaryng and ROOT. It hardly needs saying that at present these hypotheses are nothing but speculations, but they indicate directions for potentially fruitful neuroanatomical explorations.

Pursuing this line of reasoning further, one may regard (13) as a circuit diagram in which the different class nodes represent binary switches. One can then imagine that the intention to articulate a particular sound results in a specific configuration of on and off positions of the switches in the circuit. An immediate consequence of this way of looking at (13) is that whenever a class node is in an off position, no current can flow past it to any of the nodes below it in the circuit, so that the state of the switches lower in the hierarchy becomes irrelevant. The situation is equivalent to that resulting from delinking a class node from the nodes it dominates.

When an articulator node switch is thrown into the off position, we assume that no instructions are transmitted to the articulator. In this case, the articulator will persist in the position to which it was instructed to proceed during the preceding timing slot, or it may continue to move in the direction of that position, subject to the effects of gravity and other external forces that might be acting on the articulator, or, as suggested previously, the articulator may move to its neutral position. In any event, the behavior of an articulator under these circumstances is determined by physiological or physical factors that are independent of the speaker's linguistic intentions.

There are further implications of looking at (13) as a switching circuit. Perhaps the most striking of these implications emerge when we examine from this point of view the production of the two major classes of speech sounds: the consonants and the vowels.

Vowels in all languages are executed with the tongue body; that is, they always involve the dorsal articulator. The lips usually also participate in the production of the vowels, although there are languages (the examples usually cited since Trubetzkoy, 1939, are from the Caucasian languages: Adyge, Kabardian, Abaza), in which the lips play no role in differentiating vowels. The participation of the tongue blade in the production of vowels is quite rare; the "retroflex" vowels of certain Dravidian languages and of English seem to be the major attested examples of vowel sounds that are coronal. Vowel production may or may not involve active participation of the soft palate. A minority of languages have nasal vowels; all languages have nonnasal vowel. Moreover, there are languages (e.g., certain African languages) in which the various laryngeal features are fully exploited in the production of vowels, as discussed in Halle and Stevens (1971).

In the production of consonants, there is a marked difference between the set of features executed by the larynx and the soft palate, on the one hand, and those executed by the tongue blade, tongue body, and lips, on the other hand, that is, by the articulators dominated by the class node Place. As noted previously, in many languages, when a consonant is produced, only one of these Place articulators is active in the production of consonants. Thus, in English, when a labial consonant is produced, only the lips are actively involved and no role is played by the tongue body and blade. And the same – *mutatis mutandis* – goes for consonants produced with the tongue body, like [*k, g,* ŋ], and those produced with the tongue blade. This complementarity does not extend to nasalization or to features executed by the larynx: Consonants are or are not nasal, regardless of which role the three place articulators play in their production, and the same is true for voicing and aspiration. In (16), this fact was expressed by means of a pointer connecting the ROOT node with a particular articulator.

I should note here that the situation with English consonants is not universal. There are many languages (e.g., Russian) in which consonants involve the simultaneous participation of two articulators, and in Kinyarwanda (Sagey, 1984) there are consonants produced with simultaneous activation of three Place articulators. Formally, such sounds are represented in the fashion illustrated in (16), except that instead of a single pointer there are multiple pointers from the ROOT node to the different articulators involved.

When a particular articulator is linked to the ROOT node by the pointer, the articulator executes the feature(s) specified at the ROOT. The articulator may or may not also execute some of the terminal features it dominates. For example, in English, none of the terminal features is specified for labial or dorsal (= velar) consonants, but for coronal consonants the terminal features [anterior], [distributed], and [lateral] must be specified.

By distinguishing phonemes in which a place articulator has specified terminal features from those in which it does not, we can account for the well-known fact that in vowel harmony languages the consonants, for which the terminal features are not specified, are transparent to the propagation of such terminal features as

[back], [round], and [advanced tongue root]. It has been observed that in harmony processes (Kiparsky, 1985) the harmonic feature cannot be propagated across a phoneme for which the feature in question has been specified. Since consonants do not normally block backness harmony and roundness harmony in languages like Finnish or Turkish, it must be assumed that these features are not specified for consonants. Support for this analysis comes from the treatment in Turkish of the special palatal stops for which the feature of backness must be specified: Such stops block the propagation of backness harmony (Clements & Sezer, 1982).

The terminal features tell us what configuration a given articulator is to assume during the production of a particular sound. Articulators differ in terms of the variety of configurations they are capable of assuming. The soft palate is capable only of being lowered or raised. By contrast, the tongue body and the larynx have a varied repertory of configurations. This difference, of course, is explained primarily on anatomical grounds: The muscles controlling the tongue allow a great variety of configurations, whereas those of the soft palate do not. In our formalism, these differences are reflected in the number of terminal features dominated by a particular articulator.

It is, of course, obvious that articulators come to occupy one position or another only as a consequence of some muscular action. In Halle (1983) I have made concrete suggestions about how particular feature specifications are translated into activities of particular muscles, and I have tried to show that what little electromyographic evidence there is does not radically contradict the proposed account. The theoretical framework that I have sketched in this section is considerably richer than that underlying the attempt in Halle (1983). It provides, therefore, many new openings for further investigations into the questions raised there.

Notes

1. In line with results of Halle and Stevens (1971), the feature [voiced] utilized in the preceding discussion, is replaced in (13) with the feature pair [stiff vocal cords] and [slack vocal cords].
2. A lateral is an *l*-type sound.

References

Archangeli, D. (1984). Underspecification in Yawelmani phonology and morphology. Ph.D. dissertation, MIT.

Clements, G. N. (1985). The geometry of phonological features. In C. Ewan & T. Anderson (Eds.), *Phonology Yearbook*, Vol. 2 (pp. 223–52). Cambridge University Press.

Clements, G. N., & Sezer, E. (1982). Vowel and consonant disharmony in Turkish. In H. Van der Hulst & N. Smith (Eds.), *The Structure of Phonological Representations* (Part II, pp. 213–55). Dordrecht: Foris Publications.

Goldsmith, J. (1979). *Autosegmental Phonology*. New York: Garland Press.

Halle, M. (1978). Knowledge unlearned and untaught: What speakers know about the sounds of their language. In M. Halle, J. Bresnan, & G. A. Miller (Eds.), *Linguistic Theory and Psychological Reality* (pp. 294–303). Cambridge, Mass.: MIT Press.

Halle, M. (1983). On distinctive features and their articulatory implementation. *Natural Language and Linguistic Theory, 1,* 91–105.

Halle, M. (1985). Speculations about the representation of words in memory. In V. Fromkin (Ed.), *Phonetic Linguistics* (pp. 101–14). Orlando, Fla.: Academic Press.

Halle, M., & Stevens, K. N. (1971). A note on laryngeal features. *MIT RLE Quarterly Progress Report,* No. 101, 198–213.

Jakobson, R. (1938). Observations sur le classement phonologique des consonnes. Reprinted in *Selected Writings,* Vol. I (pp. 273–9). The Hague: Mouton.

Jakobson, R., Fant, G., & Halle, M. (1952). *Preliminaries to Speech Analysis.* Technical Report #13. Cambridge, Mass.: MIT Acoustics Laboratory.

Kahn, D. (1976). Syllable-based generalizations in English phonology. Ph.D. dissertation, MIT.

Kiparsky. P. (1985). Some consequences of lexical phonology. In C. Ewan & J. Anderson (Eds.), *Phonology Yearbook,* Vol. 2 (pp. 85–138). Cambridge: Cambridge University Press.

Levin, J. (1985). A metrical theory of syllabicity. Ph.D. dissertation, MIT.

Liberman, M. (1975). The intonational system of English. Ph.D. dissertation, MIT.

Mascaro, J. (1983). Phonological levels and assimilatory processes. Unpublished paper, Autonomous University, Barcelona.

McCarthy, J. (1979). Formal problems in Semitic phonology and morphology. Ph.D. dissertation, MIT.

McCarthy, J. (1982a). A prosodic account of Arabic broken plurals. In I. R. Dihoff (Ed.), *Current Approaches to African Linguistics.* Dordrecht: Foris Publications.

McCarthy, J. (1982b). Prosodic templates, morphemic templates, and morphemic tiers. In H. Van der Hulst & N. Smith (Eds.), *The Structure of Phonological Representations* (Part I, pp. 191–223). Dordrecht: Foris Publications.

Mohanan, K. P. (1983). The structure of the melody. Unpublished paper, University of Singapore.

Pierrehumbert, J. (1980). The phonology and phonetics of English intonation. Ph.D. dissertation, MIT.

Sagey, E. Walli. (1984). On the representation of complex segments and their formation in Kinyarwanda. Unpublished paper, MIT.

Sagey, E. (1986). The representation of features and relations in nonlinear phonology. Ph.D. dissertation, MIT.

SPE = Chomsky, N., & Halle, M. (1968). *The Sound Pattern of English.* New York: Harper & Row.

Steriade, D. (1982). Greek prosodies and the nature of syllabification. Ph.D. dissertation, MIT.

Steriade, D. (1986). A note on coronal. Unpublished paper, MIT.

Trubetzkoy, N. (1939). *Grundzuege der Phonologie.* Second edition (1958). Goettingen: Vandenhoeck and Ruprecht.

Van der Hulst, H., & Smith, N. (1982). *The Structure of Phonological Representations.* Dordrecht: Foris Publications.

Yip, M. (1982). Reduplication and CV skeleta in Chinese secret languages. *Linguistic Inquiry, 13,* 637–61.

PART IV   Studying the lexicon

Much of the early work on psycholinguistics at the Center for Cognitive Studies focused on the psychological reality of grammar. The influence of Chomsky was strong and broad, and his interest in syntax permeated the thinking of many of the psycholinguists at Harvard. Somehow, in the enthusiasm over the experimental results on the psychological reality of grammar, the semantics of language was neglected. George, however, has never been one to travel a well-worn road and he soon changed course, turning from an interest in syntax to an interest in the mental lexicon. This new interest has occupied him up to the present. By now, George had left Harvard for The Rockefeller University. Philip Johnson-Laird outlines their joint work on the lexicon that began at the Institute for Advanced Study in Princeton, New Jersey, and found an *outlet at* Rockefeller in a monumental book, *Language and Perception*. Keith Stenning, a student of George's at Rockefeller, traces the changing concerns of semanticians in the last fifteen years. Susan Carey first met George at the Center for Cognitive Studies as a graduate student, and when George was at Rockefeller, she participated in his exploration of the development of the child's lexicon. Her chapter chronicles this joint work and the work that has grown out of it.

13   On opening the dictionary

Philip Johnson-Laird

Introduction

In the late 1960s, I was teaching psychology to undergraduates in their final year at University College, London. After three years of diverse courses, there was a danger that they would lose sight of the subject as a whole, and so each lecturer ran a seminar designed to help them pull their ideas together. One of the students in my seminar had to go into hospital to have a baby shortly before the final examinations. I suggested that she should read *Plans and the Structure of Behavior*; it would provide an excellent framework in which to integrate her thoughts about psychology. Soon after the baby was born, I went to visit her in the hospital. Mother and child were doing well, but nevertheless I was anxious; she was the brightest student in the seminar, and the recent event might have deflected her from revision. (Such is the egoism of teachers.) I need not have worried. She was sitting up in bed, notes and books all over the counterpane, the baby fast asleep in the crib next to her, and she was plainly working very hard. What had she thought of *Plans*? Well, she explained, it had all seemed rather obvious.

At first, I was amazed and annoyed; here was this highly intelligent young woman telling me that one of the classics of cognitive psychology was superfluous. I could hardly express my feelings in the circumstances, and so I carried them away with me. My student duly graduated with a first class degree; I was still bothered by her error of judgment. Only then did I realize what should have been clear from the start. The book had been published nearly a decade earlier, and its ethos had so thoroughly perfused the intellectual ambience that students absorbed it at second or third hand without realizing it. I myself was one of those second hands. No wonder my student had found it so obvious; she had heard it all before.

Plans was a striking example of a prescience typical of George Miller's career. My concern in this brief memoir is with another instance – the psychological analysis of the meaning of words – but in this case the world has not yet quite caught up with Miller. He opened up the mental dictionary; later we wrote a

186

book together about it, which he sometimes jokingly referred to as "Son of *Plans.*" I am going to recount something of the genesis of its ideas.

Verbs of motion

Your head is stuffed full with words, yet you are able to find the right word for the right job with amazing facility. When Miller first began to think about this problem, psycholinguists were preoccupied with comprehension. It yields problems enough, but the issue of how you retrieve the right meaning for a word that someone uses in speaking to you seemed at least to be tractable; you identify the word and then mobilize the psychological equivalent of "selectional restrictions" (Katz & Fodor, 1963). When you want to *describe* something, however, you must find words that correspond to the percept, image, or idea, that you have in mind, and it was not obvious how you even start to search for them. Miller made one crucial but surely correct assumption; you normally encode your experiences, not in words but in something more remote from them – a conceptual representation of some sort. Hence, the symbols of language must be stored in memory in a form that is easily retrievable in order to describe these conceptual representations. His first investigations of this problem included a major study of the semantics of motion verbs (Miller, 1972).

Miller chose verbs because predication is so important a function of language and because anthropologists had established a foothold on nouns with their componential analyses of kinship terms. To restrict the study to a manageable size, he chose only those verbs that have a meaning implying movement from one place to another. His aim was to find the semantic components underlying their meanings, and to understand how they fitted together, in order to sketch the broad outlines of the semantic domain.

Few people can read the list of over 200 verbs that Miller selected without being daunted by the task of spelling out their semantic organization. No one at that time had attempted such an analysis; most extant semantic theories either finessed the problem of lexical meaning (see, e.g., Thomason's introduction to Montague, 1974) or got by on a handful of examples (see, e.g., Quillian, 1968; Katz, 1972), though one honorable exception was Bierwisch's (1967) analysis of spatial adjectives. Miller's strategy was, first, to assume that there is a generic concept of motion and, second, to pursue an analysis of the verbs by paraphrasing them in terms of it and other concepts. The generic concept corresponds reasonably closely to the sense of *travels* in *The ball travels across the room. Travels,* in turn, can be paraphrased as *changes location.* One verb is thus paraphrased in terms of others, which correspond to more primitive concepts. Miller referred to the procedure as the method of "incomplete definitions." It calls for sensitivity and skill in the use of language, but those familiar with his writings know that he lacks for neither (as befits a man who had originally set out to make a career as a novelist). But the method is sometimes misunderstood, and it is vital to get straight the nature of the intended exercise.

Miller's aim was to discover the concepts underlying the mental dictionary. He proposed to analyze a set of semantically similar verbs and to reveal their interrelations by the entailments of incomplete definitions. For example:

> He raised his hand.

entails:

> He made his hand move up.

which in turn entails:

> He caused his hand to move up.

Since an incomplete definition is not wholly synonymous with the word it defines, it cannot necessarily be substituted for that word without doing violence to the meaning (and syntax) of the sentence. Yet it does reveal the concepts implicit in a word.

Miller had no intention of making any claims about how the underlying concepts are mentally represented or about their role in the processes of speaking and understanding. He wanted to explain what the conceptual system contains, not how it works. Indeed, the information might be represented by a semantic network, by a set of meaning postulates, by a mental dictionary with entries that decompose meanings into semantic primitives, or by some other system yet to be formulated. The concepts, however, should characterize a speaker's judgments about the meanings of the words and about the similarities and differences among them. The analysis should be more systematic and more informative than a good dictionary in revealing the *content* of the concepts that are used to cope with experience.

The results revealed a coherent organization of motion verbs based upon a number of semantic components. Among the major classes of components were the following, which I have illustrated with typical incomplete definitions:

Medium:	*He swims* is paraphrasable as *He travels through water*.
Instrumental:	*He motors* is paraphrasable as *He travels on land by vehicle*.
Direction:	*He enters the house* is paraphrasable as *He travels into the house*.
Causative:	*He moves the chair* is paraphrasable as *He causes the chair to travel*.

Miller corroborated these intuitive analyses by giving naive subjects sets of verbs, each presented in an illustrative sentence, and asking them to sort these sets into categories on the basis of their similarity in meaning. The subjects tended to sort together those verbs to which he had ascribed the same components (see also Miller, 1969, for other techniques for analyzing such data). He had used altogether some twenty formulaic definitions based on twelve primitive concepts to provide incomplete definitions of 217 motion verbs. As he himself wrote: "The result has been a structural description of how one suburb of the lexicon might be organized, but it says nothing about any mechanisms whereby such a structure could be realized or exploited" (Miller, 1972, p. 367).

Language and perception

George Miller generously invited me to spend the year 1971–2 with him at the Princeton Institute for Advanced Study. Shortly after I arrived, I read a draft of the paper on verbs of motion. The approach it took seemed to be the only way in which to map out the architecture of the concepts underlying the lexicon. The intriguing problem was the extent to which other domains could be delineated by the same methods. I pointed out one or two places where certain economies might be made – the concept of "allowing" something to happen seemed to be equivalent to "not causing it not" to happen – and Miller and I set out to write a short paper on the perceptual foundations of certain concepts.

Thus began my education in semantics, and indeed in the cognitive sciences as a whole, for Miller's genius was ultimately to take us on a grand tour through many topics and disciplines. At the time, however, I was absorbed by the challenge and the excitement of writing a paper with a colleague of extraordinary originality and erudition. We soon established a working regimen. We would discuss a current problem at length, go to our typewriters to write our separate sections, and then exchange and comment on our respective manuscripts. Of a draft of Miller's, I would make a few minor criticisms. Of a draft of mine, he would say, "It just needs to be put through my typewriter," and it would come back to me the next day like a long-lost relative who has made a fortune and been educated. I could still discern the dim outlines of the original, but it had meanwhile acquired a cogency, a style, and a panache and scholarship quite beyond its initial pretensions.

Our paper grew rapidly in length, and when it had reached some 140 pages, it dawned upon us that we had taken on a book-sized problem. As it turned out, *Language and Perception* (henceforth, *L & P*) was a very large book, and still it did not solve all of the problems that we had set ourselves. Yet, it was more than a beginning.

Our goal was to create a comprehensive psychological theory of lexical meaning – to create, in a word, a "psycholexicology." Our strategy was to try out a theory, to push it for all it was worth and, when it collapsed, to revise it. Our travails are faithfully recorded in the book. On rereading it, I was reminded of a familiar experience in climbing a mountain; when you have reached what you thought was the summit, you see yet another peak looming above you, waiting to be surmounted. (Writing the book was like that, too.) Although we warned our readers early on of our "revisionist" strategy, more than one of them failed to make it to the top and, as a consequence, misperceived the purview of the final theory.

We began with those aspects of perception likely to provide a basis for some of the concepts that enter the mental dictionary. The *idéologues* of the French revolution, inspired by Locke's empiricism, had essayed a semantic analysis of words into their primitive, allegedly perceptual, components. This analysis, they believed, would establish which ideas were *sensible* and which were not, and society could then be rebuilt on solid foundations. The logical positivists attempted a similar, though logically more sophisticated, program of research. It too failed, and so we knew from the outset that language could not be reduced to perceptible predicates (see *L&P*, p. 8). Yet, language does contain at least some concepts of this sort. An alternative approach, much favored then and now by practitioners in artificial intelligence, was to treat semantics solely as an exercise in the conceptual relations among words. This approach also fails, because it takes no account of reference. Yet, there are conceptual relations among words. A perceptually based analysis might allow us to start to bring together conceptual relations and reference.

Since people talk about what they perceive rather than how they perceive it, a major problem for us was to develop a coherent way in which to characterize the contents of the perceptual world, that is, the output of perception that is available to other psychological processes. This problem remains strangely neglected, perhaps because it does not fall squarely into the domain of perception or of any other faculty. We tackled it by reviewing what was known about perception and building up a list of representative predicates that people can ordinarily attend to and make judgments about. Some were sensory such as *red*, and others were more truly perceptual, such as *vertical*. Ideally, the visual predicates needed to be related to the output of a vision program, that is, to be mapped onto a three-dimensional representation of the visual world so that descriptions of scenes could be constructed out of them. We could not even begin to carry out this task, because there were no such vision programs. All we could do was to assume that "at some stage in the recognition process there is a component that is functionally equivalent to the application of a set of perceptual tests" (*L&P*, p. 136). What we lacked was an algorithmic theory of perception, such as the one subsequently developed by Marr (1982), and hence we could not identify the primitives of the system with certainty.

There are at least two reasons why any project to found language on a perceptual basis is bound to fail. First, there are many predicates that cannot be reduced to perceptions of any sort. We analyzed several of them in detail, including the concept of ownership. You can perceive evidence of ownership, but not the relation itself, which depends critically on the concept of permissibility. Second, there are concepts that, though they may relate to perception, go beyond it. Consider, for example, the notion of causation. Michotte (1954) demonstrated that you can have a direct phenomenal perception of causation; you can see that one object collides with another and causes it to move. Yet, this percept is not identical to the concept of cause: "The *concept* of cause seems to imply that the state of the world would have been different if the antecedent event had not occurred, but are worlds-that-might-have-been perceptual objects?" (*L&P*, p. 99). Of course not. We worked for a long time to uncover the conceptual roots of the everyday notion of causality; we never succeeded in devising any satisfactory way of testing our analysis, probably because causation appears to function like an unanalyzable primitive in daily life (as it does in many semantic theories). If our analysis is correct, however, the concept of possibility underpins causation, and possibility depends, in turn, on a presumably innate ability to envisage states of affairs that might have been.

Other concepts that go beyond perception are those of mental processes themselves, such as remembering, planning, and decision making. At this point, the vexed notion of a *procedure* entered the scene. I say "vexed" not because we found it troublesome, but because it caused, and continues to cause, problems for others. An effective procedure is a finite set of instructions for carrying out some task; the brain is presumably a device that runs many such procedures. We began to compile a list of the procedures needed by the conceptual system. The ones that particularly interested us were those of visual search, recognition, and labeling, but we were also interested in their analogs in memory when you search for something, identify it, or label it. These procedures had a twofold status for us. On the one hand, they enable the conceptual system to work, and so, by examining them, we could gain some insight into how it related to the perceptual system. On the other hand, they are themselves the objects of verbal descriptions; the lexicon contains a rich set of psychological predicates.

If perception could not establish the general relations between words and the world, we needed a conceptual theory to do the job. Our first step was to treat the comprehension of an utterance as a form of information processing. What it constructs is, in turn, some sort of procedure. But this procedure is not one that, if executed, would assess the truth value of the utterance. Such a theory is wholly unworkable; verification is only one of several conceptual operations a person might try to perform as a *consequence* of understanding a sentence, and there are other intractable problems for such a theory (*L & P*, p. 122). Moreover, the procedure that is constructed does not represent the meaning of the sentence;

rather, it is based on the meaning of the proposition expressed by its utterance in a specific context. The procedure specifies a mental process – which, depending on the circumstances, might call for a perceptual test, the retrieval of information, its storage, or a number of other operations – but the procedure might never be executed at all, as when you do not even try to answer a question.

What is the meaning of a word, such as "book," when it is uttered in the sentence "That is a book"? We could readily see what it is *not*; it is not the particular book that is designated, or a perception of the book, or the class of objects that "book" can refer to, or a disposition to assert that a certain object is a book, or the speaker's intention to designate a particular entity, or a part of environmental circumstances that causes a speaker to use the word, or a mental image of a book, or the set of verbal associations with "book," or the procedure that people learn in order to verify that some object is conventionally labeled a book. Of course, granted that comprehension yields a procedure, the interpretation of a word must contribute components to that procedure, and these components must derive from a knowledge of books. Part of that knowledge is how to identify an object as a book, but there is much more to such knowledge (*L & P*, p. 129). The *concept* of books goes beyond the merely perceptible because it concerns the functions and purposes of books – matters of human intentions and aspirations – and because it contains connotative information that relates the concept to others. Thus, we arrived at our final account of language, which was a theory based on concepts, in part innately determined, and the procedures that use them.

Armed with this theory, we opened the dictionary once more and set out to investigate a representative fragment of its contents. Our plan was to lay out the semantic organization of the mental lexicon; our assumption was that speakers shared intuitions about lexical concepts; our method was to exploit our own intuitions using incomplete definitions fortified by a few informal tests. We selected a variety of domains, which included:

> objects
> persons
> color
> kinship
> spatial relations
> temporal relations
> causality
> motion
> possession
> vision
> communication

We would take apart the meanings of the words in a domain and then move on to the next domain informed by our previous findings. When at last we had finished, we found that we had analyzed well over 2,000 words. It seemed a lot until we recollected that the average seven-year-old picks up that number of words effortlessly in about a hundred days (Templin, 1957).

Our discoveries were of two sorts. The first were those that concerned overall structure. The mental dictionary does fall, as many theorists had supposed, into "fields" of semantically related words, and what underpins each semantic field is a general core concept, such as *travel,* based on a tacit theory of the domain. Certain other important concepts crop up in every semantic field. The most notable of them are space, time, possibility, permissibility, causation, and intention. The field provides the domain of discourse, and these further concepts provide the framework of ideas in which one thinks about experience. They modulate the core concept so as to embody a variety of relations, and many of the resulting concepts have been dignified by a word of their own. The following incomplete definitions illustrate the ubiquitous role of cause in verbs of motion, possession, and vision:

> She propelled the ball: She did something that caused the ball to travel.
> She gave the ball to him: She did something that caused him to possess the ball.
> She showed the ball: She did something that caused it to be possible to see the ball.

And likewise for intention:

> She chased the ball: She intentionally traveled after the ball in order to catch it.
> She stole the ball: She intentionally took possession of the ball without permission and with no intention of returning it.
> She searched for the ball: She intentionally looked (in some places) in order to see the ball.

To avoid the looseness of such paraphrases, we developed an extensive semantic notation to capture our analyses more formally.

The second sorts of discoveries were numerous small-scale insights into the meanings of individual words – discoveries that collectively revealed something of the exquisite subtlety of the mental dictionary. I can mention only a few of these vignettes:

– There is at least one everyday notion that calls for a recursive definition: if you *own* something, you can transfer your ownership to someone else, and when you do so, you transfer the right of transfer too.

– Many verbs contain an intentional component, for example, *emigrate, buy, search.* Many verbs lack this component, for example, *move, get, see.* At least one verb, however, contains a component denying intentionality: you cannot, in the conventional sense, *lose* an object intentionally.

– It is commonly claimed that the verb *buy* expresses a converse of the verb *sell.* The claim is not strictly correct because of the locus of the intentional component. It can be true that *I am buying some chocolate from a vending machine,* but false that *The vending machine is selling me some chocolate.*

General knowledge directly enters the meanings of words at several points. One example arose in our analysis of the spatial preposition *at*, which cost us much effort. We had started with the common assumption that its meaning could be specified in geometric terms. In fact, it hinges on the notion of a region of interaction: one says *x is at y* only if x is in the region within which x's (whatever they may be) normally interact with y's (whatever they may be) in their normal way (whatever that might be). Hence, *John is at the typewriter* is an unsuitable description if he is facing away from it.

There are many, many more of these vignettes. On a number of occasions since the publication of the book, both Miller and I have had the unfortunate experience of listening to a speaker labor to make a point already refuted by one of them.

Conclusions

I have so far tried to refrain from the Whiggish impulse to judge old ideas in the light of new knowledge. Here, finally, it is appropriate to make such judgments; if not, the temptation is, at any rate, irresistible.

If a theory is concerned only with comprehension, it may postulate that there is no special set of semantic primitives and that a grasp of the implications of utterances depends solely on, say, meaning postulates in which all words enter as equals (Kintsch, 1974; Fodor, Fodor, & Garrett, 1975). This idea seems less plausible if the theory is to explain how people describe states of affairs; many different representations of the world can be described with the same word, and many different words can be used to describe the same representation. The theory is bound to specify how these mappings are established, and, granted that they are many-to-many, they must be mediated by components at a lower level than individual words or scenes. A system of conceptual primitives of the sort that we specified might enable speakers to find the right word with the maximum speed and the minimum fuss. The problem, however, is that there is little evidence in favor of a process of decomposition into such primitives. It was this consideration that lay behind our careful insulation of conceptual decomposition from matters of performance (*L & P,* p. 326). It may be that an alternative formulation of performance, perhaps in terms of parallel distributed processing or the "chunking" of information (cf. Miller, 1956, 1986a; Newell & Rosenbloom, 1981) can solve this problem.

The issue of decomposition raises further questions. Why is there a need for incomplete definitions? Why can one go only so far in capturing a word's underlying concepts in the vocabulary of natural language? The fact is that mental dictionaries are very different from printed dictionaries. Dictionaries on the shelf, like certain semantic theories, often contain nothing but words; they are notoriously circular. Dictionaries in the head may contain many primitive concepts for which we have no everyday words, because they do the tacit work of relating language to reality. Likewise, mental dictionaries do not consist of vast sets of independent entries. Children do not acquire their vocabularies as independent, insulated items (Miller, 1977); adults do not have to search their entire vocabulary every time they describe something. Words are related to one another, and these relations may also call for ineffable concepts. We developed a psychologically motivated set of primitives, relating our choices to what we knew about the psychology of cognition, but we had no methods with which to tap into the ineffable system.

A decade later, the central arguments of *Language and Perception* still seem correct. A psychological theory of meaning must pull together accounts of the semantic relations among words, such as one finds in psychology and artificial intelligence, and accounts of reference and truth conditions, such as one finds in formal semantics. We were led, seemingly ineluctably, to a procedural solution to this problem. Perhaps we should have developed a computational model of the procedures that we envisaged. Such an undertaking was not strictly necessary for the development of the theory, but it has proved helpful in thinking about how a word can have a mental representation that enters into many different procedures. The procedural approach, indeed, still seems the only feasible way in which to characterize the mental processes underlying the communication and representation of meaning.

Envoi

George Miller opened up the mental dictionary. Others, including myself, were privileged to look into it over his shoulder. It is not yet a closed book. But since he continues to work on it with undiminished enthusiasm (see, e.g., Miller, 1986b), it will surely yield more secrets.

References

Bierwisch, M. (1967). Some semantic universals of German adjectivals. *Foundations of Language, 3,* 1–36.

Fodor, J. D., Fodor, J. A., & Garrett, M. F. (1975). The psychological unreality of semantic representations. *Linguistic Inquiry, 4,* 515–31.

Katz, J. J. (1972). *Semantic Theory.* New York: Harper & Row.

Katz, J. J., & Fodor, J. A. (1963). The structure of a semantic theory. *Language, 39,* 170–210.

Kintsch, W. (1974). *The Representation of Meaning in Memory.* Hillsdale, N.J.: Erlbaum.

Marr, D. (1982). *Vision: A Computational Investigation in the Human Representation of Visual Information.* San Francisco: Freeman.

Michotte, A. (1954). *La perception de la causalité,* 2nd ed. Louvain: Publications Universitaires de Louvain.

Miller, G. A. (1956). The magical number seven, plus or minus two: Some limits on our capacity for processing information. *Psychological Review, 63,* 81–97.

Miller, G. A. (1969). A psychological method to investigate verbal concepts. *Journal of Mathematical Psychology, 6,* 169–91.

Miller, G. A. (1972). English verbs of motion: A case study in semantics and lexical memory. In A. W. Melton & E. Martin (Eds.), *Coding Processes in Human Memory.* Washington, D.C.: Winston.

Miller, G. A. (1977). *Spontaneous Apprentices: Children and Language.* New York: Seabury Press.

Miller, G. A. (1986a). Where in the world is the information? Computers in Everyday Life: GTE Foundation Lecture Series, Brown University. Mimeo, Department of Psychology, Princeton University.

Miller, G. A. (1986b). Dictionaries in the mind. *Language and Cognitive Processes, 1,* 171–85.

Miller, G. A., Galanter, E., & Pribram, K. (1960). *Plans and the Structure of Behavior.* New York: Holt, Rinehart, and Winston.

Miller, G. A., & Johnson-Laird, P. N. (1976). *Language and Perception.* Cambridge, Mass.: Harvard University Press.

Montague, R. (1974). *Formal Philosophy: Selected Papers.* New Haven, Conn.: Yale University Press.

Newell, A., & Rosenbloom, P. (1981). Mechanisms of skill acquisition and the law of practice. In J. R. Anderson (Ed.), *Cognitive Skills and Their Acquisition.* Hillsdale, N.J.: Erlbaum.

Quillian, M. R. (1968). Semantic memory. In M. L. Minsky (Ed.), *Semantic Information Processing.* Cambridge, Mass.: MIT Press.

Templin, M. C. (1957). *Certain Language Skills in Children: Their Development and Interrelationships.* Minneapolis: University of Minnesota Press.

14   Lexical development – the Rockefeller years

Susan Carey

In the early 1960s, George Miller and Jerome Bruner taught a course at Harvard – Social Sciences 8, one of the core offerings in social science. Social Sciences 8 started with the empiricist–rationalist debate, with readings from Locke, Hume, and Kant, moved on to Durkheim and Freud, then to Piaget and Chomsky. As a biology major, I took the course to satisfy my social sciences requirement; the next semester, I switched to psychology as a major and began working as a research assistant in the Center for Cognitive Studies. My personal course of intellectual development was set in motion by George and Jerry.

At the time, though work at the Center was defining the new field of cognitive psychology, it enjoyed too little respect *within* the psychology department at Harvard, still dominated by S. S. Stevens and B. F. Skinner. A conversation I had with Stevens several years later, after George had left for Princeton, brought home how difficult this must have been. Smitty was pressing me about what cognitive psychology was, and in particular, what had happened to George, who after all had the demonstrated capability to do really important work in psychophysics. Smitty said that as far as he could see, all George was interested in was *words* (sneering tone of voice). This interest had captured Jeremy Anglin, who also had some flair for psychophysics, and was also capturing me, and it was even remotely possible that I could do some decent work in psychophysics. Of course, Smitty was goading me, trying to pick a fight that I was all too happy to engage him in, but he was also serious. There was no way that he would let on that he understood that the lexicon is a window onto the packaging of human concepts, that debates about the meanings of words have been at the core of the empiricist–rationalist debate at least back to the time of Plato, and that it was becoming clear that the lexicon was to play a larger and larger role in theories of syntax. Throughout his career, George's interest in words took him to all of those concerns, and others. But my job here is to provide a glimpse of just one small part of George's work on the lexicon, the work on lexical development.

George had already told the tale of his school of developmental psychology, opened in 1972 with himself as the sole pupil. *Spontaneous Apprentices* (Miller,

197

1977, henceforth *SA*) is an autobiographical account of the years that followed, in which he describes the reasons for studying lexical development, the projects undertaken, and the reasons he abandoned the effort. In this brief chapter, there is little I can add to George's profound and charming book-length case history of a piece of ordinary "insignificant" science. So what I will do instead is write an idiosyncratic essay on what has happened in the field since George abandoned it, and how what has happened is related to the concerns he had in the mid-1970s.

As George states in *SA*, he opened his personal school of developmental psychology because he saw the study of lexical development as one source of experimental test of the Miller and Johnson-Laird theory from *Language and Perception*. He had two rather vague ideas about how watching vocabularies grow could test the theory: First, just as Chomsky's syntactic theories provided a detailed description of the end state that poses the problem for syntactic development, so too the Miller–Johnson-Laird theory of lexical structure provided a detailed description of the end state of lexical development. Though one cannot study the development of something without characterizing that something, the problem is to derive developmental predictions from an account of the end state of development. Only with such predictions can developmental data test the theory. The second idea concerned developmental predictions. The Miller–Johnson-Laird theory is componential; the components (and their interrelations) that organize lexical domains are outlined. What was wanted was evidence for the psychological reality of the proposed components and structures. Early stages in the acquisition of any lexical domain could provide such evidence in two different ways: (1) The child's incomplete or incorrect hypotheses could reveal that hypothesis testing proceeds over the proposed base of componential primitives, and (2) lexical entries that are more complex on the Miller–Johnson-Laird analysis could be shown to be acquired later than those in proceeding over the proposed base of primitives. These are, of course, the two sources of evidence for any putative componential analysis that Eve Clark spelled out in an important paper (Clark, 1973). Miller's proposed program of research required such evidence to be forthcoming. This is not the place to review in detail the fate of research programs searching for data of these sorts (see Carey, 1982, for a complete discussion). As Miller says (*SA*, p. 117), the assumption that the components of adult competence will appear as components of child development fails. Also, using this assumption to test any particular lexical hypothesis requires an accurate account of a child's lexical entry for any given word. George's lament, "it seemed so difficult to get inside children's heads and see the world and language through their eyes" (*SA*, p. 9), points to two crucial problems. Methodologically, the problem is that many factors, such as response biases and non-linguistic strategies for coping in difficult situations, enter into a child's response to any particular instruction or query; locating a lexical entry in a pattern of responses is not easy. The difficulty is compounded by the fact that the child's conceptual system sometimes differs from the adult's, so the problems of translation between incommensurate systems may arise (Carey, 1985; Kuhn, 1982).

In describing the structure of lexical domains, Miller and Johnson-Laird showed the complexity that the learner must master. Of course, just what of the Miller–Johnson-Laird structures the child must learn is an empirical question. Of course, he or she must learn the mapping between words and concepts, but it is possible that many of the conceptual structures are themselves innate. Even so, there is an enormous learning problem. Research on infants reveals them to be sensitive to many perceptual and conceptual distinctions – indeed, just about any that have ever been probed. Thus, the potential hypothesis space for word meanings is indeed huge, and we find ourselves faced with the Quine–Goodman problem of constraining induction. Students of lexical development have increasingly turned to problems of the constraints on word learning – what considerations limit the child's earliest hypotheses?

There have been two kinds of proposals about constraints on word meanings: (1) constraints that would limit induction about the meaning of any word and (2) constraints that would limit inductions about the meanings of only some classes of words. In what follows, I discuss examples of proposals of each kind. For any putative constraint we want to know what work it could do, the evidence for it, whether it is innate (as opposed to induced in the course of earlier experience with language), and whether it is language specific (i.e., whether it is a constraint on inductions about *word meanings* per se or induction in general).

Constraints on the meaning of any word

For examples of the first kind of constraint, take two related proposals: Eve Clark's "principle of contrast" and Ellen Markman's "assumption of mutual exclusivity." In an elegant paper, Clark (1986) argues that language learners assume that every two forms contrast in meaning; this is the principle of contrast. Her argument is applied to any forms in language; here I concentrate on its application to lexical items. If learners make this assumption, several predictions about languages and about language learning follow. About language – there should be no synonyms within a given dialect, for learners will be seeking contrasts in meanings and so create different meanings for different words. Clark argues that this prediction is true and that any two words that are apparently synonyms (e.g., "cop" and "policeman") have different privileges of occurrence. Clark takes a difference in privilege of occurrence (due to register, connotation, or whatever reason) as equivalent to a difference in meaning. A second prediction is that established words have priority over words coinable by productive rules of word formation. For example, just as "*goed" is preempted by "went," so too "*longness" is preempted by "length." A third prediction is that innovative coinages will not be used in place of established words with identical meanings, but rather will fill only lexical gaps. Clark argues persuasively that both of these latter predictions are also true.

Parallel sorts of evidence suggest that the principle of contrast constrains early word learning. Young children, too, coin innovative words only to fill gaps in their lexicons (although these words may in fact express meanings for which there are words in the language that the child does not yet know). There is evidence that bilingual learners go through an early period in which they reject apparent synonyms (e.g., "casa" and "house"), doggedly keeping to one word from one of the two languages for each meaning they can express (Ervin-Tripp, 1974; Fantine, 1974; Taeschner, 1983, cited in Clark, 1986). Presumably, this period ends when the child understands that there are two languages involved, for the principle of contrast operates only within a given language. Clark also cites the process of narrowing down overextensions as additional words in a lexical domain are learned. If the child has been using "dog" to refer to all animals, when "horse" is learned the extension of "dog" is narrowed. Finally, there is also experimental evidence that the principle of contrast constrains early word learning. Many studies have shown that if a new word is used to refer to an array of items, only one of which has no known label, the child assumes that the word refers to that one (Dockrell, 1981; Hutchinson, 1986, Golinkoff et al., 1985). In a different paradigm, Markman and Wachtel (in press) showed the principle of contrast operating when novelty is not an issue. They taught new words for parts of objects or for the substances of which objects are made. The important manipulation was whether the child already knew a word for the object itself. For example, a new word might be used to refer to a part of an unfamiliar object (e.g., the mouthpiece on a snorkel) or to the substance of which it is made (e.g., synthetic rubber). Alternatively, the new word might be used to refer to a part of a familiar object (e.g., the claw of a hammer) or to the substance of which it is made (e.g., steel). In five different studies, they found that when three-year-olds already knew a word for the object itself (e.g., "hammer"), they were significantly more likely to interpret the word as referring to the part or substance than they were when they did not know a word for the object itself (e.g., "snorkel"). According to the principle of contrast, when children already have a word for a kind of object, they assume that a word applied to an object of that kind cannot refer to the object itself, and so consider different hypotheses (e.g., unnamed parts, substance).

All of these observations suggest that children honor the principle of contrast. As Clark realizes, the principle of contrast alone will not explain all of these observations. "Dog" and "animal" contrast in meaning after all, and in learning new lexical domains, if the child thought that "dog" referred to all animals, "horse" to all large animals, and "cow" just to cows, the principle of contrast would be honored. Therefore, the principle of contrast cannot account for the narrowing of the extensions of overgeneralized words as new words in the domain are learned. Similarly, in the Markman and Wachtel studies, the child might well posit subordinate or superordinate categories of the objects for which one category name is already known. Early in language acquisition children apparently honor an even stronger constraint: They make what Markman calls the "assumption of mutual exclusivity." Children not only assume that there are no synonyms in a given dialect, they make the much stronger assumption that the extensions of two words from a single domain do not overlap. This constraint is patently false about language in general (it rules out words like "dog" and "pet" or "dog" and "animal"), so if this constraint is part of the early language learning system, it must be jettisoned.

To sum up, it is clear what work the contrast assumption (and the stronger assumption of mutual exclusivity) can do. In a scene represented in terms of concepts, most of which have known labels, the contrast assumption guides the search for the meaning of a newly heard word. Evidence for a posited constraint can be of two sorts. First, in conditions in which the constraint would help learning, learning should proceed as predicted. Evidence of this kind is provided by the studies of Dockrell, Golinkoff et al., Hutchinson, and Markman and Wachtel. Second, there presumably will be conditions in which the constraint would impede learning, in which case we should have evidence that learning is difficult for the child. Evidence that children resist learning synonyms can be of the second type. Also, Markman's assimilation of the child's difficulty in learning class inclusion hierarchies to the mutual exclusivity constraint is an argument of the second type.

Let us grant, for the sake of argument, that children's inductions about word meanings are constrained by the assumptions of contrast and even of mutual exclusivity. Two questions now remain. Are these constraints language specific? And are they part of the innate language-learning mechanism, or are they induced by experience with language?

The first question is easy to answer. These constraints are language specific in that most inductive inferences we make are not constrained in this way. Note that being referred to by a certain word is a property of a given object (or kind of object). That is, being called "dog" is a property of dogs. The mutual exclusivity constraint is that being called "dog" precludes being called anything else. The contrast constraint is that the meaning of "dog" cannot be the same as the meaning of any other word. Now consider hosts of other properties of dogs – such as having a certain part (e.g., a nose) or being capable of a certain behavior (e.g., searching for a missing object). Having one of these properties does not preclude having other related properties. Nor does having one of these properties preclude the existence of other properties distributed across objects in exactly the same way. Quite the contrary; most properties of objects are richly correlated: Learning that an object has one property licenses the projection of many other properties to that object. If we learn that an unknown object has a nose, we infer (properly) that it has many other parts (e.g., lungs, a mouth, eyes, ears, blood vessels, a brain). If we learn that an object can search for something lost, we infer (properly) many other capacities that it has (perception, memory, self-initiated motion, intentional behavior, etc.). The contrast constraint and the even stronger mutual exclusivity constraint are special to inductions about the relations between meanings and linguistic forms. Induction is generally not so constrained.

Now turn to the question of whether these language-specific constraints are innate. Learnability considerations suggest that they are. It is the very beginning learner who needs the most help in acquiring the lexicon. Indeed, the mutual exclusivity constraint, not honored by the language as a whole, is an early constraint that must be given up. It is given up by age three. The evidence we have also favors the position that these constraints are innate. The novelty paradigms have been used with children under two, and the evidence from rejection of synonymy in children learning two languages also comes from children under two.

Constraints that apply to only some classes of words

So far so good. Clark and Markman have identified closely related constraints that do considerable work for the young word learner and have provided evidence that one or another of these constraints does guide early word learning. However, the assumptions of contrast (or of mutual exclusivity) barely scratch the surface of the problem of mapping words to concepts for a very familiar reason. Imagine that the child hears "that's a cup" when the speaker is indicating a brown plastic cup half-filled with coffee. Suppose further that the child knows of no word to refer to any aspect of this situation, so the principle of contrast is of no help. "Cup" could refer to brown, plastic, coffee, being half-full, the front side of the cup and the table, the handle, any undetached part of a cup, the particular cup, the particular cup at that particular moment in time, the number one, any cup, and so on for an infinitude of possibilities. The child's hypotheses must be highly constrained to converge on the correct meaning efficiently. This point loses force if it can be shown that the young infant does not find many properties of the world salient. That is, although it is true that any given object has an infinite number of properties (this very cup is not 5 feet wide, not 6 feet wide, not 7 feet wide, etc.), maybe only a small subset of these properties are salient, or even accessible, to young infants as the basis for induction. If this is the case, then specifying the innate feature space would be the first step in stating substantive constraints on word meanings. Unfortunately, studies of habituation in infants show them to be sensitive to any feature of the world we have yet probed – color, size, shape, number, prototype structure in classes of two-dimensional figures, aspects of physical causality, and so on. Therefore, when it comes to word meanings, young children do face a substantial induction problem. To specify the constraints on lexical induction, one must provide an ordering of properties that the child posits as candidates for meanings of newly heard words.

Markman and Wachtel's studies on objects, substances, and parts motivate a substantive constraint. The assumption of mutual exclusivity does not explain the tendency for the child's first hypothesis when a word is used for an unfamiliar object, with unfamiliar parts, made of an unfamiliar substance, to be that the word refers to the whole object, not the substance or a part. Markman suggests a second constraint, the "taxonomic assumption." The child's first hypothesis is that a word refers to a taxonomic category of an object; only if such a word is already known does mutual exclusivity lead the child to search for a nontaxonomic meaning of a newly heard word. Markman and Hutchinson (1984) showed that sorting under instructions to group together the items described by a word (even a novel word in a novel domain) induces taxonomic sorting, compared to neutral instructions (e.g., "put the ones that are alike together"), in which case thematic sorting dominates. The main problem with the taxonomic assumption is that it is difficult to spell out what a taxonomic relation is. Markman defines a taxonomic relation as one in which the members are grouped together on the basis of similarity, rather than on the basis of other types of relations (e.g., causal or thematic relations). But on this definition, "red things," "plastic things," and "things I like" would be taxonomic categories. Also, these studies concern taxonomic categories of physical objects – what role does the object's being a physical object play?

Soja and her colleagues (Soja, 1987; Soja, Carey, & Spelke, in preparation) have examined this latter question. Soja wanted to know whether young children's first hypothesis about a newly heard common noun is that it is a sortal term for physical objects. Thus, it is not the taxonomy assumption alone she was after, but also the role of the ontological type, "physical object." One might wonder why this hypothesis is even worth testing. After all, we already know that children's early common nouns refer to kinds of physical objects (e.g., Nelson, 1973). But do we actually know that? We know that their first common nouns ("doggie," "cracker," "book," etc.) refer to kinds of physical objects in our lexicons, but we do not know how they function in the child's lexicon. These words could refer to shapes in the child's lexicon (e.g., "doggie" means dog-shaped, "cracker" means cracker-shaped, "book" means book-shaped). Or they might be even more unnatural from the point of view of the adult lexicon. Quine (1969) suggested that early nouns might function most like mass nouns in the child's conceptual system – that is, "book" refers to a kind of book stuff, any given book being a piece of book stuff. He hypothesized that until the child learns the syntax of quantification (determiners, plurals, and quantifiers such as numbers, "some," and "another"), the child's conceptual system does not make the distinction between kinds of objects and kinds of stuff. Finally, even if children's early nouns have the same meanings for young children as they do for us, we do not know whether these meanings were the first hypotheses the child entertained. Thus, Soja set out to see whether children do distinguish between physical objects and nonsolid substances, and whether children's first hypotheses about the meanings of newly heard words are affected by this ontological distinction. Her paradigm was simple, involving two kinds of trials. In one, the child is shown an unfamiliar molded solid object made of an unfamiliar substance (e.g., a brass pyramid with rounded edges), and the experimenter says, "See what I have here; this is my blicket." The child is then shown three pieces of the same substance (e.g., brass) and another of the same kind of object, made of another substance (e.g., a plastic pyramid). The question is, "Which is the blicket?" (See Fig. 14. 1a.) Soja used subjects just turning two (mean age, 2:1). Many were still in the one-word stage; few commanded much noun phrase syntax (determiners, adjectives, quantifiers). The subjects thought that the new plastic pyramid was the blicket, not the pieces of brass. So far this does not tell us much about the question we are asking. All we know is that the child sees similarity in shape and number as relatively important to how one uses "blicket," and color and texture as relatively unimportant. We do not know that the blicket's status as a physical object plays any role whatsoever. The crucial information comes from parallel trials, depicted in Figure 14.1b. The child is shown some new nonsolid substance, such as Nivea skin lotion with Grapenuts cereal in it. It is arranged in a shape as distinctive as the shapes of the objects in the first kinds of trials. Again, the child is told, "See what I have brought you. This is my moak." Then the child is given a choice of the same substance, now arranged in three little blobs of nondescript shape, or a new substance (say, Prell shampoo) arranged in the original shape. When asked to pick the moak, subjects pick the same substance. In this case the child finds similarity in shape and number relatively unimportant, and similarity in color and texture relatively important.

What can we conclude from this study? First, contrary to Quine's conjecture, presyntactic infants do conceptualize the world in terms of solid physical objects and nonsolid substances. Further, their first hypothesis about the meaning of a word applied to a physical object is that it refers to objects of that type; their first

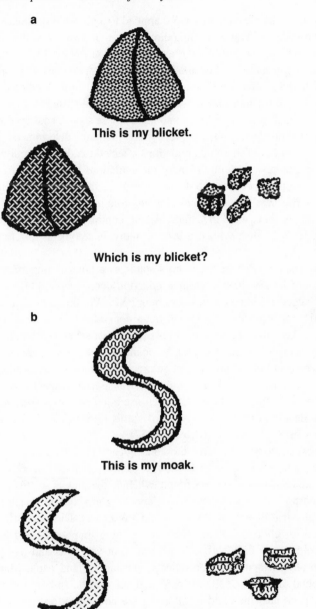

a

This is my blicket.

Which is my blicket?

b

This is my moak.

Which is my moak?

Figure 14.1 (a) and (b).

hypothesis about the meaning of a word applied to a nonsolid substance is that it refers to substances of that type. Soja did her study in two ways. For one group of subjects, the original introducing event was as in Figure 14.1 ("this is my blicket; this is my moak"). For another group, syntactic cues were added that were consistent with the word's referring to the object in the first case ("this is a blicket") and to the nonsolid substance in the second ("this is some moak"). Furthermore, she divided her subjects into those whose spontaneous speech showed that they commanded some noun phrase syntax, including determiners, and those who did not. Neither of these manipulations affected the data (the children were not at ceiling; there was room for these manipulations to make a difference, at least in the mapping between words and nonsolid substances). There is no evidence that in this case syntactic cues play any role in constraining the two-year-old's hypotheses about word meanings. Again, contrary to Quine, the child does not have to learn English syntax to learn to individuate objects differently from substances.

We do not know whether the word's status as a noun is important to these results; we know only that the child's induction does not seem affected by the noun's subcategorization as a mass or count noun. We do know that noun subcategorization as a proper or common noun does affect word learning by this age. Katz, Baker, and Macnamara (1974) found that seventeen-month-old girls (and twenty-four-month-old boys; see Macnamara, 1982) used the absence of an article (proper noun) or the presence of an article (common noun) to infer whether a newly heard noun referred to an individual or a type, respectively. We also know that by ages three and four, children use noun subcategorization as mass or count in deciding whether newly heard words refer to unfamiliar objects or unfamiliar nonsolid substances (Brown, 1957).

Soja's posited constraints have the consequence that the child should have difficulty learning words that refer to solid substances, such as "wood," "metal," "plastic," and "glass." Soja has found evidence that this is so. First, analyses of natural corpora show that these words appear relatively late, much later than words for physical objects and for nonsolid substances. Dickinson (in preparation) probed for children's comprehension of these four words and found that three-year-olds knew only "glass," whereas four-year-olds and five-year-olds knew them all. In their study on objects, substances, and parts, Markman & Wachtel found different results for parts and substances. In both cases, mutual exclusivity prevented the child from taking the new word to refer to a type of object if a label for that type of object was already known. However, when the intended referent was a substance, three-year-olds did not provide clear evidence that they took it as a substance either. When it was a part, it was clearly so interpreted even by three-year-olds.

To sum up, we have evidence for two specific constraints: Nouns (or words) applied to physical objects are sortal terms for those objects; nouns (or words) applied to nonsolid substances are sortal terms for those substances. The two questions we raised about the contrast constraint (and the mutual exclusivity constraint) now arise. Are these constraints innate, and are they special to language?

Again, the only information we have concerning the innateness of these constraints is how early we can find evidence that infants honor them. Soja's subjects were two and did not induce these constraints from knowledge of count/mass syntax. It is likely that they are innate. But what about being language specific? Unlike the case of the contrast constraint and the mutual exclusivity assumption, where a minute's reflection showed them to be language specific, there is a very real possibility that these constraints are conceptual, not specifically semantic. That is, the infant's conceptual system may carve the world up into physical objects (indeed, Spelke, 1983, has shown that this is so) and non-solid substances, and may be prepared to make all kinds of inductions about types of physical objects and types of nonsolid substances, including inductions about labeling. Conversely, just as they resist positing word meanings that are solid substances, they may be unwilling to project any properties on the basis of type of solid substance or spatial arrangement of nonsolid substances. Thus, it is an empirical question whether these constraints have a language-specific component. What this question comes down to, experimentally, is whether the projection of any newly learned property would show the same pattern as the projection of a newly learned label. Wiser (in preparation) and Soja (1987) have data on this point, showing that at least at age three, one of the constraints is language-specific. What they did was to compare patterns of inductive projection of weight with patterns of inductive projection of a new word. In each trial, the child was shown two unfamiliar objects made of two different unfamiliar substances. On some trials (weight trials), the child felt both objects and was told, "This one is heavy and this one is not." On naming trials, one of the objects was named for the child: "This one is called a 'blicket' and this one is not." Subjects were then shown two new objects with the shape and material reversed (see Fig. 14.2). In the weight trials, when asked to predict which one was heavier, three-year-olds judged different kinds of objects with the same material as the target to be the same as the target. In naming trials, when asked which one was called a "blicket," the same subjects judged objects of the same shape, but of different materials, to be the same as the target. At least by age three, substance projections over solids can be made, even when both the object types and solid substance types are all unfamiliar. In this situation, if the label of the object is at issue, the child goes with object type. But if the issue is whether the object is heavy or not, the child goes with substance.

It is clear from this discussion that many different constraints, indeed, many

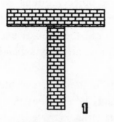
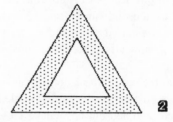

Naming Trial: This (object 1) is a blicket;
this (object 2) is not.

Weight Trial: This (object 1) is heavy;
this (object 2) is not.

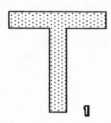
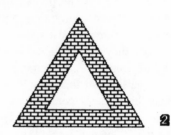

Naming Trial: Which one is the blicket?

Weight Trial: Which one is heavy?

Figure 14.2

different types of constraints, will converge to ensure the word-learning wizardry
of young children. It is also clear that the methodology of choice for characterizing the constraints is that with which George ended *SA*, namely, the experimental teaching of new words and assessment of the first hypotheses children
entertain about their meanings. George was aware of the irony of the situation;
his laboratory had figured out what to do just as it was to be closed down.
Luckily, the lesson was not lost to the field as a whole.

References

Brown, R. (1957). Linguistic determinism and the part of speech. *Journal of Abnormal and Social
    Psychology, 55,* 1–5.
Bruner, J. S., Goodnow, J. J., & Austin, G. A. (1956). *A Studying of Thinking.* New York: Wiley.

Carey, S. (1982). Semantic development, state of the art. In L. Gleitman & E. Wanner (Eds.), *Language Acquisition, State of the Art.* Cambridge, England: Cambridge University Press, pp. 347–89.

Carey, S. (1985). *Conceptual Change in Childhood.* Cambridge, Mass.: Bradford Books.

Clark, E. V. (1973). What's in a word? On the child's acquisition of semantics in his first language. In T. Moore (Ed.), *Cognitive Development and the Acquisition of Language.* New York: Academic Press.

Clark, E. V. (1986). The principle of contrast: A constraint on language acquisition. In B. MacWhinney (Ed.), *Mechanisms of Language Acquisition.* Hillsdale, N.J.: Erlbaum.

Dickinson, D. (in preparation). Children's understanding of material kinds.

Dockrell, J. E. (1981). The child's acquisition of unfamiliar words: An experimental study. Ph.D. dissertation, University of Stirling, Scotland.

Ervin-Tripp, S. (1974). Is second language learning like the first? *TESOL Quarterly, 8,* 111–27.

Fantini, A. E. (1974). *Language Acquisition of a Bilingual Child: A Sociolinguistic Perspective (to Age 5).* Brattleboro, Vt.: Experiment Press.

Golinkoff, R. M., Hirsh-Pasek, K., Lavallee, A., & Banduini, C. (1985). What's in a word?: The young child's predisposition to use lexical contrast. Paper presented at the Boston University Conference on Child Language, Boston.

Hutchinson, J. E. (1986). Children's sensitivity to the contrastive use of object category terms. Paper presented at the Stanford Child Language Research Forum, Stanford University, April 4–6.

Katz, B., Baker, G., & Macnamara, J. (1974). What's in a name? On the child's acquisition of proper and common nouns. *Child Development, 45,* 269–73.

Kuhn, T. S. (1982). Commensurability, comparability, communicability. *PSA 1982,* Vol.2.

Macnamara, J. (1982). *Names for Things,* Cambridge, Mass.: Bradford Books.

Markman, E. M., & Hutchinson, J. E. (1984). Children's sensitivity to constraints on word meaning: Taxonomic vs. thematic relations. *Cognitive Psychology, 16,* 1–27.

Markman, E. M., & Wachtel, G. (In press). Children's use of mutual exclusivity to constrain the meanings of words. *Cognitive Psychology.*

Miller, G. A. (1977). *Spontaneous apprentices.* New York: Seabury Press.

Miller, G. A., & Johnson-Laird, P. N. (1976). *Language and Perception.* Cambridge, Mass.: Harvard University Press.

Nelson, K. (1973). Structure and strategy in learning to talk. *Monographs of the Society for Research in Child Development, 38* (1–2), Serial No. 149.

Quine, W. V. (1969). *Ontological Relativity and Other Essays.* New York: Columbia University Press.

Soja, N. (1987). *Constraints on Word Meaning.* Ph.D. Dissertation, Massachusetts Institute of Technology.

Soja, N., Carey, S., & Spelke, E. S. (in preparation). Ontological constraints on word meanings.

Spelke, E. S. (1983). Cognition in infancy. *MIT Occasional Papers in Cognitive Science,* No. 23. Cambridge, Mass.: MIT Center for Cognitive Science.

Taeschner, T. (1983). *The Sun Is Feminine: A Study on Language Acquisition in Bilingual Children.* Berlin and New York: Springer.

Wiser, M. (in preparation). Objects and substances; weight and names.

15 Methodical semanticism considered as a history of progress in cognitive science

Keith Stenning

> If you are interrupted while painting a wall, when you return, the wall will provide an unmistakable reminder of how far you had gone and where you should resume.
>
> Miller (1965, p. 426)

Introduction

To begin with

Put logic, linguistics, psychology, and computer science together and you get cognitive science. The inventory is a truism in the 1980s, even if the plan is sometimes in dispute. This chapter is a remembrance of where the bits came from. Logic, linguistics, psychology, and computer science came, like so many other disciplines, from taking philosophy apart.

As any child knows, taking things apart is easier than putting them back together. I have a recurrent image: Frege and Wundt, as two little boys in shorts, kneel over the philosophical mechanism, saying: "It's not working right. It'll have to come apart; we're not going to be able to resist for long. And if it's never quite the same when it's back together – well, they didn't want it back broken, did they?"

Some current controversies about how it all goes back together bear a resemblance to some of the controversies that tore it apart a century ago – in particular, controversies about the role of semantics in the enterprise. From my own little corner, I cannot always escape the feeling that some members of the team are trying to put it back broken.

Specifically, the term "methodological solipsism" has, following Putnam's coining and Fodor's adaptations, become a popular label for an argument that is supposed to establish that psychology is the study of narrow psychological states that are characterized without reference to semantic relations. I propose "methodical semanticism" as a banner for the opposing argument that psychology

210

cannot be pursued by describing purely narrow psychological states, and that it therefore crucially consists of the study of semantic relations. Furthermore, its history is the history of this hard-won realization.

To take our disturbed painter as an example, any account of his mental processes will have to refer to his wall (and its paint and . . .). If our solipsist objects that it is only his beliefs about his wall – the representations of it that he has in his head – that can function in his mental processes, we can see that this is a mistake. For him, just as for us, those representations function in the way they do because they are interpreted as referring to his wall. Give him reason to change his interpretation and his behavior will change even though the same memory representations remain.

The study of semantic knowledge of language presents problems not presented by the study of syntactic knowledge, but that is not because of some inadequacy of current conceptions of semantics nor because semantics is ineffable. It is because the object of semantic knowledge is broader. To eschew semantics is to return to a solipsistic psychology of the 1870s or to a view of psychology that many philosophers of mind seem never to have revised.

To give an account of how psychology, linguistics, and philosophy did relate through these issues in some work of the 1970s, and how they should relate in the 1980s, it is helpful to allude to the several earlier stages of cognitive science's dismantling and reassembly process. In order to get to the 1970s, I will sketch my own view of the psychological landscape inherited from the 1950s and 1960s, which is the topic of other chapters in this volume. This sketch will review, if briefly, much earlier attitudes to semantic issues, attitudes of the 1870s. The schism between psychology and philosophy/logic that took place then is marked by imperialistic attitudes on both sides. The intent was not just mutual division but also mutual conquest. Both parties' fiendish plans foundered on semantic issues. In the 1970s, attempts to bridge this schism were made in work both on lexical and on logical semantics.

A comparison of a psychological with a philosophical work on lexical semantics – *Language and Perception* (Miller & Johnson-Laird, 1976) with *The Meaning of "Meaning"* (Putnam, 1975) – will serve to illustrate the bridge's problems. Logical semantics I will treat through my own work on text comprehension, its relation to work in linguistics and logic, and to psychological work with different conceptions of semantics.

Recent history

In "The Magical Number Seven," Miller (1956) provided, as succinctly as conceivably could be done, a demonstration that a theory of mind must postulate processes of interpretation and the construction of representations. The semantic information capacity of human short-term memory cannot be measured without recourse to the subjects' interpretation of the codes that pass through that bottleneck into mental history. To a reasonable first approximation, anything can represent anything. We must know what the seven items are interpreted as representing in order to make any estimation of what memory preserves and what it consigns to oblivion. We must study these codes and their interpretation in order to understand practically any cognitive accomplishment. Much of the intervening years have been taken up for psychologists by repeated demonstrations of the existence of such codes and, more charitably, by detailed analyses of a few cases.

"The Magical Number Seven" ends with the question "What are the codes?", which I shall call the "second question." It begins with the question "Is there a common source for the limitations of short-term memory and of absolute judgment tasks?" This, the "first question," has received less attention in the ensuing years, and indeed has been widely seen, though not, I think, by its author, as having been dismissed in the negative by the discovery that short-term memory is item, not information, limited. I now believe that the first question will have to be taken up again (more of that presently), but in 1969, when I began work as George's graduate student, my main preoccupation was with the codes rather than their representations.

The codes used to illustrate the independence of memory capacity from the information content of its contents were artificial codes, explicitly learned and consciously deployed. They were also cases of pure symbolic compression – binary numerals into hexadecimal, with no change in the semantic type of the represented. After "The Magical Number," the studies of phonological and syntactic coding showed that the natural codes described by linguists were also to be seen in operation in subjects' perceptual performances. Here there is a semantic shift. The type of the encoding is not the same as the type of the encoded – an acoustic pattern is encoded, perhaps as a phoneme, perhaps as a syntactic structure, perhaps as a meaning, or perhaps as all of these.

The classification of information processing into syntactic and semantic deserves more careful attention than it has received, and certainly more than it can receive here. In completed formal theories, the distinction is clear, easily drawn in all cases, and fundamental. Usually, there are only two relevant levels. In the sorts of chains of processes that psychologists necessarily treat, the distinctions are often opaque, difficult to apply to cases, and fundamental. There are generally several relevant levels and a syntax–semantic distinction between adjacent pairs of levels. Hearing a sentence and comprehending its meaning constitutes a paradigmatic semantic encoding. But equally, though not similarly, to hear a sentence and derive a parse tree for it is to perform a semantic encoding; a parse tree is a different type of thing than an acoustic pattern.

Certainly, there are differences to be observed. The relation between words and the objects they are about is one of denotation. The relation between an acoustic pattern and a parse tree is that between abstraction and instantiation. But both relations are to be contrasted with the relation between 1100 binary and 12 decimal.

Methodological solipsists observe that computational processes proceed by virtue of the syntactic form of the symbols with which they compute, and without recourse to their semantic interpretation. They conclude that computational processes cannot access semantic properties of the referents of the symbols they manipulate. In one sense this is trivially true, but in the important senses it is materially false. Any computational process that directs its activity by decisions based on the consistency of information *under a given semantic interpretation* accesses semantic properties of the referents of the symbols it manipulates. All the classical demonstrations of top-down processing have this characteristic. If we read

> Paris in the
> the spring

as a well-formed noun phrase, it is because our sentence perception mechanisms have decided that the evidence for one "the" will have to be ignored if the symbols are to be consistently interpreted as an English noun phrase.

Once codes became the objects of interest, the evidence for them was everywhere (e.g., Miller & Nicely, 1955; Miller & Isard, 1963). They could be seen in the relation between input and output – but could they be caught in the act? Transformational grammar, by its very form, suggested an opportunity for showing a formal mapping that could be translated into operations whose occurrence could be observed in the time course of language digestion.

For all sorts of reasons that become clear in hindsight, that most acute of all of the human senses, the answer turned out to be "no." Despite early seductive suggestions to the contrary, the mapping is not computed in the way the formalism suggested. Although many of the structures posited by transformational grammar could be observed by static techniques, the operations were not revealed in the dynamics, because those dynamics were driven by semantic phenomena that overlay and cut across them.

Transformational grammar suggested a candidate set of encoding processes that turned out to be either masked or subverted by semantic phenomena – semantic in the tables and chairs sense. Now, twenty years later, psycholinguistics has told us quite a bit about the processes involved. Some psychologists saw the early psycholinguistic work on syntax as a formalist aberration because they did not understand that in psychological terms the processes involved were semantic in the broader sense. They were processes by which subjects make judgments and encodings of things at one level on the basis of judgments or experiences of things at another level.

How does one recover from a syntactic disappointment, and where does one go in search of semantic satisfaction? People experience language primarily as a semantic phenomenon, and that is why they developed an explicit theory of it as a semantic phenomenon earlier and more fully than as a syntactic one. Ironically, logic – the theory of language as a semantic phenomenon – is the very approach that developed the tools required for syntactic description. One might suppose that logic would provide just the codes that the psychologist would jump at. But there were formidable historical barriers to such a leap. The efflorescence of logic with Frege, and of the experimental approach to the mind with Wundt, coincided with the splintering of psychology from logic and philosophy.

Both of these avenues of development adopted a solipsistic attitude to concepts, with attendant restrictive attitudes to semantic issues. Frege's logicism and his leanings toward a proof-theoretic development of logic saw semantics as something one could "catch on to" but not objectify (Van Heijenoort, 1967). Wundt, at least in his experimental psychology, sought to explain how a solipsistic subject could construct the conceptual world from sensory atoms. Both avenues of development eventually rejected these restrictions.

Although philosophers and psychologists may acknowledge these rejections within their own disciplines, they often behave as if the other discipline had remained frozen since 1870. The problems with bridging the gap in the 1970s are well illustrated by a philosopher who would appear to have psychologists adopt a solipsistic concept of "concept" for their theories of knowledge of meaning, and by some psychologists who would seem to believe that logic is a syntactic theory of inference.

Studying knowledge of meaning

"The Magical Number's" representational theory of mind focuses attention on semantic issues. Representations represent under semantic interpretation. For the first time in the history of such theories, their rear is protected from vicious regress by a bedrock of computation. Our attention is free to follow the chain of semantic ascent. We can study the influence of the adoption of particular semantic interpretations on the course of conceptual action. To approach the semantic (in the full tables and chairs sense) side of peoples' knowledge of language, there are two major alternatives. One investigates either lexical semantics or logical semantics. Both approaches to bridge building were actively pursued during the 1970s. George chose the lexical approach.

Meanings of words and knowing meanings of words

Transformational grammar had proved an inappropriate avenue of approach to full-blooded semantic issues. Perception is psychology's traditional contribution to the study of relations between the subject and the world. George realized that, construed in the right way, perceptual theories could be seen as one of psychology's contributions to semantic issues. One thing perceptual theories lacked was a formal framework in which to systematize the relations between percepts and concepts. Perhaps computational ideas could provide such a framework. Here he was back on his own ground.

As one whose acquaintance with George's work had begun by reading "The Magical Number" and the papers on applications of information-theoretic ideas to memory and language, I had not appreciated, before arriving in New York, the degree to which his intellectual roots were centered in the psychophysical and perceptual traditions. I had been an undergraduate at an old university with a new Psychology Department, and although I knew some of the history of epistemology, I had had an almost totally ahistorical brush with psychology. It was a moving discovery that before Miller there was Stevens, and before Stevens, Boring, and before Boring, Titchener, and before Titchener, Wundt. I was adamant that philosophy and psychology were to be engaged, but knew practically nothing about their history of separation. Perhaps George's motivation in writing *Language and Perception* had much to do with ameliorating the ignorance of a younger generation of scientists like myself, not by writing psychology's history but by consolidating its results. Having done more than anyone else to get psychologists to look beyond their discipline to mathematics and linguistics, I think George sometimes felt that they had begun to overlook the breadth of language and psychology. The great tradition of perception and psychophysics had always held out the hope that the results of the study of perception could lead inward to the understanding of conceptual processes and knowledge. Not just knowledge in a narrow syntactic domain, but the full panoply of experience. Never forget the first question of "The Magical Number"!

My own knowledge of the writing of *Language and Perception* is both direct and indirect. During the period when George was writing, I had frequent discussions with him about topics that appear in the book. He was, however, charitably dark about there being any book. That made it much easier for me to sort out my own ideas, not having to wonder how they sat with *Language and Perception*. After finishing a thesis and discovering the book half complete, I had to reconstrue my memories of all of those discussions in light of the discovery. One particular theme of the discussions was classification, which plays a central role in the book's theory.

Language and Perception. Language and Perception asks, what constitutes people's knowledge of the meaning of words, and how does the contribution of psychology to an answer fit in with the neighboring disciplines of philosophy and linguistics? Unlike syntactic knowledge, which might take the form of rules relating language to language, people's knowledge of meaning must relate language to the world. One way in which this happens is by perception. Words are often related to open-ended classes of exemplars, and though our knowledge of the exemplars of "table" may be less determinate than our knowledge of the exemplars of "sentence," it poses the same sort of problem of describing infinite or open-ended domains with finite means. Perceptual tests offer one mechanism for the implementation of the necessary rules.

For anyone with any philosophical memory at all, these ideas must ring bells – warning bells. They immediately sound like verificationalism, and I remember predicting, after my first reading of the manuscript of *Language and Perception*, that the charge of verificationalism would be laid against the work. I did not feel the accusation justified. The whole book is a search for a framework that gives credence to perceptual experience without falling into the verificationalist trap. But criticisms can be unjustified and inevitable, and I regret that my baleful prediction was proved correct.

Language and Perception proposed an approach to lexical meaning in which the relation between perception and conception is like the relation between biologists' keys and their taxonomies. A key provides immediately applicable tests that are sufficient for identification of an individual's taxon *in a context*. Move from Scotland to England and a new key may be necessary, even to identify the same species. This species may require different tests because it must now be distinguished from a different range of possibilities in the new environment. Even staying in Scotland, two keys may use completely disjoint sets of tests for the same species and may be equally adequate. The taxonomy is what lies behind all of the keys and acts as an adequacy constraint on them, and behind the taxonomy generally, there lies still more theory about taxonomies and organisms in general.

According to this picture of word meaning, even words for high-level taxonomic groupings and theoretical entities may have key tests associated with them. We have quite good perceptual tests that we use to decide which things are living things. We have quite a bit of intuitive theory about what those things ought to be like. There are difficult cases; viruses and sponges threaten different aspects of our expectations. But even such theoretically central concepts as "ability to reproduce" have keylike tests associated with them. They aren't good tests for a field guide because they call for too much patience in the naturalist.

Language and Perception thus works through the "Magical Number's" insight that it is the adoption of a semantic interpretation of perceptual data that determines the course of conceptual activity. A concept is not to be identified with the narrow psychological state constituted by the concept's syntactic specification for a single environment. Concepts have cross-environment identities and are open-ended in that they may receive new syntactic specifications in new environments.

So stout a volume must do with so slim an exegesis. The seriousness of *Language and Perception*'s attempt to bridge the divide between philosophy and psychology can be brought out by some comparisons with Putnam's much slimmer but more or less contemporaneous philosophical essay. The comparison is illuminating because it shows a philosopher accepting the 1870s solipsistic rendering of concepts as "narrow mental states" – accepting it despite his own arguments – and hence being forced to miscast the relation between philosophy and psychology. It is psychology's century long clamber out of this solipsistic pit that *Language and Perception* so eloquently surveys.

The Meaning of Meaning's concept of concept. Although Putnam is more sympathetic than many to the empirical study of meaning and the knowledge of meaning, this essay nevertheless left psychology with the solipsistic concepts that psychology has struggled so hard to reject, and was taken up – in ways that I feel sure its author does not sympathize with – to become a peculiar proposal for regress in cognitive science. I will try to show that one can accept the main point of Putnam's argument, revise its concept of "concept" (which Putnam himself acknowledges is outmoded), and come out with a theory of knowledge of meaning that is less divorced from philosophical questions about meaning – a theory that is familiar to readers of *Language and Perception.*

Putnam conceived of the study of meaning and knowledge of meaning as being in a conceptual mess specifically in relation to the study of syntax and knowledge of syntax. He saw the trouble as running so deep as to infect the foundations of the traditional view of the relation between meanings, concepts, extensions, and intensions. According to the traditional view, meanings, or intensions, are concepts, and concepts are in the mind. Intensions determine extensions, which are, for "tables" and "chairs," in the world. Putnam's central observation is that whatever it is that most knowers of many words know about their meaning, that something does not determine the extension of those words in the world. He cites as an example the fact that he knows the meanings of "elm" and "beech," but he can't classify things as elms or beeches. In particular, he can't tell elms from beeches. He claims that this shows that his concept of "elm" is the same as his concept of "beech," roughly "a sort of deciduous tree," and although his concepts are the same, he well knows that the meanings are different. He concludes that meaning has an indexical element and that concepts do not. Therefore meanings are not concepts. What fixes the extension of "gold" is that it is that substance there (says Putnam, pointing to a sample he is "sure of").

I am genuinely puzzled here. The essay starts by noting that "traditional philosophers of mind" employ this restrictive, "solipsistic" attitude to concepts. Having reduced this view to the appropriate rubble, Putnam does not abandon it. After this reduction, what better candidate is there for negation?

Concepts are ways of sorting things into exemplars and nonexemplars that are deployed by a person in an environment. Their full specification demands specification of much that is in the mind, but also of much that is in the world. Concepts can come with samples as an integral part. It seems that one can shed this particular restrictive program and incorporate Putnam's insights into a theory of knowledge of meaning that does not make it so hard to account for the intertwining of knowledge of semantic markers and knowledge of extension.

Let's get the philosopher back into an environment. Take Putnam's elm example. His concept of an elm is, he assures us, identical to his concept of a beech. This is surely false modesty. Evidence internal to the essay suggests that part of Putnam's concept of an elm is that elms are not beeches, and part of his concept of beeches is that they are not elms. In short, he believes that they are both *species* and that they are distinct species, and he knows that exemplars of distinct species are distinct. There's no doubt that this could show up in his classificatory abilities. I suspect that he has a reasonable but not infallible grasp of how different-looking species of deciduous trees can be, and still be the same species. Faced with a beech and an elm (an easy pair), his grasp would be sufficient to know that they are different species. Given evidence that one was a beech (perhaps from an expert's label affixed to it), I think he would assign it to the category of non-elm, whereas he might judge the other to be non-beech and maybe-elm. Even this modest discriminatory ability suffices to show that Putnam's concepts of beech and elm are not identical. Philosophers sometimes know more than they let on. I am not suggesting that Putnam's concept of elm is identical to the meaning of elm – just that his concept isn't solipsistic, and that it is rather closer to the ideal than he appears to realize.

Although our knowledge of extensions is incomplete and sometimes erroneous, the philosophical concentration on the final stages of discrimination between the smallest categories of natural taxonomies gives a misleading impression of our semantic competence. The reason we are content to acknowledge that Putnam knows the meaning of elm is that he knows it names a species of tree. Knowing this, and what he knows about species and about trees, actually allows him to make all but the finest discriminations of elms from the rest of the furniture of the universe. It also allows him to discriminate "elm" from other words such as "hardwood," "sapling," and "plank."

Psychologists are interested not only in people's knowledge of stereotyped information about extension but also in how their knowledge of what Putnam calls "semantic markers" combines with their knowledge of the world to allow them to determine extensions as far as they do, and to fail where they do.

One of the questions that arise is how the "samples" that are part of people's concepts interact with their linguistic knowledge. The answer has to do with the sortals under which the samples are brought. This is not the place to discuss it, but there is philosophical substance to the question of how this can be. It is not so easy to separate philosophical questions from psychological questions – a sign that perhaps we are beginning to put it back together. To a psychologist interested in these issues, Putnam's "traditional philosopher of mind" can seem rather like a contemporary phlogiston theorist. One source to which such a sleeping beauty should be directed is *Language and Perception*.

Meanings of texts and knowing meanings of texts

For an approach to the study of knowledge of meaning, my own inclination was, and still is, toward the logical rather than the lexical. With this shift of focus from content to form, we experience a shift of psychological focus from perception to memory.

Already in 1969, there had been a number of demonstrations that the codings we impose on text are not sentence based. I suppose Bartlett had shown the way, and it had been continued by others (Bransford & Johnson, 1972; Sachs, 1967). These demonstrations were generally hostile to the episodic approach to memory and the systematic statement of encoding schemes. These approaches concentrated on the inferencing that is necessary to establish implicit connections between sentences. But there is another prior, and neglected, problem about what happens when connections are established even when they are established explicitly. For all of the talk about construction and reconstruction, these theorists had little to say about what was constructed. I wanted to see if logic could be of any help in specifying what people did construct and reconstruct as they understood and remembered texts. Given two explicitly connected logical forms, one containing an antecedent and the other an anaphor, how were they put together?

Linguists' and psychologists' anaphors. As we consume language, as you are consuming this text, we must relate what is new to what has gone before. This process presents unique challenges to sentence-based logical and linguistic theories and a unique psychological opportunity. Because information arrives incrementally in conveniently identifiable quanta, text provides the psychologist with a bench on which to study the accretion of new knowledge onto old. No other sources of information come with their own notation.

One class of structures that tie what is new to what has gone before are antecedents and their anaphors. The treatment of anaphors brings to light deep-seated differences between the interests of psychologists and linguists. The linguist contrasts what is anaphoric with what is deictic – what points to other language as opposed to what points at the world. For the psychologist, text is a convenient stimulus medium, but only one example of the process of the accretion of knowledge. A psychologist must connect new language indifferently with preceding language or with nonlinguistic experience. What is crucial for the psychologist is the contrast between what is new and what old information it must be connected to.

These interests lead the linguist to focus on explicitly "reduced" anaphors like pronouns – anaphors that appear to wear their anaphoric status on their sleeve. For the psychologist interested in text, full noun phrases have to be related to earlier structures just as much as do pronouns, and it is an open question whether the relation is mediated by the world or by linguistic structures. In the most primitive case in which an antecedent refers to a referent and a succeeding anaphor refers to the same referent, there seems to be little call for mediation of the relation by a linguistic relation between the antecedent and the anaphor. All that is required is a theory of how the antecedent refers to its referent and an account of how the anaphor refers to its referent, and we will then automatically have an account of how they both refer to the same referent. This can be thought of as the minimal account in which anaphoric relations play no part. The maximal account is then the "replacement theory," in which the anaphor is seen as literally substituting for a repetition of its antecedent. In this maximal account, the relation between antecedent and anaphor does all the work.

The minimal account dismisses anaphors as linguistically uninteresting. The maximal account, typical of early transformational grammar, gets into trouble when the antecedent cannot function the same way in the anaphor's position. The antecedent's occurrence, along with other events, has changed the circumstances so that the anaphor can function the way it does. The antecedent has had many effects at many structural levels, and the question is, at what level in all of these structures can we get the best explanation of the link between antecedent and anaphor? Candidates are cautioned that there may not be one answer.

In the early 1970s, linguists were already interested in anaphors, but for apparently quite different reasons. Many of the examples brought by the generative semanticists against the standard theory and its extensions involved quantified antecedents and their anaphors. The standard theory had avoided any consideration of the semantic properties of noun phrases (they were still analyzed as referential entities with an indexing semantics). The generative semanticists found semantically awkward examples but were interested in them for grinding syntactic axes about the form of the syntactic component of grammars. They did not seem very concerned about the descriptive semantic problem.

The most cursory glance at the range of anaphors in text revealed a variety of diabolically difficult, far-reaching logical problems. Introductory first-order logic exercises were not an adequate preparation for this radical translation task. The most obstinate and most central example emerged quite rapidly. An indefinite introduction of a new item into a story followed by a definite back reference to the item is a fundamental structure in expository text: "Freda had a cat. The cat was a tabby." But under standard logical analyses, the first statement contains no reference to a cat for the second sentence's subject noun phrase to refer back to. So much the worse for standard logical analyses, one might conclude. Some had suggested that the indefinite article was ambiguous and that it had a "specific" or "referential" reading. That was okay as a label for the problem, but no one had any proposals on how to give a semantic treatment of the difference between "the cat" and "a cat" (specific). The whole appeal of logic as a basis for a theory was that it had a well-worked-out semantics for suitable fragments. To introduce hand waving again meant that one might as well not introduce the logic in the first place.

Getting hold of logic from the right end. Inasmuch as introductory logic was any preparation for the problem, it suggested that these connections should be mediated by variable binding. "There was *something* that was Freda's and that *something* was tabby." This didn't seem to get the truth conditions right, and there were cases, notably plural antecedents, in which the type of quantifier binding the antecedent wasn't even the same as that of the one binding the anaphor. "Freda had cats. They were tabbies." The more I inspected the readings available for all sorts of noun phrases as a function of their determiners and their contexts, the more peculiar the logical design of English seemed. There was, of course, a large store of philosophical examples of interesting problems. The task was to collect them, to examine how they operated in multisentence texts, and to try to systematize them. Logicians often took the attitude that if you wanted a system, you'd better invent one. This psychologist thought that there ought to be one to be found.

Either English was just wantonly ambiguous in its logical structure or the classification principles were wrong. Ambiguity itself was not unexpected: Lexical polysemy is rife in natural languages but is intuitively unavoidable. If we have many concepts and not as many words, polysemy is inevitable and has many advantages. But determiners are different. I considered only about six; quite enough they were too. If the fundamental distinction in logic is between universal and existential quantifiers, why should both of the English articles in both singular and plural appear to function as both types of quantifier? These are among the commonest items in the language, and the number of potential interpretations in some texts explodes accordingly. Four is not a large number of items to add to a language to clear up such fundamental confusion. Something was wrong with the framework.

The realization of what was wrong came slowly. Obviously, people didn't really experience all of these alternatives in the contexts in which they lurked. As they went along they built something, and within that something the new phrases received an unambiguous interpretation. Moreover, what they were building in the storylike examples that I found myself constructing was not what logic was invented to describe. In logic, we construct proofs. Proofs are reformulations of what is already there in a shared set of assumptions. Stories are just the opposite. They are the provision of a set of assumptions for the hearer, who didn't know of them, by the speaker, who did.

When one learns logic, one generally learns logical forms and some inference rules. Only later is the apparatus of semantic interpretation introduced. What was needed was not some "natural logic" but a natural application of logic to the task at hand, and since the task was not the customary one, the application had better be rather different. Logicians, focusing on validity, that which is true in all possible interpretations, are not generally interested in what is contingently true in particular interpretations, but with my story listeners, that was just what they were interested in – what is in this domain, and what properties do these things have?

Why were all of the examples storylike? Because in stories all of the context construction is done explicitly; when the speaker and hearer are assumed to share no episodic knowledge beforehand, everything must be done explicitly in the text. An indefinite phrase introduces a set of an element(s) into the domain – whatever set makes the minimal addition to the interpretation that will keep that interpretation a model of the text thus far. A subsequent definite anaphor quantifies over this set. Such was my attempt at a system in the jungle in 1975. Since then, logicians and linguists with more formal acumen than myself have proposed alternative approaches to capturing various subsets of examples familiar to me from my specimen collecting. Kamp (1981) uses partial models; Richards (1983) uses complex terms. I confess to finding assessment of the formal approaches as hard as the logicians themselves do. For my own purposes, the insight that texts that allowed the extraction of unique models were psychologically special seemed solid enough to allow me to go in search of psychological consequences. This much would not evaporate on the discovery of the next awkward example. The search for an experimental entrance required a clear view of the status of models.

New stories aren't just new. They're also sometimes untrue. The newness is what is crucial to this enterprise; their fictional status is quite irrelevant. Because this sort of discourse semantics *defers* comparison between text and world, some have taken it to be an exercise in "psychological" semantics (e.g., Johnson-

Laird, 1983*)*. Psychological in the sense that it is taken to relate language to mental entities rather than nonmental things. I do not know what is the right account of fictional discourse *(*that is a hard and interesting problem that may have many answers or maybe none*)*, but that is quite irrelevant to the current issue. One can decide at the end of a text whether it is true of the world; in just the same way, one can judge the truth of a sentence at its end and not always before. Of course, it often doesn't come to that. Subjects in text comprehension experiments generally don't go through any comparison of the texts with real-world objects. They extract a representation that is interpreted as a constraint on possible models of the text. Even when such representations turn out to be the end of the process, they can be understood for what they are only through their possibilities of interpretation of the world. The topic is how the standard semantic relation is represented: the topic is not some nonsemantic relation between language and mental representation.

From abstract objects to psychological experiments. Choosing to see semantics as a relation between language and "mental models" is, of course, another example of methodological solipsism. To see the peculiarity of this program, it is helpful to look at the status of the other type of abstract object that appears in a classic semantic theory – the sentence – and its place in psychological theories of language use.

The sentence is an abstract object with a hierarchical and sequential structure. Relatively crude behavioral observations are sufficient to reveal the importance of this class of abstract objects for theories of language use. It is much more difficult to say how people instantiate these structures – how the structures are represented and processed. That is what psycholinguistics is all about. From the earliest results, this much was clear. There are several different ways in which these objects are represented and processed. At superficial levels, they have properties that resemble their acoustic manifestations. At deeper levels, they appear to behave in a treelike fashion. It is no explanation of how they are implemented to say that there are mental sentences.

Similarly, models are abstract objects – mappings of linguistic vocabulary items onto nonlinguistic elements. Again, it is possible to use relatively crude behavioral observations to show that models are important for linguistic behavior. (Some examples will be given presently.) It is most of the psychologist's task to say how these abstract structures are implemented in mental processing. We surely should not expect there to be one answer. It is certainly no explanation to say that there are mental models. This is just where the work begins.

If this outbreak of solipsism runs against the concepts of model theory, so does it run against psychological method. The reason language is the "royal road to the mind" is that we have externalized representations of abstract structures and these structures are also implemented internally. Much of our knowledge of the nature of the abstract objects implemented in the mind has come from the study of these externalized codes by logicians and linguists. That knowledge provides a starting point for the investigation of their mental implementation. To mistake the statement of the problem for its solution is like thinking that one has arrived by buying a ticket.

The necessity for these clarifications did not occur to me until much later. The immediate need was for evidence that models were implicated in textual processing. We could see that the conventions of expository text interpretation impose a model on sentences that in themselves provide no warrant. We could also see that texts that block the imposition of these conventions and prevent the reader from extracting a unique model are difficult to process, and that it is this failure to specify a model rather than any of several other superficial features that is the cause of the problem. The sorts of failures possible are of many different types, some more fundamental than others. In my search for an experimental path to the study of model implementation, I could not, for a long while, find a way of studying the sort of failure that is most interesting because it is most fundamental. Indeterminacy of reference was what I wanted to study, but the conventions of expository text seemed to make it impossible to find texts that were indeterminate but well formed. With hindsight I think this was because I was looking for "natural" texts and was unwilling to give my subjects enough help in providing constraints on their interpretation, to make the texts natural.

A glance at images. An experimentally easier but analogous form of the indeterminacy issue is provided by texts that underdetermine spatial relations between a set of objects. If our theory is that subjects seek to interpret a text as defining a model, and to represent it by representing that model, then the way to demonstrate our theory is to deny subjects some of the information that is needed for such a construction and to observe how this affects their performance. We are here entering the imagery versus propositional representation debate, but from a perspective different from the usual one.

Instead of supposing that mental images have unknown properties and going in search of unknown structures in the unknown mind, we can pursue Bishop Berkeley's observations and ask what would follow if pictures were used as representations. Spatial images demand the specification of spatial relations. If subjects do use such representations, it does not automatically mean that they will stop in their tracks if the relations are not supplied, or that they will supply the relations by default and then be unable to remember that they were not given them. Perhaps they can supplement their chosen representation with annotation as to which information is information with an extrinsic source and which is supplied by the system itself. It is nevertheless possible to predict different error patterns according to whether subjects use a representational system that forces the specification of spatial relations or, alternatively, one that allows them to remain indeterminate.

Here was a tractable experimental setting and a respite from quantifiers. Subjects could read natural route directions that were sometimes indeterminate as to whether a turning was right or left (e.g., "Go down the street to the bridge and turn up the hill"). Their memory showed that they did supply the default in order to construct a maplike memory. In fact, they most often supplied the default "right." They were also quite good at remembering that they had supplied the information, showing that they had something more than a map (Stenning, 1977). We may conceive of this as a propositional system of representation and as one involving an imagelike data structure. It gives a precise meaning to the latter idea and shows that the debate has been, for the most part, singularly ill-defined. This approach gives a general and precise specification of the contrast between different types of representational systems that it seeks to distinguish and derives clear-cut evidence about the type of system people use in this task. To continue to argue about whether the system is propositional or imagistic is to indulge in semantics in a sense that even this author does not recommend.

Taking models away from readers. Presenting information indeterminate with regard to spatial relations is only a special case of the general contrast between texts that specify or do not specify unique models. A fragment of a language may simply not include spatial relations, and so interpretations of that fragment may require no specification of spatial relations. Referential relations are different and more fundamental to the specification of models. In a domain of two objects, in which one is red and the other not, and one is square and the other not, any adequate interpretation of these properties onto the predicates "red" and "square" will have to specify whether the red thing is square or not.

The conventions of expository text conspire to make it difficult to avoid such specification. If we are told that there is a butcher and later that there is a baker, it is quite difficult to construct the text so that we suspend judgment as to whether these two men are one and the same. This makes it difficult to experiment on the consequences. I finally realized that the only course is to tell the subject exactly why this information is not provided – to construct a setting in which the producer of the text didn't have the information: "Imagine that the author of the texts you will see is sampling objects from a nonidentical pair of objects in a box, and that brief glimpses of them suffice only to give information about two of the objects' properties." Subjects who read "There is a small black. There is a small white. There is a black square. There is a white circle" at no time experience any referential indeterminacy. They can always infer referential relations within the text. It turns out that this costs them little compared to readers for whom those relations are explicit: "There's a small black. It's square. There's a small white. It's a circle." Not so the poor subjects presented with "There is a small black. There is a small square. There is a small white. There is a white square. There is a black circle." They experience an indeterminacy at sentence 2 that is not finally resolved until sentence 5. Nowhere are there any complex sentences, nor in the whole text is there a large amount of information, but these latter texts are at the readers' limits of comprehension and therefore of memory. When the information that allows resolution of the indeterminacy arrives, subjects take a long time reorganizing their memory, but afterward they resume their normal processing speed. Allow them to extract a unique model and they continue as if nothing had happened (Stenning, 1986). It's just like taking candy from a baby.

Questions of interpretation versus questions of representation. Establishing determinate spatial and referential relations between the referents of a text appears to be crucial to the construction of representations for the text. Is this because of the nature of the particular representational schemes used? Or is it a very general property of possible schemes?

Suppose we take the four items "Swiss," "dentist," "customer," and "father" and impose on them an interpretation, among the indefinitely many, whereby they describe a set of four people. Under another interpretation, they describe a single individual who is a paternal Swiss dentist buying something. We could represent either interpretation in indefinitely many ways, and any representation of one would serve as a representation of the other. In order to use a representation, we need to interpret it, and if we are using it in memory, we had better interpret it the same way we did when we constructed it if we are to remember the right thing.

If we define our subjects' task as recall of the verbal items, their choice of interpretation and representation is free. Such tasks are exercises in associating items: So long as the grouping can be read from the representation, it does not matter whether the grouping is a grouping of properties or of individuals (or of sounds, for that matter). Classical verbal learners thought of their experiments as observing the formation of such neutral associations: Any particular semantic interpretation would be imposed on this neutral associative grouping. The other picture is one in which only the adoption of a particular semantic interpretation captures the episodic association. This is the "Magical Number's" picture. Contemporary semantic network theories are like the classical theory in that the networks themselves still stand in need of semantic interpretation, and little of such work has addressed semantic issues.

Since 1980, we have been engaged on an experimental program aimed at these questions. We know that choosing to impose the "set" rather than the "individual'' interpretation on the same items makes a great difference in the time required to encode them. But there are also certain fascinating patterns common to both processes. We have the tools to investigate these issues. We have had them for many years. Their deployment is a slow and methodical business.

That first question

In this framework, which demands highly detailed analysis of the representation of particular interpretations, bottom-level questions of representation are close to the "Magical Number's" first question: Is there a common explanation of the limitations of absolute judgment and immediate memory? Absolute judgment *is* an immediate memory task; the only difference between it and relative judgment is that the subject must remember the "comparison stimulus" for a period of time. The "Magical Number's" limitation appears whenever absolute judgment is psychophysically pure. This invites the conjecture that it appears wherever no semantic recoding is available. Given physical (or sensory) magnitudes on a single dimension, adequately representable by real magnitudes, perhaps there is no possibility of any recoding. The contents really are information limited.

How does this speculative view transfer to classical immediate memory tasks? We know that the contents of the items in memory can be used to recode indefinite amounts of information. But suppose we take a subject who is not using any recoding strategy. Suppose the items simply stand for themselves. Then why should the items be limited to seven? Well, the obvious speculation is that it is our ability to find the item that limits the number of items we can hold, and it seems not at all impossible that this limitation is the same as the one that allows us to address only seven psychophysical magnitudes. Whatever substrate we use to represent intervals on a pure psychophysical dimension may be the same substrate that we use to represent the identities or whereabouts of the items that represent the codes we hold in immediate memory.

In our gruesomely detailed analyses of short-fat-Polish-bishop-and-short-thin-Swiss-nurse knowledge, we begin to see evidence of particular dimensions, such as order of arrival, being used to represent semantic features such as the identity of the property dimension on which matches and mismatches of property between two objects occur. When our subjects forget that the only match was on the stature dimension, they are most likely to recall short-fat-Polish-bishop-and-tall-fat-Swiss-nurse, thus moving the match from the second property dimension to the first. Here we are observing a stage of representation during which time of arrival, or perhaps sequence of arrival, represents highly abstract characteristics of the information presented. It is somehow fitting for a first example to be one in which the substrate memory used appears to be a representation of time.

We have not answered the first question of the "Magical Number" in the last thirty years of psychological research. But we can thank its author, among others, for the context in which it has been possible to become a little clearer about the difference between his first question and his second, and therefore about the determining role of semantic interpretation in the course of mental processes.

References

Bransford, J. D., & Johnson, M. (1972). Contextual prerequisites for understanding: Some investigations of comprehension and recall. *Journal of Verbal Learning and Verbal Behaviour, 11,* 717–26.

Johnson-Laird, P. N. (1983). *Mental Models.* Cambridge: Cambridge University Press.

Kamp, H. (1981). A theory of truth and semantic representation. In J. A. G. Groenendijk, T. M. V. Janssen, M. B. J. Stokhof (Eds.), *Formal Methods in the Study of Language,* Vol. 136 (pp. 277–322). Amsterdam: Mathematical Centre Tracts.

Miller, G. A. (1956). The magical number seven plus or minus two, or, some limits on our capacity for processing information. *Psychological Review, 63,* 81–96.

Miller, G. A. (1965). Computers, communication and cognition. *Advancement of Science,* pp. 417–30.

Miller, G. A., & Isard, S. (1963). Some perceptual consequences of linguistic rules. *Journal of Verbal Learning and Verbal Behaviour, 2,* 217–28.

Miller, G. A., & Johnson-Laird, P. N. (1976). *Language and Perception.* Cambridge: Harvard University Press.

Miller, G. A., & Nicely, P. (1955). An analysis of perceptual confusions among some English consonants. *Journal of the Acoustical Society of America, 27,* 338–52.

Putnam, H. (1975). The meaning of "meaning." In K. Gunderson, (Ed.), *Language, Mind and Knowledge,* Vol. 7. Minneapolis: University of Minnesota Press.

Richards, B. (1983). Anaphora, descriptions and discourse representations. *Synthese, 54,* 209–33.

Sachs, J. S. (1967). Recognition memory for syntactic and semantic aspects of connected discourse. *Perception and Psychophysics, 2,* 437–42.

Stenning, K. (1977). On remembering how to get there: How we might want something like a map. In A. M. Lesgold, J. W. Pellegrino, S. W. Fokkema, & R. Glaser (Eds.), *Cognitive Psychology and Instruction* (pp. 101–10). New York: Plenum Press.

Stenning, K. (1986). On making models: A study of constructive memory. In T. Myers, K. Brown, & B. McGonigle (Eds.), *Reasoning and Discourse Processes* (pp. 165–85). London: Academic Press.

Van Heijenoort, J. (1967). Logic as calculus and logic as language. *Synthese, 17,* 324–30.

PART V Cognitive neuroscience

Cornell University Medical College is up the block from the Rockefeller University. When Michael Gazzaniga arrived at Cornell, he and George began a series of conversations and seminars. Unlike many cognitive psychologists, George did not have a closed mind about the importance of the brain. Indeed, if the study of language and the astounding linguistic abilities of humans taught him anything, it was that one must ultimately approach psychology from a biological perspective. Here Gazzaniga discusses the early conversations that he had with George and the formation of the Cognitive Neuroscience Institute, today a viable center for the study of the relation between mind and brain. George was instrumental in its formation and still sits on the governing board. In his chapter, Hirst, who spent several years with George at Rockefeller and was an early attendee of the Gazzaniga–Miller seminars, explores the history of the relation between cognitive psychology and neuroscience, especially in the context of memory research.

16   Life with George: the birth of the Cognitive Neuroscience Institute

Michael S. Gazzaniga

Introducing George Miller to clinical states of mind was my pleasure during the late 1970s. After arriving at Cornell Medical College and experiencing the white-out of medical dress, I reached for the phone the first afternoon and called George. There was no one at Cornell who remotely resembled a psychologist, and I was in desperate need of someone who knew what a theory was all about. Propinquity governed once again, since George was also the closest psychologist.

I had never talked to or met the man before 1976, and I quite frankly did not know what to expect. As a general rule, I don't like meeting legends. Either they have removed themselves from the business of establishing new personal relationships or they are not what their metroself appears to suggest. (The concept of the "metroself" was introduced to me by Richmond Crinkley and serves well the problem of distinguishing the personal reality of a public person from his or her public reality, or "metroself.") When you are in a public business, and scholarship, alas, is that, the metroself can begin to drive the personal self and effectively run and ruin lives. When someone works only on the metroself and never on the real joys of a personal life, disaster ensues. But George put my worst fears to rest.

Shortly thereafter, we began to meet regularly after work at the bar in the Rockefeller Faculty Club. We talked about everything from neglect to neologisms. It was on one of those evenings that he coined the term "cognitive neuroscience"; shortly thereafter, we formed our small but lovable enterprise. What he meant by cognitive neuroscience was to emerge – slowly. What we already knew was that neuropsychology was not what we had in mind. Tying specific functions to lesioned brain areas was not going to be our enterprise. The bankruptcy and intellectual impoverishment of that idea seemed self-evident, especially with the advent of new brain-imaging techniques that revealed how much else was always damaged following what had previously been thought to be focal damage.

They used to say that Jack Benny, the world's funniest man, was the best

230

audience in the world. Everyone loved to try his stuff out on Jack. If George is in an audience, he is usually asleep. If he *is* the audience, that is, if you are one on one, he is the best. It is like having an ongoing editor as one pours out one's story. He asks questions that elicit more, but then as you hear yourself, you begin to edit as silly formulations slide off his deadpan expression. There is not much new in this world, and certainly not much new about the psychological nature of human beings. What passes for discovery these days tends to be an individual scientist's rediscovery of some well-established phenomenon. Most of these have come and gone, and George knows all of them. Yet, on the hundredth trip to the well, one is overjoyed to see a glimmer in his eye. Perhaps there was something to that last idea!

We started exchanging stories, mine about episodes in the clinic and his about new experimental strategies. I would tell him about patients with high verbal IQ's, as measured by the Wechsler Adult Intelligence Scale *(WAIS)*, who lacked a grammar school child's ability to solve simple problems like the raven's Progressive matrices. He would tell me about people who talk a good game but really have nothing to say. He would also say that psychologists do not yet have anything resembling a theory of intelligence or mind. He urged the continued collection of dissociations in cognition, as seen in the clinic, in the hope that a theory would emerge from these bizarre facts.

I took him on my rounds one day and showed him a range of phenomena from perceptual disorders to language disorders. He had never seen anything like it and commented afterward that the neurologic patient was really what many psychologists were looking for. After all, he observed, psychologists try to break brains by making college sophomores work fast or by presenting stimuli rapidly so that errors are made. In the clinic, the errors pour out of largely highly responsive systems with little or no effort.

One patient we saw was a distinguished executive in New York who had fallen down a staircase after consuming too many martinis. He was reported to be globally aphasic, which means that he would not understand much, if anything, and would speak only a little. As we arrived in his room, the computer tomography technicians were fetching him for a scan, so we tagged along. The technician asked Mr. C to slide over to the gurney, to which he replied "Yes, sir." Once positioned and rolling down the hallway to the scanner, the technician inquired about his comfort. "Are you feeling Ok?" "Yes, sir," said Mr. C. After arriving at the scanner, the patient was again slid off the gurney onto the table and was again asked if he felt alright. "Yes, sir," said Mr. C. The scan took place and Mr. C was returned to his room by the technician. The technician, who was familiar with my interests, turned to me and asked why we were interested in this patient. He felt that there was nothing wrong with him. I turned to the patient and said, "Mr. C, are you the king of Siam?" "Yes, sir," he replied with great assuredness. George grinned and observed that getting anywhere with anything is simply a matter of asking the right question.

We started the formal aspect of our effort in cognitive neuroscience with a year-long lecture series. To pay for this, as well as for some of our subsequent ventures, George and I applied for and received funding from the Sloan Foundation for a training grant. They were in the midst of their "Particular Program in Cognitive Science," and the application seemed a reasonable way to incorporate the brain sciences into the topic of cognition. Mike Posner spent much of his time with us in an attempt to bring together the fields of brain science and cognitive science. There was plenty of talent on both sides of the fence that doggedly divides these two disciplines. Emilio Bizzi, Floyd Bloom, Steven Hillyard, Russ Develois, John Marshall, and Rodolfo Llinas talked about the brain and Dave Premack, Leon Festinger, Roger Shepard, Edgar Zurif, and Donald MacKay talked about cognition. When Mike Posner summarized it all for us, it became clear that an integrated field of cognitive neuroscience was a goal, not a reality. The beauty of each separate contribution was best dealt with individually.

As it worked out, George and I were called upon to write something about cognitive neuroscience. We took to the mails. One evening in late May 1978, we were having drinks, and as the second martini was taking hold, I asked him, "Just what is it cognitive science wants to know?" He looked at me, alerted for action, and then said, "Let me think about that." The following week, the guiding ideas behind our Cognitive Neuroscience Institute took form:

To: Michael S. Gazzaniga
From: George A. Miller
Re: "COGNITIVE SCIENCE [sic]"
An intense undergraduate, in the sharp panic of an identity crisis, rushed to his professor: "I don't know who I am. Tell me, who am I?" The professor replied wearily, "Please, who's asking the question?"

The story flashed to mind recently when a friend, who watches science with the eyes of a biologist, asked: "What do cognitive scientists want to know?" Anyone capable of posing such a question must already know the answer. To know is to have direct cognition of. Obviously, scientists of cognition want to have direct cognition of having direct cognition. Any etymologist could tell you that. Indeed, the very phrase "cognitive science" invites a scholarly disquisition on the Latin verbs *scire* (whence "science"), *gnoscere* (whence "know"), and *cognoscere* (whence "cognition").

Habits of mind that lead one into biology, however, are not satisfied by verbal play. They demand serious answers. What do cognitive scientists want to know?

Who knows? Trying to speak for cognitive science, as if cognitive scientists had but one mind and one voice, is a bum's game.

Nevertheless, certain facts are beyond dispute. Somewhere out there is a group of people who, at appropriate tribal gatherings, regard themselves as cognitive scientists. Moreover, some of them edit journals like *Cognitive Science*. And recently a philanthropic foundation announced that it would contribute $15,000,000 to advance cognitive science. No wonder that even biologists are curious to know what cognitive scientists are up to. People, meetings, publications, money – given these trappings, can content be far behind? There must be something that cognitive scientists are trying to understand.

What would a biologist accept as an answer? Something deep is called for. My friend is not asking about computers, or simulations, or logical formalisms, or the latest methods of psychological experimentation – none of that ancillary horseshit that fills so much of the conversation of cognitive scientists. A deeper answer is that cognitive scientists want to know the cognitive rules that people follow and the knowledge representations that those rules operate on. But this language – cognitive rules, knowledge representations – is precisely the kind of smoke that started my friend looking for a fire.

Let us begin with a question that we can answer: What do biologists want to know? Biologists want to discover the molecular logic of the living state. What is the molecular logic of the living state? Simple. It is the set of principles that, in addition to the principles of physics and chemistry, operate to govern the behavior of inanimate matter in living systems. (That is an almost direct quotation from the introduction to a biochemistry textbook.)

Is this the kind of answer a biologist expects when he asks what cognitive scientists want to know? If so, perhaps we can construct an answer based on this model of what an answer should be. Because I am a little slow at these games, however, I shall take three steps to get where I am going.

First, I will substitute psychologists for biologists. No substitution seems required for molecular logic; I assume that "molecular" in this context means "susceptible to analysis," and is not limited to the analysis of matter into chemical molecules. And then I will substitute conscious for living, because I consider consciousness to be the constitutive problem for psychology, just as life is the constitutive problem for biology. Now I have achieved the following: Psychologists want to discover the molecular logic of the conscious state.

So far so good. But now what do we mean by molecular logic of the conscious state? Let's see if substitution leads anywhere: the set of principles that, in addition to the principles of physics, chemistry, and biology, operate to govern the behavior of inanimate matter in conscious systems. These substitutions say little more than that psychology is the next step in the positivistic hierarchy of sciences. The result sounds pretty good to me, but can I follow through? That is to say, the biochemist whose formulation I have borrowed as my model had a large and impressive textbook full of biological principles to illustrate what he was talking about. What do I have?

One thing I do not have is behaviorism, because most behaviorists are dedicated to the proposition that consciousness is irrelevant to the science of psychology. Another thing I do not have is artificial intelligence, because computer si ·ulations have no need for the psychological distinction between living and nonliving sys.ems, for that matter.

What I seem to have is a way of looking at psychology, a criterion to keep in mind while thumbing through psychological handbooks. It might be formulated like this: Any behavior that is unaffected by the state of consciousness of the behaving system is of no concern to psychology. Dreaming, for example, is a concern of psychology, because if you wake up – if your state of consciousness changes – dreaming is affected.

This reminds me of the opposite side of a challenge I have been giving my students for many years. I challenge them to give me any psychological principle that I cannot violate by a simple act of will. I have always seen this challenge as a devastating criticism of psychology as a science, and I have consumed many of my intellectual watts looking for inviolable principles – for limitations on short-term memory, for example, or sensory thresholds, or what have you. But always without success. Any lay subject who refuses to cooperate in my experiments can violate my conclusions. Now, however, I would simply change my value judgment. The ability to violate some principle by an act of will is now the critical test that the principle in question is one that is relevant to psychology.

A basic problem for this kind of psychology, however, is the characterization of different states of consciousness. If it is too difficult to differentiate a hungry consciousness from a thirsty one, we can postpone those refinements until we have some of the cruder differences under control: the difference between awake and asleep, say, or between asleep and hypnotized, or between hypnotized and anesthetized. These differences are important because, if we hope to follow the formulation we reached by substitution, we must have reliable ways of knowing whether states of consciousness have changed. Only then can we begin to study the effects of those changes on behavior.

I assume that most psychologists conform to this general proposition without stopping to think about it. When they publish the result of a rote memorization experiment, for example, the reader is generally safe in presupposing that the subjects were awake during the learning trials and that different results would have been obtained if they had been asleep. That presupposition is regarded as too obvious to bother mentioning. But perhaps we need to grab hold of a few obvious facts like that in order to provide a firm foundation for scientific psychology?

In most respects, our search for principles governing conscious systems would not change the research we do, although it might change the way we talk about it. The major place I would expect a change would be in those situations where what people do and what they say about what they do are different. Such situations have in the past been used primarily to illustrate the unreliability of introspective reports. Under the new regime, they would provide prime opportunities to explore how the state of consciousness is related to behavior, a question that could not even be raised if consciousness and behavior had always been correlated.

All of this could be elaborated in some detail, although psychologists are still a long way from any catalogue of principles comparable to those of biochemistry. The problem, however, is that my friend did not ask what psychologists want to know. He asked what cognitive scientists want to know.

A second set of substitutions can be tried, therefore. Suppose we substitute states of knowledge for the conscious state. Then we obtain: Cognitive psychologists want to discover the molecular logic of states of knowledge, where the molecular logic of states of knowledge refers to the set of principles that, in addition to the principles of physics and chemistry, govern the behavior of inanimate matter in knowledge systems. Reference to biological and psychological principles is here omitted, for the computers can instantiate knowledge systems; computers need obey no biological or psychological principles.

The criterion for looking at research would now become: Any behavior that is unaffected by the state of knowledge of the behaving system is of no concern to cognitive science. If you turn off the power in a computer, for example, the consequences will not depend on the state of knowledge of the computer, so they would be of no concern to cognitive scientists. I suspect that this criterion distinguishes rather sharply between those kinds of information that are imposed on the machine by its program and those imposed by its fixed architecture. This boundary can vary from one information processing device to the next, and the boundary of cognitive concern would vary correspondingly. I am not sure this is a happy result for cognitive scientists, since it seems to constrain the principles we can find to particular systems. For each system, a new science.

I have no desire to dissuade anyone who wants to develop cognitive science along these lines, but neither do I have any desire to join with them. I would prefer to take a different line, defining still another science more narrowly. So I will now take a third step, as follows: Cognitive neuroscientists want to discover the molecular logic of epistemic systems, where the molecular logic in question this time is the principle that, in addition to the principles of physics, chemistry, biology, and psychology, governs the behavior of inanimate matter in epistemic systems. (The term "epistemic system" is negotiable; I use it as a placeholder for something better.) A further substitution is possible: animate for inanimate in the final clause. I am unclear whether it would make any real difference.

By including the requirement that cognitive neuroscience is concerned only with living, conscious systems, we cut artificial intelligence free to develop in its own way, independent of the solutions that organic evolution happens to have produced. Now our concern is for a subset of conscious systems, and the criterion is whether or not the system's state of knowledge affects its behavior – what Pylyshyn has called its "cognitive penetrability." Perhaps cognitive penetrability should be paralleled by conative or affective penetrability, but since I don't really know what I am talking about, I will not try to pursue the contrasts.

One problem I feel with this formulation may be worth mentioning. Since the search is for principles that govern behavior, the definition presumably commits cognitive neuroscientists to the goal of predicting and controlling behavior. The inclusion of psychological principles, where "psychological" is defined in the way suggested earlier, allows for a considerable degree of mentalism in the methodology of cognitive science. A British psychologist named David Lieberman has recently argued that this is precisely the stance psychologists ought to take: behavioristic goals, but allowing introspective evidence. I agree with Lieberman that this describes the position of most cognitive psychologists at the present time, but it bothers me – it seems schizoid. If I could think of something other than behavior that cognitive principles would govern, I would opt for that, but everything I think of as an alternative is of questionable identifiability – that is, most mental contents are too hypothetical to let us observe what governs them. I know that this is the kind of trouble scientists don't get into unless they ask for it, but nevertheless I shall continue to ponder it in my own muddle-headed way.

It should be clear by now that I really don't have an answer to the question, what do cognitive scientists want to know? But I think that cognitive neuroscientists want to know something that is reasonably interesting, and that there really might be some promise in following up systematically the implications of the definitions that we arrived at by substitution into our biological model.

Unbelievable as it may seem, I attempted a response. It was spring.

To: George A. Miller
From: Michael S. Gazzaniga
Re: Exemplars of Cognitive Neuroscience
O.K., your claim is that our task is to understand those processes active in living systems that can exert control over the comings and goings of a variety of mental

constituents that make up a cognitive agent. (Put differently, is it also fair to say that the defining qualities of a cognitive system are coincident with an information processing disorder?) Alternatively, it is our task to understand cerebral software, the programming stuff that orchestrates the spatial–temporal patterns of the neural network.

First, has your definition of cognitive neuroscience moved the ball down the field? I think it has. Consider what others have said about what cognition is, usually using other terminologies. Sperry, for example, used to argue that consciousness is an emergent property of the spatial–temporal interaction of the neuronal system subserving the phenomenon. He maintained that these emergent mental properties feed back, as it were, and control the activities of the system that produced it. To me this position is a neuroscientist's way of saying cognitive act.

MacKay's hypothesis on what the cardinal feature of a cognitive system is goes like this: "the direct correlate of conscious experience is the self-evaluating, supervisory or metaorganizing activity of the cerebral system and it is this system that determines norms and priorities and organizes the internal state of readiness to reckon with the sources of sensory stimulation." That strikes me as a rather passive description of the conscious process and it takes on more of the character of a "jobber" or "dispatcher." He does not characterize the system as one that tries to penetrate the organism's natural tendency to reflexively respond to a command.

If I am right, your definition has advanced at least my understanding of some issues and has clearly stated that the task is to discover the rules that govern the epistemic system – the one living system that governs the biologic system. When thinking about that, I am maintaining that the epistemic system is supraordinate to the biologic system. Is that what you were driving at?

At any rate, you have set us to the task of actually trying to figure out the principles of not only how cognitive systems announce their products to consciousness, but also the criterion that a cognitive system is a process that can supersede the cerebral architecture. How else can we illuminate this dynamic other than by studying disruptive brain states? In some sense the cognitive neuroscientist is trying to trick out of the organism insight into that puzzling problem. But before raising some problems from studies on brain-damaged patients, let me make one other observation that I think needs up-front analysis.

The kind of analysis one would bring to understanding a New Yorker as opposed to understanding New York would be quite different. The kind of analysis one brings to understanding a serial system as opposed to a parallel system also seems to me to be quite different. Before we proceed with an intelligent analysis of cognitive function, do we have to face up to the issue as to whether or not the system is in fact competing for the attention of the person? If we agree that this is a reasonable model, crudely put at this point, then it seems to me how one approaches problems in brain disease that merit consideration for a theory of cognition becomes quite different.

Let me now consider a brain disease situation that speaks to this notion of what constitutes a cognitive system. There can be in brain disease relatively discrete disruptions of one of the system properties of the cognitive agent. It is common, for example, to study patients with memory dysfunctions. On one level of analysis they are unable to (1) retain new information and (2) combine two new elements into a fresh concept. Looking into the pathophysiology underlying these disorders, one finds that both diffuse and focal disease states correlate in this psychologic disarray.

It is only on deeper probe that one begins to see differences at the psychologic level. Patients with focal disease possess a dense inability to transfer information from short-term to long-term memory, although lavishly assisted in their recall performance by cueing (e.g., categorical headings embedded in a long word list). On the other hand, patients with diffuse disease are not assisted by this cognitive strategy. Their recall performance stays down on the floor.

What are we to do with these observations? First of all, are we to dismiss the diffuse disease patients as still embodying a cognitive system? Has their agency been lost? If not, what is it about them that characterizes them as a member of this species? I don't have an answer.

It seems to me that brain-diseased patients tell us immediately that we must bring more specificity to the definition of "cognitive penetrability" as a criterion for a cognitive system. I have the strong feeling that there is a real insight here, but a nagging feeling that we can too easily dismiss a lot of cognitive agents.

To which George replied:

To: Michael S. Gazzaniga
From: George A. Miller
Re: There's a long, long trail awinding
Since you accept, at least tentatively, my definition of cognitive neuroscience, our next task is to try to put it to work. I want to restate the definition, but first I want to get rid of "epistemic system." Let me begin by pointing in the general direction I had in mind.

Organic Knowledge Systems. A "knowledge base" is any tangible collection of signals that are arranged according to some accepted coding scheme in order to represent a given body of information. A knowledge base coupled with an information processing system for using it (for storing, retrieving, erasing, comparing, searching, etc.) is a "knowledge system." Obviously, a knowledge base is useless except as part of a knowledge system that (unlike libraries or computers) is governed by biological and psychological principles, i.e., a living, animate, agentive knowledge system.

Definition of Cognitive Neuroscience. Cognitive neuroscientists attempt to discover the molecular logic of organic knowledge systems, i.e., the principles that, in addition to the principles of physics, chemistry, biology, and psychology, govern the behavior of inanimate matter in living knowledge systems.

The Cognitive Criterion. It follows from this definition that any behavior unaffected by the state of knowledge of the behaving system is of no concern to cognitive neuroscience.

Implications of Definition. This definition is compatible with various approaches to cognitive neuroscience: (1) Evolution of knowledge systems. For example, the evolutionary shift from genetically stored knowledge to knowledge acquired from experience. (2) Ontogenesis of knowledge systems. For example, the neural basis of personal memory. (3) Psychology of knowledge systems. For example, the effects of attention, as indicated by evoked potentials, perhaps, on knowledge-governed behavior. (4) Neurology of knowledge systems. For example, the correlation of different types of brain disease. And so on. None of these approaches is novel – which means that we could have something to say about each of them.

A philosophical objection to this approach is that, by introducing successive definitions of biology, psychology, and cognitive neuroscience in this manner, we have made it reductionistic. That is to say, the principles sought by the cognitive neuroscientist are also principles of psychology, and the principles sought by psychologists are also principles of biology. Since I have always thought of scientific psychology as a branch of biology, this objection carries little weight with me. It would carry greater weight, however, with such distinguished scientists as B. F. Skinner or H. A. Simon.

Implications of Criterion. A central question in your memo of June 1 might be phrased as follows: What are the operational implications of the claim that "any behavior unaffected by the state of the behaving system is of no concern to cognitive neuroscience"?

Several things occur to me when you press this button. First, Zenon Pylyshyn should not have to assume responsibility for this phrasing of the criterion. As I understand his notion of "cognitive penetrability," it is intended to discriminate between the fixed "architecture" and the modifiable programs for a mental computer. We, on the other hand, are trying to distinguish what cognitive neuroscientists want to know from what they leave to others. It is not clear to me, in my ignorance of Pylyshyn's ideas, whether these two distinctions coincide, so the only line I can try to develop is our own.

Second, I see two obvious ways to apply the criterion: (1) Change an organism's state of knowledge and try to demonstrate a resultant change in its thinking or behaving. Or (2) leave the organism's knowledge alone, but vary the materials used in a task to see whether thought or behavior changes as a function of their familiarity.

If I have understood your example, the case of a patient with diffuse brain disease illustrates one of the difficulties of applying the criterion in manner (1), since it is apparently impossible to change such a patient's state of knowledge, his memory-governed behavior was of no concern to cognitive neuroscience. For such a patient, therefore, it would be necessary to apply the criterion in manner (2) – essentially, to change the contents of the questions asked until we find something the patient does remember. Does this answer the disturbing question raised at the close of your memo?

Third, I would think of this criterion as something to guide us, as authors, in picking and choosing what studies to write about and how to organize them. I see nothing wrong with confessing that this is the criterion we used (if, indeed, we did), but it does not seem to me to be something that we must rub the reader's nose in.

Levels of Description. One of the biggest problems I have in trying to get my thoughts straight about cognitive neuroscience is that different people work at different levels of description, and no one pays attention to how his level is related to descriptions at other levels. I assume this degree of incoherence is possible because the different levels are only loosely related, which, if true, is an interesting observation in its own right.

The closest discussions I have seen of the level problem have come from the MIT Artificial Intelligence Laboratory, where I assume that Minsky and Marr have been the guiding lights. It is forced on anyone who works with computers, I guess. For example, in P. H. Winston's *Artificial Intelligence* (Addison-Wesley, 1977) eight levels of description of the operation of a computer are distinguished: (1) transistors, (2) flip flops and gates, (3) registers and data paths, (4) machine instructions, (5) compiler or interpreter, (6) LISP, (7) embedded pattern matcher, and (8) intelligent programs. D. Marr and T. Poggio (A theory of human stereo vision, *Proc. Royal Soc. London,* 1977) bring this closer to neurology when they distinguish four levels of description that should apply both to computers and to brains: (1) transistors and diodes, or neurons and synapses, (2) assemblies made from elements at level (1), e.g., memories, adders, multipliers, (3) the algorithm, or scheme for computation, and (4) the theory of the computation.

Clearly, most neuroscientists today are gung ho for level (1); neurotransmitters are hot stuff. I have also encountered a little work at level (2) – e.g., Mountcastle's description of columnar assemblies – so I assume there is more that I don't know about. Level (3) is as abstract as any neuroscientist had dared to dream about – maybe it has been achieved in such cases as Vince Dethier's analysis of flies. Level (4) has been neglected, and Marr and Poggio propose that it is the responsibility of artificial intelligence to provide general theories by which the necessary structure of computation at level (3) can be defined.

I hold no brief for either of these analyses, but I do agree with them that anything as complicated as a nervous system can be understood at several levels. And the logic of levels is such that they must be only loosely connected to one another – otherwise they would not be distinct levels. Moreover, the processes described at level N could probably be achieved by many higher processes at level N + 1 – so a description at level N is never really an explanation of what is really going on at level N.

Problem. What do levels have to do with our definition of cognitive neuro-science? This is not a rhetorical question – I really need an answer.

For example, a particular drug known to affect synapses in a given way (manipulation at level 1) is observed to affect behavior governed by the patient's general knowledge of spatial relations (a consequence at level 4). It meets our criterion (applied in manner 2) for inclusion in cognitive neuroscience. But to include it is not to understand it! Help!

Years have intervened, and we wrote a different chapter. But the idea that neuroscience needed cognitive science has prevailed. I put it that way because that, after all, is what is at stake. The molecular approach in the absence of the cognitive context limited the fashionable neuroscientist to pursuing answers to biologic questions in a manner not unlike that of the kidney physiologist. Although such approaches represent an admirable enterprise, they do, when put in that light, make it impossible for the neuroscientist to attack the central integrative questions of mind–brain research.

The Cognitive Neuroscience Institute has taken all of this to heart. We plan yearly meetings. We were going to have more, but once a year is enough. We invite distinguished scientists from neuroscience and cognitive science to a far-off place and have them sit and think together for a week. None come to the meetings with the answers. We avoid inviting such people. Instead, we collect together people who want to know how to connect cognition with brain processes. The meetings are a pure delight, and tangible progress is being made. We have had two on the problem of memory, with the first effort representing the Institute's first monograph. Four more monographs are in the works. But our anxiousness and worry about the questions we badgered each other with went, ultimately, to make up the flavor of the Cognitive Neuroscience Institute. It continues to plug away, and we both love it. Yet, the concept and the means would not be without the modest but driving force of George Miller.

17 Cognitive psychologists become interested in neuroscience

William Hirst

Cognitive neuroscience is a nascent field of study emerg ng out of the growing dialogue between cognitive psychologists and neuroscientists (LeDoux & Hirst, 1986). I first heard the term when George Miller and Mike Gazzaniga were meeting over martinis at the Faculty Club of The Rockefeller University. At the time, I viewed the label in political rather than intellectual terms. It implied an acceptable common ground between cognitive psychology and neuroscience, something neither neuropsychologists nor physiological psychologists consistently provided. The work of physiological psychologists more actively embraced the concepts of learning theory rather than cognitive psychology, and neuropsychologists often narrowly confined their interest to the description of behavior in brain-damaged patients, without considering other areas of neuroscience or the implications of their work for cognitive psychology.

Cognitive psychologists have not always appreciated the need to talk to neuroscientists. As the field of cognitive psychology was finding its way in the late 1950s and early 1960s, many cognitive psychologists took pains to distinguish their endeavor from neuroscience, echoing the philosophical principles of functionalism (Fodor, 1983; Putnam, 1975). Putnam (1975), in enunciating the functionalist approach, argued that there is a level of discourse between behavior and brain akin to software in a computer. Although a computer's behavior depends on its hardware, it can be captured and described more effectively at the software level. The software mediates between hardware and behavior. It can be independent of the hardware, inasmuch as a program developed on an IBM mainframe can be easily transferred to a Sperry UNIVAC. Simon (1969), in his elegant book *The Science of the Artificial*, followed up on this point and assigned to cognitive psychologists the job of describing the ''software.'' For both Putnam and Simon, models of the mind can be devised independent of any consideration of the nature and function of the brain. Neisser (1967), who helped define the problems and boundaries of the field in his classic book *Cognitive Psychology*,

I would like to thank the NIH for Grant NS 17776 for support and Edward Levine, Martha Farah, and David Stark for their comments.

also effectively dismissed the need to consider the brain. After reiterating the analogy between the study of psychology and the development of software, he continued:

The same point can be illustrated with quite a different analogy, that between psychology and economics. The economist wishes to understand, say, the flow of capital. The object of his study must have some tangible representation, in the form of checks, gold, . . . but these objects are not what he really cares about. The physical properties of money, its location in banks . . . is of little interest to him. Psychology, like economics, is a science concerned with the interdependence among certain events rather than with their physical nature. (pp. 6–7)

Feelings about the role of neuroscience in cognitive psychology were quite strong. As a graduate student at Cornell, I took a seminar from Eric Lenneberg, a major proponent of what was to become known as "cognitive neuroscience." I distinctly remember both Neisser, my advisor, and J. J. Gibson, another prominent cognitive psychologist on the faculty, being puzzled by my interest. Gibson, in particular, thought that cognitive psychology had nothing to learn from the study of the brain. He used to lecture Eric about the lessons to be derived from Lashley's work, and Eric used to rebut with the claim that things had changed quite drastically since Lashley's time. Neisser was less vociferous about his opinions but showed little interest in the brain. Eric, who considered himself a cognitive psychologist, complained about being isolated.

Although feelings like those I experienced in graduate school still exist, the mood among cognitive psychologists has changed significantly. A recent paper that I reviewed for a cognitive psychology journal spent the first few pages arguing that the study of brain-damaged patients, the topic of the paper, could provide basic data for understanding normal cognitive functioning. Another reviewer suggested, and the editor concurred, that this defense was unnecessary: Everyone now agreed that cognitive psychology could learn from neuroscience.

Why have cognitive psychologists' attitudes changed during these past few years? The shift has not occurred because a strong conceptual argument has been mounted against the basically philosophical concerns of Putnam, Fodor, and Neisser. To be sure, several contemporary philosophers, particularly Patricia and Paul Churchland (See Churchland, 1986; Churchland, 1984), are constructing arguments for combining cognitive psychology and neuroscience into a single discipline. But most psychologists have probably never heard of, let alone read, the Churchlands' work. The changed attitude of cognitive psychologists to neuroscience has probably grown out of the success of neuroscience in clarifying issues important to cognitive psychologists.

Scientists are, by and large, a pragmatic lot. If they were more introspective, there might not be any need for philosophers of science. But most scientists do their work without much consideration for the hidden assumptions and the philosophical commitments that they make. Each discipline has a set of what are considered important and tractable questions. They are the "hot" issues of the day. A cognitive psychologist interested in memory, for instance, may want to learn why recognition is much better than recall or why visual material is remembered much better than verbal material. Such issues may ultimately be of interest to neuroscientists, but neuroscientists' day-to-day concerns are much more focused. They may want to know what areas of the brain mediate memory or which brain areas are connected to which other areas. Answers to these questions may provide solutions to the cognitive psychologists' questions about memory, but providing these answers is not the neuroscientists' immediate aim. Generally, for both neuroscientists and cognitive psychologists, if a method or idea clarifies an issue of importance to their field, they use it and leave the philosophical implications to someone else.

One area in which the attitudes of cognitive psychologists toward neuroscience have changed markedly is the field of memory. As we shall see, some aspects of the neuroscience of memory have had more of an impact on the cognitive psychology of memory than others, and the nature of the interaction between neuroscience of memory and psychology of memory has changed with time.

Working with cells

Biological models of memory

Memory is the means by which people have access to the past. A large variety of both inanimate and animate objects could be said to have memory to some degree. A spring will return to the same resting place after it is squeezed, a bird will be able to locate hundreds of spots in which it hid food, and a computer can retrieve billions of bits of information on command. Clearly, any biological theory must explain how the brain brings an image of the past to the "footlights of consciousness." A theory must do more than this, however.

Human memory is unlike the memory of a computer, a bird, or a spring. It has properties and works according to principles that make it unique. Unlike a computer, a human being easily forgets past events, and when he or she does remember one, the recollection is often inaccurate. Unlike a bird, human spatial memory cannot retain the hiding places of hundreds of objects. Unlike a spring, the past is not always reproduced exactly, but for many, there is a flexibility and adaptability of human memory that makes the "memory" of a spring almost not a memory at all.

Any model of human memory must explain not only how the past can be reproduced or reconstructed in the present but why human memory has the properties it has. This two-pronged aim is a tall order, one that biological models of human memory have had trouble achieving. A truly reductionistic theory of memory would map a psychological model into a cellular or even biochemical model. By and large, most reductionistic theories of memory claim that the memory trace is spread over the brain. The brain is thought of as a network of connected neurons in which certain neurons more readily activate or inhibit some neurons over others. From this perspective, a memory trace could be represented as a network of weighted connections between neurons (McClelland & Rumelhart, 1986; Rumelhart & McClelland, 1986).

Although many neuroscientists agree that any model of memory must be couched in terms of neuronal potentiation and the strength of connections between neurons, a specific proposal involving biochemical actions at the cellular level has been hard to realize. A single fleeting experience can often be retained for years. I learned of the assassination of John F. Kennedy from an announcement broadcast over a PA system at my school. I was in art class. The announcement lasted only a few seconds, yet this small event has left an indelible and vivid memory (Brown & Kulik, 1977). It is not enough to say that various neuronal connections or potentiations responsible for my present memory were made at the time of the announcement. Neurons are constantly dying, dendritic and axonic connections are constantly in flux, and there is no evidence that neuronal potentiation changes that occur with stimulation last for more than a few hours, let alone for decades (Black, 1986).

Of course, individual connections or potentiations are probably not responsible for a specific memory. Rather, a memory is a result of a complex pattern of connections and potentiations among neurons. A memory may be so multiply encoded in a network that the death of cells or a change in connections may have little effect on the basic configuration of the trace. A full understanding of the nature of the memory trace and how humans remember may rest not in studying neuronal potentiation or dendritic growth, but in studying the state of a network with a trillion trillion connections. When viewed this way, modeling of memory becomes quite daunting.

The awesomeness of this task increases when one realizes that retention is just the beginning of the difficulties for the neuroscientist. As already noted, a biological theory of memory must not only explain retention, it must also account for the kind of retention seen in humans – where emotional material is remembered better than affectless material, where it helps if the material is meaningful, where images are remembered better than words. It is not surprising that cognitive psychologists have devoted little effort to the literature on the biology of memory.

Some neuroscientists have argued that this problem of complexity can be sidestepped, at least to some degree, by studying memory in simpler organisms. Aplysia, for instance, possesses relatively few neurons – about 10,000 (as compared to the 1,000,000,000,000 neurons in the human brain) – and its neurons are quite large, making experimental analysis relatively easy. By examining few but large neurons, one could hopefully see the effects of learning on the neural structure and thereby discover the neural mechanisms of learning. Kandel and his colleagues have doggedly pursued the study of learning in aplysia, with quite satisfactory results (Kandel, 1979). Conditioning aplysia to aversive stimuli, they have been able to trace from initial stimulus to conditioned response the biochemical changes that take place with learning. They offer an elegant model and, at first glance, seem to provide a complete blueprint to the underlying neural mechanism of memory.

Although most cognitive psychologists know of Kandel and his work, it is rarely mentioned in the literature and has had no impact on their theorizing. Klatzky (1980), for instance, does not mention Kandel in her introductory book on memory, and it does not figure in such widely cited theoretical papers as Craik and Lockhart (1972). This neglect is not surprising. First, it is not clear that Kandel's model tells one much about memory. Kandel's model concerns learning – more specifically, associative conditioning, habituation, and sensitization. The principles of learning may underlie those of memory, and one may have to start with the simple before moving to the complex. Nevertheless, cognitive psychologists have long expressed skepticism about the idea that learning has anything to do with memory (Neisser, 1978). Interestingly, some neuropsychological evidence supports this skepticism. Human amnesiacs who have profound memory problems as a result of brain damage can acquire aversive conditioning even though they cannot describe the learning experience (Weiskrantz & Warrington, 1979). This dissociation suggests that a neurological model of learning may not bear directly on the form that a neurological model of memory should take.

There is a second and deeper reason for cognitive psychologists' neglect of work with invertebrates. Even if the model were of memory and not learning, it might be located at the wrong level of discourse. If I wanted to know why one bar of metal breaks under little pressure while another holds fast even under strong pressure, I could consult quantum mechanics and produce reams of equations. This explanation, however, might not be easily understood by even the most sophisticated physicist – who, after all, can easily grasp reams of equations. Fortunately, a much simpler explanation is possible: One bar is rigid, the other is not. The rigidity explanation is the appropriate level at which to address the question. The recourse to quantum mechanics, although correct, does not illuminate the issue. The equations are simply too difficult and too far removed from the issue of concern.

Network models

The issue of levels of discourse has been raised in the recent debate over the new generation of network models of memory. In the 1940s, McCulloch and Pitts (1943) tried to capture neuronal networks in an abstract model consisting of nodes and weighted connections between nodes. The stronger the connection, the larger the weight. The virtue of translating the biological model of connected neurons into a mathematical one is obvious. One may not be able to determine whether memories are represented by the interconnections of neurons, but one can explore whether a network, as defined by nodes, connections, and weights, can serve as a basis for learning and memory. Although early network models were too weak to account for known phenomena of learning (Minsky & Papert, 1969), the current crop of networks models are quite powerful (see McClelland & Rumelhart, 1986; Rumelhart & McClelland, 1986, for discussions of recent work).

In this new generation of models, there are three layers of nodes – input nodes, output nodes, and hidden nodes mediating between the input and output nodes. Orthographic features, for instance, are clamped to the input nodes and phonological features are clamped to the output nodes. Investigators then explore whether the network learns to read after being shown examples of the correspondence between words and the sound patterns of the words. By "learning" I mean that the weights change from a random pattern to a pattern that allows the network to "read" text that it had not encountered before. Recent work by Sejnowski and Rosenberg (1986) suggests that such sophisticated learning is possible.

As long as networks are treated as physiological models, questions about levels of explanation do not arise, but many of the proponents of distributive memory networks want their models to be taken as psychological theories. For instance, McClelland and Rumelhart (1985) argue that distributive memory networks supply a theory of category representation that differs substantively from either the prototype theory or the exemplar theory. An event is not directly recorded in the network; rather, the weights are changed. Exemplars of a category, therefore, are not directly recorded, but have a cumulative effect on the strength of the connections in the network. One cannot point to either the individual exemplars "in" the network or to a prototype of the category. Instead, the category is represented by an abstract pattern of connections.

Although McClelland and Rumelhart argue that their model is an alternative to other psychological models, other investigators (e.g., Broadbent, 1985) have raised the levels issue. They hold that questions concerning the physical mechanism of a psychological entity or process involve a different level of discourse than questions concerning the nonphysical properties of the entity or process. The notions of category, exemplar, and prototype are psychological concepts. It is entirely possible that a category may be represented at a psychological level as a prototype and at a physiological level as weighted connections. McClelland and Rumelhart (1985) may be able to translate their model into already existing psychological terms – no mean feat in itself – but without the psychological terms in the first place, it is unclear whether one would understand the network's psychological import. For instance, one may not be able to predict whether categories have rigid or fuzzy boundaries when represented by weighted connections without first actually running a simulation of the model and "empirically" determining the answer. In the end, why the network produced fuzzy boundaries may be as mysterious as why human categories have fuzzy boundaries.

The role of network models – and, by extension, cellular models – in psychology is far from clear. In expressing his opposition to network models as psychological theories, Broadbent (1985) stated: "It is unfortunate that the level of evidence to which [McClelland and Rumelhart] appeal is from a different level of explanation, and therefore irrelevant to the undoubted merits of the distributed approach" (pp. 191–2). McClelland and Rumelhart (1985b) responded:

It should be said that the decision between our particular formulation and those implicit in the [alternative psychological models] will not be made on the basis of general considerations about what level of theories psychologists should or should not be interested in. Ultimately, the worth of our formulation will be determined by how useful it is at explaining the facts of memory storage and retrieval and to what degree it leads to new and fruitful insights. (p. 196)

Working with brain-damaged patients

The levels issue is often avoided in the study of brain-damaged patients, which may explain in part why neuropsychology (or the study of brain-damaged patients) has attracted more attention from cognitive psychologists than empirical work on cellular theories of memory. Indeed, at least some experimental psychologists have always shown an interest in brain-damaged patients. Bartlett (1932), for instance, cited Henry Head's work on aphasia with respect. Nevertheless, the role that the study of brain-damaged patients may play in cognitive psychology is still evolving. It has grown from an ancillary field of only passing interest to cognitive psychologists into a central subdiscipline. This new role is especially true for the study of patients with organic amnesia but also holds for other areas of interest, such as the study of patients with attentional, perceptual, and motor disorders.

Working for the neurologist

The study of amnesia started to burgeon in the late 1950s with Milner's reports on H.M., who received a bilateral hippocampectomy for the correction of epilepsy (Milner, 1959; Milner, Corkin, & Teuber, 1968). H.M. evidenced a dense anterograde amnesia following surgery. He could remember events that occurred before surgery, could retain new events for 10 to 15 seconds or longer if given an opportunity to rehearse, but could not retain any information for longer periods of time.

At the time when research on H.M. was proceeding, cognitive psychologists were developing a model of memory that serendipitously provided a precise way to describe the problems of H.M. Atkinson and Shiffrin (1968) had separated memory into three distinct components – sensory register, short-term store, and long-term store. Short-term store retained information for about 15 seconds unless control processes, such as rehearsal, continued to refresh the memory. Long-term store could retain information for an indefinite period of time (a few minutes to years). Information flowed from the outside world into the sensory register to short-term store and then finally long-term store. Information had to go through short-term store to get to long-term store. H.M. apparently had intact long-term store, in that presurgical memories could still be retrieved. He also had an intact short-term memory, given his digit span. He could not, however, move information from short-term store to long-term store.

The work on H.M. was originally published in medical journals, such as the *Psychiatric Research Bulletin* (Milner, 1959) and the *Journal of Neurology, Neurosurgery, and Psychiatry* (Scoville & Milner, 1957). At the time, there was no outlet for work on the psychology of brain-damaged patients other than medical journals. Neurology had once consisted mainly of the case studies of brain-damaged patients with careful postmortem examination to determine the location of the lesions. The original work with H.M. fits nicely into this tradition. The surgery supplied a means of specifying the location of the lesion, and the analysis of the behavior provided a means of mapping the behavioral deficit to the brain damage. In the original study, all of the references were to other neurological works. There were no references to experimental or theoretical psychological studies of memory.

At around the time of the first studies of H.M. (the mid-1960s), the field of neuropsychology was losing its institutional home base. Although it was still treated as a subdivision of neurology, neurologists were becoming more interested in the anatomy, physiology, and biochemistry of the brain. Neuropsychology was becoming a poor relative, a less than universally admired subdivision. Neuropsychological studies were still published in medical journals, but fewer pages were allocated. Publishing in experimental psychology journals was not a ready option. The results of neuropsychology experiments might bear on issues of central interest to readers of these journals, but the methodology was quite different. For some bizarre reason, journals are usually aligned with a methodology rather than a set of issues. Despite the success of the research with H.M., editors of experimental psychology journals were not ready to devote scarce journal pages to neuropsychology.

This atmosphere gave birth to *Neuropsychologia,* the first journal devoted solely to neuropsychological work. Something magical happens when a subdiscipline gains its own journal. It acquires its own mouthpiece and begins to develop an identity of its own. Interestingly, the founders of the journal must have realized that their main constituents, apart from neuropsychologists themselves, were cognitive psychologists because they included on their editorial board scholars such as Noam Chomsky and Jean Piaget.

At this time, neuropsychology was still not incorporated into cognitive psychology. The work with H.M. and other amnesiacs did not go unnoticed, but it was treated lightly. Even though Craik and Lockhart (1972) claimed that Milner's work with H.M. provided "persuasive" evidence for a component model of memory, they did not bother to address this source of evidence when arguing against the model. Klatzky (1980), in her popular text on memory, devotes only two paragraphs to work with amnesiacs.

Cognitive psychologists clearly felt more comfortable writing about laboratory experiments than about experiments with brain-damaged patients and did not feel compelled to account for neuropsychological results if they contradicted their theoretical position. Nevertheless, they could not help seeing the relevance of this evidence to the debate over whether memory was unitary or multicompartmental. Thus, the fleeting references. Familiarity breeds contentment, however.

Working for the cognitive psychologist

Those psychologists who study brain-damaged patients do so because they believe that a breakdown in functioning proceeds in an organized fashion with brain damage, revealing the components and processes of the mind. The work on H.M. supported this conjecture because it showed an orderly breakdown in cognitive functioning – orderly at least in terms of the contemporaneous memory models of cognitive psychology. Its success brought new life to the study of amnesia.

Milner's background was in traditional experimental psychology; the next stage in amnesia research was led in America by a cognitive psychologist, Laird Cermak, teamed with a clinical neuropsychologist, Nelson Butters; in Britain it was led by a trio consisting of a neuropsychologist, Elizabeth Warrington, a physiological psychologist, Larry Weiskrantz, and a cognitive psychologist, Alan Baddeley. These researchers dominated the field of amnesia research during the 1970s (see Hirst, 1982, for a review). The study of brain-damaged patients was beginning to attract researchers trained in cognitive psychology.

Milner's original work was mainly concerned with behavioral description and brain–behavior correlations. The newer group of researchers took a more ambivalent course. They clearly wanted to describe the nature of amnesia and to play the traditional role of neuropsychologist serving the neurologist, but they also wanted the study of amnesia to bear on the problems of cognitive psychology. The amnesia research of the 1970s ingeniously combined these two goals. Investigators used the theories of cognitive psychology to guide their descriptions of amnesia, and, in turn, used the descriptions to test the validity of cognitive theories. Unlike Milner's work, cognitive psychology was woven into every stage of their research program.

With *Neuropsychologia* and a critical mass of researchers working in the field, the study of amnesia burgeoned during the 1970s. Although cognitive psychology informed most of this work, few of the experimental reports found their way into experimental psychology journals. The field of cognitive psychology was receptive to varying methodologies. For instance, the journal *Cognitive Psychology* devoted an entire issue to a computer program that understood fairly sophisticated natural language. Nevertheless, in 1975, of the 175 articles published in the cognitive psychology journals *Journal of Experimental Psychology, Cognitive Psychology,* and *Journal of Verbal Learning and Verbal Behavior,* none were on human amnesia.

Even though their research reports were not published in cognitive psychology journals, the experimental findings were unquestionably relevant to cognitive psychological modeling. The issues that amnesia experts addressed cannot be thoroughly reviewed here. Amnesia did not have to be as complete as Milner's characterization of H.M. led one to believe. H.M. may not be able to remember anything after it occurs, but other amnesiacs show some retention. This mild retention allowed neuropsychologists to probe more deeply into the nature of memory disruption with brain damage than the dense amnesia of H.M. allowed. There appeared to be better recognition than recall, increased proactive interference, and some responsiveness to cueing (Hirst, 1982).

For Warrington and Weiskrantz (1970), this characterization suggested a retrieval failure. Borrowing from interference theory, they argued that amnesiacs have trouble selecting the desired memory from among competing memories. Anything that could bypass this response competition, such as a recognition probe, could improve amnesiac memory.

Cermak and Butters (1980), on the other hand, posited an encoding failure. Building on the levels of processing approach of Craik and Lockhart (1972), they argued that amnesiacs could not benefit from deep processing. Consequently, new events were encoded shallowly and remembered poorly. The amnesiac syndrome was a consequence of this shallow encoding.

Each set of researchers devised ingenious experiments to support its position. If Butters and Cermak's characterization had turned out to be correct, amnesia would have provided an example par excellence of the consequences of shallow encoding. The study of amnesia would have shifted the weight of support offered by the work on amnesia away from the component model of memory (Atkinson & Shiffrin, 1968) to the unified model of memory posited by Craik and Lockhart (1972). Thus, amnesia research would have removed a major obstacle blocking an unqualified acceptance of the levels of processing approach.

If Warrington and Weiskrantz's position had turned out to be correct, amnesia research would have focused attention on the role of interference in memory retrieval. Cognitive psychologists occasionally try to revive this neglected aspect of memory (Baddeley, 1976), and a retrieval approach to amnesia could have renewed interest in interference theory.

I have argued elsewhere that neither approach to amnesia proved satisfactory (Hirst, 1982). Nevertheless, the flurry of work in the 1970s provided a strong foundation for future research on amnesia and demonstrated that a healthy inter-action between cognitive psychology and neuropsychology could exist.

Working as a cognitive scientist

Up to this point (the late 1970s), the study of amnesia had ridden on cognitive psychology's coattails. Students of amnesia used the work of Atkinson and Shif-frin to lend precision to their clinical descriptions, and they borrowed from the levels of processing model of memory or from interference theory to generate hypotheses about the amnesia deficit. This research seemed more concerned with verifying existing memory theories developed by cognitive psychologists than with theory development per se. This situation changed in the 1980s. The central empirical findings of this recent research are easily stated.

First, amnesiacs appear to learn motor and perceptual-motor skills at the same rate as normals, even though they may not remember the episode involving the training. Cohen and Squire (1980), for instance, trained amnesiacs to read mirror images of words. Words were either ones that subjects had never seen before or repetitions of previous words. Cohen and Squire found that the speed with which a new word was read increased for amnesiacs at the same rate as it did for normals, but that the normals' reading speed improved at a faster rate than did the amnesiacs' when the words were repetitions. That is, amnesiacs showed no deficit when they had to learn a general skill for which memory of a previous episode played little role. On the other hand, they showed a marked deficit when memory for a previous episode played a significant role, as it might for the repetitions.

The second important finding involved priming. In a priming experiment, sub-jects are usually exposed to words using a cover task and then all given another task in which the previous words figure. For instance, subjects might first be exposed to "staple" and later asked to complete the stem "sta—" with the first word that comes to mind. The prior exposure is said to prime the completion if subjects complete the stem with the old word more often than they complete a control stem with an unseen word. In a variety of studies using many different priming tasks, the priming observed in amnesiacs is as strong as it is in normals, even though recognition or recall is severely depressed. Most interestingly, if amnesiacs are asked to recall, for example, the word that they had previously studied that began with "sta," they are less likely to say "staple" than if asked merely to complete the stem "sta" with the first word that comes to mind (see Schacter, 1986, for a review).

Although the findings of normal skill learning and normal priming in amnesiacs may allow two separate explanations, most researchers have tried to account for the findings with a single explanation. A distinction is posited – X versus Y – and one argues that amnesia detrimentally affects X while leaving Y intact. Some of the distinctions, like many a good idea, are borrowed from other fields, such as the distinction between procedural and declarative knowledge in Artificial Intelligence (Winston, 1977). Other distinctions have been developed specifically to handle a set of findings – for example the distinctions between implicit and explicit memory (Schacter, 1986) or between memory with and without awareness (Jacoby & Witherspoon, 1982). At present, it is unclear which of these alternatives is best. Amnesia may leave procedural memory, implicit memory, memory without awareness, or some combination of these intact while disrupting declarative memory, explicit memory, memory with awareness, or some combination of these.

This work differs from previous work on amnesiacs in that it does not verify extant cognitive theories of memory. Rather, this study of amnesia has produced a body of data that cannot be readily accounted for by cognitive psychologists. It is forcing cognitive psychologists to expand the theories of memory and to posit components of the memory system of which they have heretofore been unaware.

The more recent finding that amnesiac recognition is relatively preserved when compared with amnesiac recall also provides some insight into the architecture of memory (Hirst, Johnson, Kim, Phelps, Risse, & Volpe, 1986). The component of memory disrupted with amnesia – be it called "episodic memory," "declarative memory," "explicit memory," or my preference, "direct memory" – could be envisioned as a global unit or module that can be disrupted uniformly. Direct memory would be treated somewhat as it is treated in faculty psychology: as a single unit that can vary in capacity as a unit. Consistent with the single-unit approach is what I call the "voltage theory" of amnesia. According to this theory, direct memory is uniformly disrupted with amnesia. The architecture and processing of memory remain intact, but the voltage has been turned down – everything is a bit dim. For instance, memory traces may be weakened with amnesia but maintain their normal structure and function. The voltage theory is consistent with the single-unit approach because it assumes that disruption can affect memory as a whole. Although amnesia may be a matter of degree, the degree is quantified over direct memory as a whole, rather than over some specific aspect of direct memory.

On the other hand, direct memory may not be a single unit but rather a composite of processes and components, any one of which may be separately disrupted. Some acts of direct memory may be easier for amnesiacs to perform than others because they rely on intact structures and processes of memory, whereas other memory acts may be more difficult because they depend on disrupted mnemonic structures and processes.

The finding that amnesiac recognition is relatively preserved when compared with amnesiac recall argues against treating memory as a whole and supports the view that memory is a composite of separate, independent processes. Specifically, the result suggests that one or more mnemonic processes more important to recall than recognition may be disrupted, whereas other mnemonic processes more important to recognition than recall may be preserved. It is not clear how to label these components in a more precise or elegant fashion, but once again, the study of amnesia is pushing theories of memory to posit components and processes of memory that current theories do not readily supply. Clearly, evidence from the study of amnesia provides a basis for constructing the architecture of the memory system. Other psychological evidence also guides such theory development, but presently, neuropsychological evidence stands on equal footing with these other more traditional sources of data.

The study of amnesia has now moved from a field ancillary to cognitive psychology – really, a subdiscipline of medicine that occasionally offered support for psychological theorizing – to one gathering primary data that shape and structure cognitive psychological theory. It is not surprising, then, that studies of amnesia rarely appeared in cognitive psychology journals when the study of amnesia was in its infancy but are now quite common. In a recent issue of the *Journal of Experimental Psychology: Learning, Memory, and Cognition,* the chief outlet for studies of the psychology of memory, three out of fifteen articles were on amnesia (1986, No. 3).

But what of . . . ?

I remember sitting many years ago in a seminar that Mike Gazzaniga and George Miller had assembled to encourage dialogue between brain scientists and psychologists. Somehow the question of drug treatment of depression came up, and one of the neurologists there, schooled in the neuroscience of the brain, wondered why drugs for depression did not immediately relieve the depression once administered. After all, they immediately corrected the neurotransmitter imbalance that was assumed to be the root of the problem. The neurologist was sincerely puzzled. George squirmed in frustration. "What of learning?" he gently suggested. The neurologist just looked at him. He knew that George was a leading scholar, and even more, a wise man. But what of learning? The neurologist later confided to me that he hadn't the foggiest idea what George was talking about. He did not realize that people learn to cope with problems of daily life and that the coping strategies they develop can become habitual, resistant to change. A neurotransmitter imbalance may initiate the depressive episode, but a biochemical correction of this imbalance will do nothing to correct the attitudes, strategies, and behavioral patterns the person learned as a result of the imbalance. The neurologist could not get beyond the cells to consider the psychological dimension.

Clearly, the dialogue between neuroscience and cognitive psychology has a long way to go. The recent interest in neuropsychology as a legitimate methodology for framing and exploring issues of cognitive psychology is encouraging. The same uphill battle about more cellular models must still be fought, if not now, then when more evidence from the neuroscientists' laboratory has accumulated. Ultimately, cognitive psychology's acceptance of neuroscience may rest on neuroscience's delivering the stuff. Perhaps Miller's and Gazzaniga's envisioned cognitive neuroscience will flourish. The ground seems more fertile than ever.

References

Atkinson, R. C., & Shiffrin, R. M. (1968). Human memory: A proposed system and its control processes. In K. W. Spence & J. T. Spence (Eds.), *The Psychology of Learning and Motivation,* Vol. 2. New York: Academic Press.

Baddeley, A. D. (1976). *The Psychology of Memory.* New York: Basic Books.

Bartlett, F. C. (1932). *Remembering.* Cambridge: Cambridge University Press.

Black, I. (1986). Commentary. In G. Lynch (Ed.), *Synapses, Circuits, and the Beginnings of Memory.* Cambridge, Mass.: MIT Press.

Broadbent, D. (1985). The question of levels: Comment on McClelland and Rumelhart. *Journal of Experimental Psychology: General, 114,* 189–93.

Brown, R. & Kulik, J. (1977). Flashbulb memories. *Cognition, 5,* 73–99.

Butters, N., & Cermak, L. S. (1980). *Alcoholic Korsakoff's Syndrome.* New York: Academic Press.

Churchland, P. M. (1984). *Matter and consciousness.* Cambridge, Mass.: MIT Press.

Churchland, P. S. (1986). *Neurophilosophy.* Cambridge, Mass.: MIT Press.

Cohen, N. J., & Squire, L. R. (1980). Preserved learning and retention of pattern analyzing skills in amnesia: Dissociation of knowing how and knowing that. *Science, 210,* 207–10.

Craik, F. I. M., & Lockhart, R. S. (1972). Levels of processing: A framework for memory research. *Journal of Verbal Learning and Verbal Behavior, 11,* 671–84.

Fodor, J. A. (1983). *The Modularity of Mind.* Cambridge, Mass.: MIT Press.

Hebb, D. O. (1949). *The Organization of Behavior.* New York: Wiley.

256   WILLIAM HIRST

Hirst, W. (1982). The amnesic syndrome: Descriptions and explanations. *Psychological Bulletin*, *91*, 435–60.

Hirst, W., Johnson, M. K., Kim, J. K., Phelps, E. A., Risse, G., & Volpe, B. T. (1986). Recognition and recall in amnesics. *Journal of Experimental Psychology: Learning, Memory, and Cognition*, *12*, 445–51.

Jacoby, L. L., & Witherspoon, D. (1982). Remembering without awareness. *Canadian Journal of Psychology*, *36*, 300–24.

Kandel, E. R. (1979). Small systems of neurons. *Scientific American*, *241*, No. 3, 66–87.

Klatzky, R. L. (1980). *Human Memory*. San Francisco: Freeman.

LeDoux, J. E., & Hirst, W. (1986). *Mind and Brain: Dialogues in Cognitive Neuroscience*. New York: Cambridge University Press.

Lynch, G. (1986). *Synapses, Circuits, and the Beginnings of Memory*. Cambridge, Mass.: MIT Press.

McClelland, J. L., & Rumelhart, D. E. (1985). Distributed memory and the representation of general and specific information. *Journal of Experimental Psychology: General*, *114*, 159–88.

McClelland, J. L., Rumelhart, D. E., & the PDP Research Group (1986). *Parallel Distributed Processing: Psychological and Biological Models*, Vol. 2. Cambridge, Mass.: MIT Press.

McCulloch, W. S., & Pitts, W. (1943). A logical calculus of the ideas immanent in neural nets. *Bulletin of Mathematical Biophysics*, *5*, 115–37.

Milner, B. (1959). The memory defect in bilateral hippocampal lesions. *Psychiatric Research Reports*, *11*, 43–52.

Milner, B., Corkin, S., & Teuber, H.-L. (1968). Further analysis of the hippocampal amnesic syndrome: A 14-year follow-up study of H.M. *Neuropsychologia*, *6*, 215–34.

Minsky, M., & Papert, S. (1969). *Perceptions*. Cambridge, Mass.: MIT Press.

Neisser, U. (1967). *Cognitive Psychology*. New York: Appleton-Century-Crofts.

Neisser, U. (1978). Memory: What are the important questions? In M. M. Gruneberg, P. E. Morris, & R. N. Sykes (Eds.), *Practical Aspects of Memory*. London: Academic Press.

Putnam, H. (1975). *Mind, Language, and Reality*, Vol. 2. Cambridge: Cambridge University Press.

Rumelhart, D. E., & McClelland, J. E. (1986). Levels indeed! A response to Broadbent. *Journal of Experimental Psychology: General*, *114*, 193–7.

Rumelhart, D. E., McClelland, J. E., & the PDP Research Group (1986). *Parallel Distributed Processing: Foundations*, Vol. 1. Cambridge, Mass.: MIT Press.

Schacter, D. L. (1986). The psychology of memory. In J. E. LeDoux & W. Hirst (Eds.), *Mind and Brain: Dialogues in Cognitive Neuroscience*. New York: Cambridge University Press.

Scoville, W. B., & Milner, B. (1957). Loss of recent memory after bilateral hippocampal lesions. *Journal of Neurology, Neurosurgery, and Psychiatry*, *20*, 11–21.

Sejnowski, T. J., & Rosenberg, C. R. (1986). *NETtalk: A Parallel Network That Learns to Read Aloud*. (Tech. Rep. No. JHU/EECS-86/01). Baltimore, Md.: Johns Hopkins University, Department of Electrical Engineering and Computer Science.

Simon, H. A. (1969). *The Science of the Artificial*. Cambridge, Mass.: MIT Press.

Warrington, E. K., & Weiskrantz, L. (1970). Amnesic syndrome: Consolidation or retrieval? *Nature*, *228*, 628–30.

Weiskrantz, L., & Warrington, E. K. (1979). Conditioning in amnesic patients. *Neuropsychologia*, *17*, 187–94.

Winston, P. H. (1977). *Artificial Intelligence*. Reading, Mass.: Addison-Wesley.

PART VI   Cognitive science

If George began studying cognitive science twenty years ago without knowing what to call it, he knew what to call it by 1980, when he moved from The Rockefeller University to Princeton University. In 1986, with the support of the McDonnell Foundation, he and Gil Harman formed a Program for Cognitive Science as well as a Laboratory of Cognitive Science at Princeton. They were not alone in this endeavor. Throughout the country, cognitive science centers, laboratories, and programs were sprouting. In some cases, Psychology Departments were dissolved and Cognitive Science Departments appeared in their place. All of this activity suggests that cognitive science may have come of age. Harman tells the Princeton story.

18   Cognitive science?

Gilbert Harman

A couple of years ago, the Princeton University psychology department conducted two searches, one for a cognitive psychologist, the other for a cognitive
scientist. The purpose of the latter search was to bring to Princeton someone who
would normally be a member of a computer science department rather than a
psychology department. George Miller was interested in having computational
linguistics at Princeton, and it had become clear that the Princeton computer
scientists had no plans to support this area. George and I were the search committee for the position in cognitive science. After much effort we decided on a
candidate, Y, and asked the Dean of the Faculty to prepare a formal offer. The
Dean was surprised. "This position has already been filled." No, the position
for a cognitive psychologist has been filled, not the position for a cognitive scientist. "I authorized only one position." You said we could hire a cognitive
psychologist and you also said we could hire a cognitive scientist. "What's the
difference? The second time, I was just confirming the one appointment."

After this was straightened out, we approached Y, who, it emerged, was unwilling to come to Princeton without at least a half-time appointment in the
computer science department. The computer scientists at Princeton are not interested in cognitive science, so that was that.

Like the Dean of the Faculty, the Princeton computer scientists consider computational linguistics and other aspects of artificial intelligence to be part of cognitive psychology rather than computer science. However, most people who pursue artificial intelligence expect to be in a computer science department and will
not come to Princeton if they are restricted to the psychology department. Furthermore, there is considerable student demand among computer science majors
for courses in artificial intelligence. Although the computer scientists at Princeton react to that student demand with the sort of dismay that I feel in reaction to
student demand for courses in semiotics or objectivism, they have agreed in
principle to include someone in artificial intelligence in the computer science
department. However, whenever we suggest someone to them, they claim the

258

person suggested is really a psychologist rather than a computer scientist (Heller, 1961).

Now, in contrast with the view of the Dean of the Faculty at Princeton and that of the Princeton computer science department, it is customary to take cognitive science as extending beyond cognitive psychology to include parts of linguistics, philosophy, computer science, anthropology, and biology. But what is "cognitive science"?

There is a temptation to identify cognitive science with the scientific study of cognition, but that is too restrictive. For one thing, although the study of language is at the center of cognitive science, it is controversial to what extent the study of language is part of the study of *cognition*. Chomsky (1965) takes linguistics to be concerned with linguistic *knowledge,* but not all linguists agree. It is better to say that cognitive science consists in the scientific study of language and the scientific study of cognition.

But even that definition is too restrictive, since it is controversial to what extent the philosophy parts of cognitive science are *scientific* studies of anything, and, similarly, many of the computer science parts might be classified as more *engineering* than *science.*

At Princeton we have just instituted a Committee for Cognitive *Studies,* echoing the name of Bruner and Miller's Center for Cognitive Studies at Harvard. This Committee is an instructional entity that helps students plan courses of study in this area. We also started a Cognitive *Science* Laboratory, which is for research. When you study it, that's one thing; when you do it, it's science.

Language

Language is the central topic in cognitive science. This is partly because language *reflects* cognition by serving as the main means of the expression of thought, so that a study of language is an indirect study of cognition. It is also possible that language *influences* cognition by influencing what concepts a person has and what thoughts will occur to him or her.

There is also a historical and more practical reason for the centrality of the study of language. Noam Chomsky's linguistics played an important role in ushering in the new "cognitive psychology" of the 1950s and 1960s. And the study of language inspired by Chomsky has proved to offer the right sort of difficulty. It is hard, but not so hard that progress is impossible. We have learned a great deal about language, and there is still a great deal to be learned. It remains possible to do good, productive research on language, for example, as described in Miller and Johnson-Laird (1976) or in Chomsky (1981).

But what kind of research? There are quite different paradigms in psychology, linguistics, philosophy, and artificial intelligence.

Psychology favors research that culminates in good controlled experiments. These experiments are supposed to yield outcomes that are "statistically significant," which means you sometimes have to repeat an experiment twenty times or more before you get an acceptable result. A typical psychological experiment might measure subjects' reaction times in certain tasks in order to judge what factors influence the subjects' performance.

An account of aspects of language or linguistic structure will be acceptable as part of psychology only to the extent that the linguistic account can figure in the design of controlled psychological experiments. In the early 1960s, when there was thought to be some reason to hope that the grammatical structure of a sentence reflected the psychological processes involved in the construction of the sentence by speakers or in the understanding of the sentence by hearers, psychologists like George Miller could take linguistics to be part of psychology, as Chomsky claimed it was (Chomsky, 1959; Miller, 1962; Miller & Isard, 1963). But Chomsky's stress (1965) on what he called the "competence–performance distinction" amounted to a denial that linguistic theories could be tested in that way. So now psychologists do not take Chomsky's generative grammar to be part of psychology.

Clearly, when Chomsky (e.g., 1986) says that linguistics is part of psychology, he does not mean that it fits in with the experimental paradigm that is characteristic of contemporary psychology. Chomsky means that the *subject matter* of linguistics is psychological or mental, since Chomsky takes this subject matter to concern the mental representation of the grammar of a particular (idealized) person's language.

In Chomskean linguistics, there is no privileged category of *evidence* in the way that there is in psychology. The linguist starts with certain information about language – these words are nouns, those are verbs, this phrase is the subject and that phrase is the predicate of such and such a sentence, this pronoun can take that noun phrase as antecedent, this sentence is ungrammatical, children learn language in a couple of years of exposure, and so forth. Theories are developed to explain this information. A plausible theory occasionally leads to the rejection of something that was initially accepted by providing a reason to think initial appearances were misleading. But nothing is especially privileged. In particular, it is not true that linguistic theories are tested only against speakers' intuitions about grammaticality. Many other intuitions are relevant, and intuitions about grammaticality are sometimes rejected as conflicting with theory.

Philosophical logic, philosophy of language, and philosophical semantics resemble this sort of linguistics in lacking a commitment to the experimental paradigm that is important in psychology. Philosophers, like linguists, do not do experiments. But philosophers are like psychologists in tending to be more concerned than linguists are with the *use* of language, for example, as in H. P. Grice's theory of conversational implication (Grice, 1975).

On the whole, philosophers are concerned with arriving at a conception of how the pieces all fit together. They are less concerned with arriving at a full, detailed theory themselves, except in special cases. They are concerned with what it is for something to be meaningful, for someone to mean something. They are concerned with the *source* of meaning: Is language meaningful because it is used to express contentful thought? If so, what gives thought its content? And so forth. Philosophers are more concerned with such general issues than with the details of the syntax and semantics of English or some other natural language.

Of course, philosophers are sometimes concerned with the details about certain words that play an important role in philosophical theory, words like "know," "true," "real," "good," and "ought." Many philosophers are concerned with what they call the "logical forms" of statements, that is, with those aspects of the forms of statements that are relevant to the logical properties of the statements. (The logical properties of statements are those properties that determine what logical, i.e., formal, implications the statements have, what other statements logically imply about them, what statements are logically incompatible with them, and so forth.)

Why are philosophers interested in these details? For several overlapping reasons. First, the soundness of certain philosophical arguments may depend on logic and on the meaning of certain key terms used in those arguments. People who disagree about these details may disagree about the soundness of the arguments. To take an oversimplified example, someone might argue for fatalism by saying, "If something is going to happen, then, necessarily, it is going to happen." In assessing that argument, it is useful to distinguish two different possible interpretations of that remark, depending (as we say) on whether "necessarily" has wide or narrow scope: *trivial interpretation*: it is necessary that (if P then P); *fatalistic interpretation*: if P, then it is necessary that (P).

Second, logic is part of philosophy, so philosophers can be interested in details of logical form because they are interested in the details of logic.

Third, philosophers are sometimes interested in logical form because they think that the logical forms of sentences can be a clue to the "ontological commitments" of speakers. Does the best account of the logical forms of statements of ordinary language reveal a commitment to events, to times and places, to properties, to possibilities? If so, then that commitment is part of the metaphysics of common sense.

I won't say much about computational linguistics in this connection, except that it, like philosophy and psychology, and unlike just plain linguistics, is concerned with the use of language, and there is a paradigmatic task: writing computer programs that do the job (parse the sentences, produce summaries, generate explanations, etc.). Many computational linguists, like most psychologists, tend to think that Chomsky's grammatical investigations are irrelevant and not a good approach to language.

Chomsky returns the compliment. The issue here is not just that there is a difference in paradigms. Each side takes its paradigm to be the more promising one for resolving issues about language, issues the one side feels are not even appreciated by the other side. The computational linguists do not see how GB theory ("Government and Binding Theory," Chomsky, 1981) can help with parsing or story understanding or the production of explanations. Psychologists do not see how the theory can lead to interesting experiments. Nevertheless, Chomsky argues that it is necessary to specify the structure of linguistic representation before there will be any possibility of understanding how language is used. Although my own sympathies are largely with Chomsky on this issue, I think he exaggerates the point. It is possible to understand many things about linguistic usage before the final syntax is laid down. Grice's theory of conversational implicature (Grice, 1975) was achieved in total ignorance of generative grammar. Various developments in philosophical semantics and in philosophical studies of logical form have influenced the theory of binding in current GB theory.

Actually, the situation is more complex. At least one computational linguist takes Chomskean theory to be directly relevant to parsing (March, 1980). Some linguists think that syntactic theory must relate more closely to the use of language and to computationally acceptable models.

Linguistics is embattled from a number of different directions. So it is, perhaps, not surprising that there has never been a department of linguistics at Princeton. Instead, we have had an interdepartmental program with members from language departments and from philosophy, psychology, sociology, and anthropology. The members from the language departments have tended to be ignorant of and skeptical of generative grammar, and this has made it difficult to build a proper curriculum in linguistics. Matters came to a head a couple of years ago when Bob Ebert resigned his chairmanship of the linguistics program and the university had to decide whether to abandon the program or continue it, either as a program in the scientific study of language or with a more "humanistic" approach via "semiotics." At the same time, George Miller and I were trying to get our program in cognitive science under way, so a decision was made to go with scientific linguistics. But it was a close call.

Cognition

Cognition includes inference, perception, memory, and learning. Psychologists are interested in how people do it, in what goes on when someone remembers something or perceives something. Philosophers have traditionally been interested in the "normative" question of when belief that results from inference, perception, memory, or learning is justified belief. Yet sometimes things seem to go the other way.

Kahneman and Tversky and their associates have studied errors in reasoning (Kahneman, Slovic, & Tversky, 1982), and Nisbett and Ross (1980) made specific proposals for improving people's reasoning. A number of philosophers who have studied this research have argued that the alleged fallacies that people make are in fact perfectly reasonable inferences in the actual situation (e.g., Cohen, 1981). I once heard Kahneman complain that philosophers are always accusing each other of fallacious reasoning but react to these psychological studies in ways that seem to imply that people never reason fallaciously.

Philosophers have this reaction in part because of a strategy that is often used for dealing with philosophical skepticism. The skeptic argues, for example, that the inference from sensory experience to conclusions about the environment is not logically conclusive, since the same experience might be the result of clever stimulation of a brain in a vat. One reply to the skeptic turns this argument on its head: Since we are justified on the basis of our sensory experience in reaching conclusions about the environment, it is possible to be justified in beliefs that are the result of inferences that are not logically conclusive.

The skeptical psychologist makes some assumptions about what inferences are justified and uses those assumptions to criticize ordinary reasoning. Some philosophers turn this around by assuming that ordinary reasoning is justified and using that assumption to criticize the psychologist's assumptions about the principles of justified reasoning.

I myself would add that it is also important not to confuse principles of logic (or principles of probability theory) with principles of inference or reasoning. These are very different sorts of things. Logic is the theory of formal or logical relations among sentences or propositions, indicating when a proposition formally implies or is implied by others and when a proposition formally contradicts others. Reasoning is a process of change in view. Principles of logic are not particularly about what beliefs a person should adopt under what conditions, nor is it easy to find any very close relation between principles of logic and principles of reasoning. I think that one reason why Kahneman et al. are so sure that they know what the correct normative principles are for belief is that they confuse these principles with the principles of logic and probability theory. It is pretty clear what are the correct principles of logic and probability theory in this sort of context; but these are not at all the sort of things that could be principles of inference or reasoning (Harman, 1986; Goldman, 1986). Ordinary people probably know very little about logic and even less about probability theory.

There are, by the way, probabilistic models of inference in which people react to new evidence by changing their old probabilities to new ones via probabilistic conditionalization (e.g., Jeffrey, 1983). But these models are not suitable for ordinary finite beings, since they are useful only if one already knows the appropriate conditional probabilities ahead of time, and the number of probabilities needed is an exponential function of the number of possible pieces of evidence one might get (Harman, 1986, chap. 3).

Shortly after Nisbett and Ross (1980) appeared, Nancy Cantor offered a seminar at Princeton on it. In a resulting review (Miller & Cantor, 1982), she and George Miller argued that ordinary people are not always trying to emulate scientists. They are often trying to reach satisfactory decisions that will not prove socially embarrassing if they should prove to be mistaken. I have wondered whether there is a difference between philosophers and psychologists in this respect. During Nancy's seminar, an interesting point of contrast between psychologists and philosophers emerged, with the philosophers being more willing than the psychologists to abandon ordinary procedures. This transpired when we discussed the extensive psychological research concerning the unreliability of interviews (summarized, e.g., in Zedeck, Tziner, & Middlestadt, 1983). The psychologists present agreed that the data are overwhelming that you actually lose information if you interview candidates for a fellowship or a job, since people are extremely bad at extracting information from interviews but think they are extremely good at it. So, interviewers end up attaching too much importance to unreliable evidence, which dilutes whatever good evidence they might have. I remarked that such considerations have led the philosophy department at Princeton to refrain from interviewing candidates for positions in the department. George reported that the psychologists do interview candidates, despite all of the evidence against doing so, and he remains in favor of it. To me, this was carrying a defense of ordinary reasoning too far. But the other psychologists all agreed with George, and indeed I have met only two psychologists who have told me that they agree with a no-interview policy, namely, Amos Tversky and Richard Nisbett.

Paradigms

People speak of a single subject or area of cognitive science because they find themselves doing research that overlaps work done by others who are in different university departments and who have different backgrounds and training. People with one kind of background find themselves talking to and interacting with people with other backgrounds, going to conferences with them, doing research with them, and teaching with them. For example, in 1985, George taught a course with a linguist (Bob Freidin) on language learning. The year before that, George and I teamed up with a computer scientist (Rich Cullingford) to teach an introductory course in the use of computers in cognitive science for faculty and students in philosophy and psychology. (I must confess that Rich did almost all the teaching in this course.) Of course, there are all sorts of interdisciplinary interactions, not just those that comprise cognitive science. But the area we call "cognitive science" does form a significant pattern of interaction.

At Princeton, this interaction has been informal until recently, except for an interdepartmental program in linguistics that has existed since the early 1960s. The linguistics program has always featured representatives from psychology and philosophy, in addition to the language departments. George and a philosopher (Scott Soames) have given semantics courses in this program, and in the 1960s I taught generative syntax as a philosophy course. Syntax is currently being taught by a linguist (Freidin) who is a member of the philosophy department because, in the absence of a linguistics department, this seemed to be the safest place for him.

Over the years at Princeton, we have had informal discussion groups in topics in cognitive science, attended by local psychologists, linguists, philosophers, and members of various other disciplines. One year, when Andrew Ortony was visiting, we discussed metaphor and analogy (taking off from the essays in Ortony, 1979). Another year we talked about Kahneman, Slovic, and Tversky (1982). One year we discussed a number of recent books – Fodor (1983), Stich (1983), Barwise and Perry (1983), and so forth.

More recently, things have become more formal, with the formation of a faculty Committee for Cognitive Studies and the Cognitive Science Laboratory. Rich Cullingford, who was visiting Princeton while working on his book (1986), helped us persuade the university to buy a Pyramid minicomputer and then did most of the teaching in the course in the use of computers in cognitive science that I have already mentioned. (We named our computer "mind," which dismayed the computer science department, whose computers have names like "tilt," "panic," and "thrash." They rejected our suggestion that their Pyramid computer be named "body.")

The university also agreed to find space for the Cognitive Science Lab and found money to bring in a series of outside speakers in cognitive studies. The speaker series meets every week now, so we have less time for the more informal discussions that we used to enjoy so much. The lab was originally planned to be located in a three-story house on Prospect Street. But because we saw ourselves using a lot of electronic equipment, especially work stations of various sorts, we became worried about handling the ongoing electrical wiring. Eventually, we rented a more modern space on Nassau Street that had previously been used by an architectural firm. Soon after we moved in this space became fairly well filled, and we have already expanded into a second floor.

While we were waiting (for over a year) to move into the lab, we found that we had already achieved a certain unity and identity simply by being on the same computer, with electronic mail to keep us in touch with each other. We tried to do all our work on the computer, so we were usually quickly available to the others. And whenever any of us were puzzled about anything, he or she would immediately send off mail about the problem and the rest of us would try to figure out the answer. Participants in this exercise acquired a certain identity based on their login name, the name used in sending them mail. Rich Cullingford was "rec," his initials. George started out as "gam" but then changed his personality to "geo."

Rich Cullingford went on to Georgia Tech (leading us to refer to him as the rambling rec), leaving George and me to run the show at Princeton. Fortunately, he left behind his student, Marie Bienkowski. Other members of the lab in its first year included Brian Reiser, a cognitive scientist in the Psychology Department, who writes his psychological theories in LISP; Steve Hanson, of Bell Communications Research in Morristown, New Jersey, who does computer statistical analysis (a.k.a. connectionism); Paul Thagard, a philosopher turned cognitive scientist who writes programs that simulate inference to the best explanation; and a number of students in philosophy, psychology, and computer science.

I quickly discovered that the main part of cognitive science is the preparation of grant proposals, an activity that is quite rare in philosophy. In the fall, George, Brian, and I took turns, producing a new proposal every week or so. So, we were ready when President William G. Bowen asked us for a short description of our research. Shortly after we gave him the description, we found out why he had asked. George got a call from Bob Jahn, then Dean of the School of Engineering. Although Jahn's main research field is jet propulsion, he has also gotten involved in an investigation of extrasensory perception (esp) and psychic phenomena – "engineering anomalies," to use his phrase. This research had been supported by the McDonnell Foundation. The foundation was interested in our cognitive science research and wanted to know if the support they were already giving to Jahn's engineering anomalies might be expanded to cover such enterprises as our cognitive science lab. We were initially leery of this idea. But we talked to Jahn and visited his laboratory, which contains several devices producing random events that a subject can try to influence. Since these devices allow the random events to occur very often, it is possible to run a huge number of trials, which can then be subjected to intensive statistical analysis. Neither George nor I is particularly sympathetic to the idea of investigating esp, but we agreed that if one was going to investigate it, Jahn's way of approaching it was a good one. George suggested that we might try to work out a proposal for a project on "mind–machine interactions." George has himself been interested in the organization and use of a computer-based dictionary with interactive video discs. We decided to go ahead. Ultimately, we teamed up to form the Human Information Processing Group, concerned with human–machine interactions with Jahn; Alain Kornhauser, who works in robotics and computer graphics; and Joel Cooper, who studies the use of computers in education. The McDonnell Foundation liked the idea and has promised us several years of support.

Now I am getting to a point that worries me. What people in cognitive science have in common is a research interest in some aspect of language or cognition. However, they differ in their ideas about what the relevant issues are and how they should be addressed. Their research paradigms are often very different.

I have already mentioned several examples of differences of paradigm for studying language or cognition. Here is another example. George was one of the early advocates of the computer model of mind and of stating psychological theories in the form of computer programs or flow charts (Miller, Galanter, & Pribram, 1960). For psychologists, the computer model promised a new kind of psychology, a new way to come up with theories that could be tested experimentally. Philosophers tended to stress a related aspect of this sort of model: It offers a solution to the mind–body problem that is compatible with a purely physical world while avoiding behaviorism. In both philosophy and psychology there is a rejection of something called "behaviorism," but this means something different in the two cases.

Psychologists discuss whether such a model can work and what the details of the model might be. Philosophers tend to suppose that it can be made to work and go on to ask whether it must nevertheless have left something crucial out, namely, consciousness, understanding, the subjective feel of experience, what it is like to see something red. For some philosophers that is a central issue, whereas psychologists may feel that they are not trying to address that issue at all.

This sort of difference in paradigm can cause trouble. Each person is inclined to think that his or her standards and interests are the right ones and that Z's work is worthless because it falls outside the relevant paradigm, that is, it misses the main point, fails to address the central issue, and commits several obvious fallacies. We would not think of dismissing work in high-energy physics in this way because it did not speak to our immediate concerns. The apparently common subject matter encourages us to make these judgments about other approaches in cognitive science.

The problem of different paradigms is not merely internal to cognitive science. It also shows up on the edges when traditional linguists reject generative grammar in favor of semiotics and when mainline computer scientists dismiss artificial intelligence as professional hocum. It shows up when people argue that esp research or semiotics is hopelessly misguided or worse.

I do not say that we shouldn't make these judgments. I make them myself, especially about semiotics! Surely, we are sometimes right when we dismiss another approach as missing the main point, committing a fallacy, being involved with empty trivialities, and so forth. But let us hope that people are not always right when they reach such dismissive conclusions, or else we will have to dismiss everything in cognitive science.

References

Barwise, J. & Perry, J. (1983). *Situations and Attitudes*. Cambridge, Mass.: MIT Press.

Chomsky, N. (1959). Review of B. F. Skinner's *Verbal Behavior*. *Language 35*, 26–58.

Chomsky, N. (1965). *Aspects of the Theory of Syntax*. Cambridge, Mass.: MIT Press.

Chomsky, N. (1981). *Lectures on Government and Binding*. Dordrecht: Foris.

Chomsky, N. (1986). *Knowledge of Language: Its Origins, Nature, and Use*. New York: Praeger.

Cohen, L. J. (1981). Can human irrationality be experimentally demonstrated? *Behavioral and Brain Sciences, 4,* 317–31.

Cullingford, R. E. (1986). *Natural Language Processing: A Knowledge Engineering Approach*. Totowa, N.J.: Rowman and Littlefield.

Davidson, D., & Harman, G. (1975). *The Logic of Grammar*. Encino, Calif.: Dickenson.

Fodor, J. A. (1983). *Modularity of Mind*. Cambridge, Mass.: MIT Press.

Goldman, A. I. (1986). *Epistemology and Cognition*. Cambridge, Mass.: Harvard University Press.

Grice, H. P. (1975). Logic and conversation. In D. Davidson and G. Harman (Eds.), *The Logic of Grammar*. Encino, Calif.: Dickenson, pp. 64–75.

Harman, G. (1986). *Change in View*. Cambridge, Mass.: MIT Press.

Heller, J. (1961). *Catch 22*. New York: Simon & Schuster.

Jeffrey, R. C. (1983). *The Logic of Decision,* 2nd ed. Chicago: University of Chicago Press.

Kahneman, D., Slovic, P., & Tversky, A. (Eds.). (1982). *Judgement under Uncertainty: Heuristics and Biases*. Cambridge, England: Cambridge University Press.

Marcus, M. (1980). *A Theory of Syntactic Recognition for Natural Language*. Cambridge, Mass.: MIT Press.

Miller, G. A. (1962). Some psychological studies of grammar. *American Psychologist, 7,* 748–62.

Miller, G. A., & Cantor, N. (1982). Critical review of Nisbett and Ross (1980). *Social Cognition 1,* 83–93.

Miller, G. A., Galanter, E., & Pribram, K. (1960). *Plans and the Structure of Behavior*. New York: Holt, Rinehart, and Winston.

Miller, G. A., & Isard, S. (1963). Some perceptual consequences of linguistic rules. *Journal of Verbal Learning and Verbal Behavior, 2,* 217–28.

Miller, G. A., & Johnson-Laird, P. N. (1976). *Language and Perception*. Cambridge, Mass.: Harvard University Press.

Nisbett, R., & Ross, L. (1980). *Human Inference: Strategies and Shortcomings of Social Judgement*. Englewood Cliffs, N.J.: Prentice-Hall.

Ortony, A. (Ed.). (1979). *Metaphor and Thought*. New York: Cambridge University Press.

Stich, S. (1983). *From Folk Psychology to Cognitive Science: The Case Against Belief*. Cambridge, Mass.: MIT Press.

Zedeck, S., Tziner, A., & Middlestadt, S. E. (1983). Interviewer validity and reliability: An individual analysis approach. *Personnel Psychology, 36,* 355–70.

Biographical information

GEORGE A(RMITAGE) MILLER

Personal

Born February 3, 1920, Charleston, W. Va. Married, two children.

Education

B.A., University of Alabama, 1940; M.A., University of Alabama, 1941; A.M., Harvard University, 1944; Ph.D., Harvard University, 1946.

Professional experience

1982–James S. McDonnell Distinguished University Professor of Psychology
1979–Professor of Psychology, Princeton University
1979–82 Adjunct Professor, The Rockefeller University
1968–79 Professor, The Rockefeller University
1976–9 Visiting Professor, Massachusetts Institute of Technology
1972–6, 1982–3 Visitor, Institute for Advanced Study, Princeton
1967–8 Visiting Professor, The Rockefeller University
1958–68 Professor of Psychology, Harvard University
1964–7 Chairman, Department of Psychology, Harvard University
1963–4 Fulbright Research Professor, Oxford University
1960–7 Co-Director, Center for Cognitive Studies, Harvard University
1958–9 Member, Center for Advanced Study in the Behavioral Sciences, Stanford, California
1955–8 Associate Professor of Psychology, Harvard University
1951–5 Associate Professor of Psychology, Massachusetts Institute of Technology
1948–51 Assistant Professor of Psychology, Harvard University
1946–8 Research Associate, Psychoacoustic Laboratory, Harvard University

269

1943–6 Research Assistant, Psychoacoustic Laboratory, Harvard University
1941–3 Instructor in Psychology, University of Alabama

Honors

1986 Guggenheim Fellow
1985 Foreign Member, Royal Netherlands Academy of Arts and Sciences
1984 Honorary Doctor of Science, University of Sussex
1982 New York Academy of Sciences, Award in Behavioral Sciences
1981–2 Editor, *Psychological Bulletin*
1981 Sesquicentennial Professor, University of Alabama
1981 Chairman, Section J (Psychology), American Association for the Advancement of Science
1980 Doctor of Science, Honoris Causa, Columbia University
1979 Honorary Doctor of Social Science, Yale University
1976 Doctorat Honoris Causa, Universite Catholique de Louvain
1976 Distinguished Service Award, American Speech and Hearing Association
1972 Warren Medal, Society of Experimental Psychologists
1971 Member, American Philosophical Society
1969 President, American Psychological Association
1963 Distinguished Scientific Contribution Award, American Psychological Association
1962 Member, National Academy of Sciences
1962 President, Eastern Psychological Association
1957 Member, American Academy of Arts and Sciences
1952 Member, Society of Experimental Psychologists
1950–5 Associate Editor, *Journal of the Acoustical Society of America*
1947–50 Consulting Editor, *Journal of Experimental Psychology*
1945 Member, Sigma Xi

Publications

GEORGE A. MILLER

Viek, P., & Miller, G. A. (1944). The cage as a factor in hoarding. *Journal of Comparative Psychology, 37*, 203–10.

Miller, G. A., & Viek, P. (1944). An analysis of the rat's responses to unfamiliar aspects of the hoarding situation. *Journal of Comparative Psychology, 37*, 221–31.

Miller, G. A., & Garner, W. R. (1944). Effects of random presentation on the psychometric function: Implications for a quantal theory of discrimination. *American Journal of Psychology, 57*, 451–67.

Garner, W. R., & Miller, G. A. (1944). Differential sensitivity to intensity as a function of the duration of the comparison tone. *Journal of Experimental Psychology, 34*, 450–63.

Postman, L., & Miller, G. A. (1945). Anchoring of temporal judgments. *American Journal of Psychology, 38*, 209–12.

Miller, G. A. (1945). Concerning the goal of hoarding behavior in the rat. *Journal of Comparative Psychology, 38*, 209–12.

Miller, G. A., & Postman, L. (1946). Individual and group hoarding in rats. *American Journal of Psychology, 59*, 652–68.

Miller, G. A., Wiener, F. M., & Stevens, S. S. (1946). *Combat Instrumentation. II. Transmission and Reception of Sounds under Combat Conditions.* Summary Technical Report of NDRC Division 17.3. Washington, D.C.

Miller, G. A., & Mitchell, S. (1947). Effects of distortion on the intelligibility of speech at high altitudes. *Journal of the Acoustical Society of America, 19*, 120–9.

Miller, G. A. (1947). The masking of speech. *Psychological Bulletin, 44*, 105–29.

Miller, G. A. (1947). Population, distance, and the circulation of information. *American Journal of Psychology, 60*, 276–84.

Garner, W. R., & Miller, G. A. (1947). The masked threshold of pure tones as a function of duration. *Journal of Experimental Psychology, 37*, 293–303.

Miller, G. A. (1947). Sensitivity to changes in the intensity of white noise and its relation to masking and loudness. *Journal of the Acoustical Society of America, 19*, 606–19.

Brogden, W. J., & Miller, G. A. (1947). Physiological noise generated under earphone cushions. *Journal of the Acoustical Society of America, 19*, 620–3.

Rosenblith, W. A., Miller, G. A., Egan, J. P., Hirsh, I. J., & Thomas, G. J. (1947). An auditory afterimage? *Science, 106*, 333–4.

Stevens, S. S., Egan, J. P., & Miller, G. A. (1947). Methods of measuring speech spectra. *Journal of the Acoustical Society of America, 19*, 771–80.

Miller, G. A. (1948). The perception of short bursts of noise. *Journal of the Acoustical Society of America, 20*, 160–70.

Miller, G. A., & Taylor, W. G. (1948). The perception of repeated bursts of noise. *Journal of the Acoustical Society of America, 20*, 171–82.

271

Miller, G. A., & Garner, W. R. (1948). The masking of tones by repeated bursts of noise. *Journal of the Acoustical Society of America, 20,* 691–6.

Miller, G. A. (1949). Voice communications: Effects of masking and distortion. In *Human Factors in Undersea Warfare.* Washington, D.C.: National Research Council, pp. 243–8.

Miller, G. A., & Frick, F. C. (1949). Statistical behavioristics and sequences of responses. *Psychological Review, 56,* 311–25.

Miller, G. A., & Selfridge, J. A. (1950). Verbal context and the recall of meaningful material. *American Journal of Psychology, 63,* 176–85.

Miller, G. A., & Licklider, J. C. R. (1950). The intelligibility of interrupted speech. *Journal of the Acoustical Society of America, 22,* 167–73.

Miller, G. A., & Viek, P. (1950). Hoarding in the rat as a function of the length of the path. *Journal of Comparative and Physiological Psychology, 43,* 66–9.

Miller, G. A., Rosenblith, W. A., Galambos, R., Hirsh, I. J., & Hirsh, S. K. *A Bibliography in Audition.* Cambridge, Mass.: Harvard University Press, 1950.

Miller, G. A., & Heise, G. A. (1950). The trill threshold. *Journal of the Acoustical Society of America, 22,* 720–5.

Miller, G. A. (1951). Speech and language. In S. S. Stevens (Ed.), *Handbook of Experimental Psychology.* New York: Wiley, pp. 769–810.

Licklider, J. C. R., & Miller, G. A. (1951). The perception of speech. In S. S. Stevens (Ed.), *Handbook of Experimental Psychology.* New York: Wiley, pp. 1040–74.

Frick, F. C., & Miller, G. A. (1951). A statistical description of operant conditioning. *American Journal of Psychology, 64,* 20–36.

Heise, G. A., & Miller, G. A. (1951). An experimental study of auditory patterns. *American Journal of Psychology, 64,* 68–77.

Miller, G. A., Heise, G. A., & Lichten, W. (1951). The intelligibility of speech as a function of the context of the test materials. *Journal of Experimental Psychology, 41,* 329–35.

Heise, G. A., & Miller, G. A. (1951). Problem solving by small groups using various communication nets. *Journal of Abnormal and Social Psychology, 46,* 327–35.

Miller, G. A. (1951). *Language and Communication.* New York: McGraw-Hill.

Miller, G. A. (1952). Finite Markov processes in psychology. *Psychometrika, 17,* 149–67.

Miller, G. A., & McGill, W. J. (1952). A statistical description of verbal learning. *Psychometrika, 17,* 369–96.

Miller, G. A. (1953). What is information measurement? *American Psychologist, 8,* 3–11.

Miller, G. A. (1953). Information theory and the study of speech. In *Current Trends in Information Theory.* Pittsburgh: University of Pittsburgh Press, pp. 119–39.

Miller, G. A. (1954). Communication. *Annual Review of Psychology, 5,* 401–20.

Miller, G. A., Bruner, J. S., & Postman, L. (1954). Familiarity of letter sequences and tachistoscopic identification. *Journal of General Psychology, 50,* 129–39.

Miller, G. A. (1954). Psycholinguistics. In G. Lindzey (Ed.), *Handbook of Social Psychology.* Reading, Mass.: Addison-Wesley, pp. 693–708.

Miller, G. A. (1955). Note on the bias of information estimates. In H. Quastler (Ed.), *Information Theory in Psychology: Problems and Methods.* Glencoe, Ill.: Free Press.

Miller, G. A., & Nicely, P. E. (1955). An analysis of perceptual confusions among some English consonants. *27,* 338–52.

Bruner, J. S., Miller, G. A., & Zimmerman, C. (1955). Discriminative skill and discriminative matching in perceptual recognition. *Journal of Experimental Psychology, 49,* 187–92.

Miller, G. A. (1956). The magical number seven, plus or minus two: Some limits on our capacity for processing information. *Psychological Review, 63,* 81–97.

Miller, G. A. (1956). Information and memory. *Scientific American, 195* (2), 42–6.

Miller, G. A. (1956). Human memory and the storage of information. *IRE Transactions on Information Theory, IT-2,* 129–37.

Miller, G. A. (1956). The perception of speech. In M. Halle, H. G. Lunt, H. McLean, & C. H. Van Schooneveld (Eds.), *For Roman Jakobson*. The Hague: Mouton, pp. 353–60.

Miller, G. A. (1956). The human link in communication systems. *Proceedings of the National Electronics Conference, 12*, 395–400.

Miller, G. A., & Beebe-Center, J. G. (1956). Some psychological methods for evaluating the quality of translations. *Mechanical Translation, 3*, 73–80.

Nicely, P. E., & Miller, G. A. (1957). Some effects of unequal spatial distribution on the detectability of radar targets, *Journal of Experimental Psychology, 53*, 195–8.

Miller, G. A. (1957). Some effects of intermittent silence. *American Journal of Psychology, 70*, 311–13.

Miller, G. A., & Friedman, E. A. (1957). The reconstruction of mutilated English texts. *Information and Control, 1*, 38–55.

Miller, G. A. (1957). A note on the remarkable memory of man. *IRE Transactions on Electronic Computers, EC-6, #3*.

Miller, G. A. (1957). Applications of mathematics in social psychological research. *Social Science Research Council Items, 11*, 41–4.

Miller, G. A. (1957). Communication and information as limiting factors in group formation. In *Symposium on Preventive and Social Psychiatry*. Washington, D.C.: Walter Reed Army Institute of Research, Walter Reed Army Medical Center, pp. 15–17.

Chomsky, N., & Miller, G. A. (1958). Finite state languages. *Information and Control, 1*, 91–112.

Miller, G. A., & Newman, E. B. (1958). Tests of a statistical explanation of the rank-frequency distribution for words in written English. *American Journal of Psychology, 71*, 209–18.

Miller, G. A. (1958). Morale and communication. In I. Galdston & H. Zetterberg (Eds.), *Panic and Morale: Conference Transactions*. New York: International Universities Press, pp. 10–56.

Miller, G. A. (1958). Speech and communication. *Journal of the Acoustical Society of America, 30*, 485–91.

Miller, G. A. (1958). Free recall of redundant strings of letters. *Journal of Experimental Psychology, 56*, 485–91.

Miller, G. A., Newman, E. B., & Friedman, E. A. (1958). Length-frequency statistics for written English. *Information and Control, 1*, 370–89.

Miller, G. A., Galanter, E., & Pribram, K. (1960). *Plans and the Structure of Behavior*. New York: Holt.

Galanter, E., & Miller, G. A. (1960). Some comments on stochastic models and psychological theories. In K. J. Arrow, S. Karlin, & P. Suppes (Eds.), *Mathematical Methods in the Social Sciences, 1959*. Stanford, Calif.: Stanford University Press, pp. 277–97.

Miller, G. A. (1961). The study of intelligent behavior. In *Proceedings of a Harvard Symposium on Digital Computers and their Applications*. Cambridge, Mass.: Harvard University Press.

Miller, G. A. (1961). Thinking, cognition, and learning. *Voice of America Forum Lectures*. Behavioral Science Series No. 12. New York: Van Nostrand Reinhold.

Miller, G. A. (1962). Decision units in the perception of speech. *IRE Transactions on Information Theory, 1962, IT-8*, 81–3.

Miller, G. A. (1962). Some psychological studies of grammar. *American Psychologist, 7*, 748–62.

Miller, G. A. (1962). *Psychology: The Science of Mental Life*. New York: Harper & Row.

Miller, G. A. (1963). Ronal Aylmer Fisher: 1890–1962. *American Journal of Psychology, 76*, 157–8.

Miller, G. A., & Isard, S. (1963). Some perceptual consequences of linguistic rules. *Journal of Verbal Learning and Verbal Behavior, 2*, 217–28.

Miller, G. A. (1963). Comments on Professor Postman's paper. In C. N. Cofer & B. Musgrave (Eds.), *Verbal Behavior and Learning*. New York: McGraw-Hill, pp. 321–9.

Chomsky, N., & Miller, G. A. (1963). Introduction to the formal analysis of natural languages. In

D. Luce, R. Bush, & E. Galanter (Eds.), *Handbook of Mathematical Psychology*, Vol. 2. New York: Wiley, pp. 269–321.

Miller, G. A., & Chomsky, N. (1963). Finitary models of language users. In D. Luce, R. Bush, & E. Galanter (Eds.), *Handbook of Mathematical Psychology*, Vol. 2. New York: Wiley, pp. 419–91.

Marks, L. E., & Miller, G. A. (1964). The role of semantic and syntactic constraints in the memorization of English sentences. *Journal of Verbal Learning and Verbal Behavior, 3,* 1–5.

Miller, G. A. (1964). The psycholinguists: On the new scientists of language. *Encounter, 23* (1), 29–37.

Miller, G. A. (1964). Communication and the structure of behavior. In *Disorders of Communication*. Research Publications of the Association for Research in Nervous and Mental Disorders, *42,* 29–40.

Miller, G. A. (1964). Language and psychology. In E. H. Lenneberg (Ed.), *New Directions in the Study of Language*. Cambridge, Mass.: MIT Press, pp. 89–107.

Miller, G. A., & Isard, S. (1964). Free-recall of self-embedded English sentences. *Information and Control, 1,* 292–303.

Mehler, J., & Miller, G. A. (1964). Retroactive interference in the recall of simple sentences. *British Journal of Psychology, 55,* 295–301.

Miller, G. A. (Ed.). (1964). *Mathematics and Psychology*. New York: Wiley.

Miller, G. A., & McKean, K. O. (1964). Chronometric study of some relations between sentences. *Quarterly Journal of Experimental Psychology, 16,* 297–303.

Miller, G. A. (1964). Man–computer interaction. In *Communication Processes*. Proceedings of a symposium in Washington, 1963. Oxford: Pergamon.

Miller, G. A. (1965). Psychology. In A. Love & J. S. Childers (Eds.), *Listen to Leaders in Science*. New York: Holt, Rinehart & Winston, chap. 14.

Miller, G. A. (1965). Computers, communication, and cognition. *Advancement of Science*, pp. 417–30.

Miller, G. A. (1965). Some preliminaries to psycholinguistics. *American Psychologist, 20,* 15–20.

Miller, G. A., Norman, D., & Bregman, A. (1965). The computer as a general purpose device for the control of psychological experiments. In B. Waxman & R. W. Stacy (Eds.), *Computers in Biomedical Research*. New York: Academic Press, pp. 467–90.

Smith, F., & Miller, G. A. (Eds.). (1966). *The Genesis of Language: A Psycholinguistic Approach*. Cambridge, Mass.: MIT Press.

Miller, G. A. (1967). *Psychology of Communication: Seven Essays*. New York: Basic Books.

Miller, G. A. (1967). Some psychological perspectives on the year 2000. *Daedalus, 96,* 883–96.

Miller, G. A. (1967). Biological origins of human speech. *IEEE International Convention Record,* 177–8.

Miller, G. A. (1967). Psycholinguistic approaches to the study of communication. In D. L. Arm (Ed.), *Journeys in Science: Small Steps – Great Strides*. Albuquerque, N.M.: University of New Mexico Press, pp. 22–73.

Anglin, J. M., & Miller, G. A. (1968). The role of phrase structure in the recall of meaningful verbal material. *Psychonomic Science, 10,* 343–44.

Miller, G. A. (1968). Psychology and information. *American Documentation, 19,* 286–9.

Miller, G. A. (1968). Encoding the unexpected. *Proceedings of the Royal Society, B. 171,* 361–75.

Miller, G. A., & McNeill, D. (1969). Psycholinguistics. In G. Lindzey and E. Aaronson (Eds.), *The Handbook of Social Psychology*, 2nd ed., Vol. 3. Reading, Mass.: Addison-Wesley, pp. 666–794.

Miller, G. A. (1969). Sprache und Denken. In O. W. Haseloff (Ed.), *Kommunikation*. Berlin: Colloquium Verlage Otto H. Hess, pp. 71–82.

Miller, G. A. (1969). A psychological method to investigate verbal concepts. *Journal of Mathematical Psychology, 6,* 169–91.

Miller, G. A. (1969). The organization of lexical memory: Are word associations sufficient? In G. A. Talland & N. C. Waugh (Eds.), *The Pathology of Memory*. New York: Academic Press, pp. 223–36.

Miller, G. A. (1969). Psychology as a means of promoting human welfare. *American Psychologist, 24*, 1063–75.

Clark, K. E., & Miller, G. A. (Eds.). (1970). *Psychology*. Englewood Cliffs, N.J.: Prentice-Hall.

Miller, G. A. (1970). Four philosophical problems of psycholinguistics. *Philosophy of Science, 37*, 183–99.

Miller, G. A. (1970). Assessment of psychotechnology. *American Psychologist, 25*, 991–1001.

Healy, A. F., & Miller, G. A. (1970). The verb as the main determinant of sentence meaning. *Psychonomic Science, 20*. 372.

Healy, A. F., & Miller, G. A. (1971). The relative contribution of nouns and verbs to sentence acceptability and comprehensibility. *Psychonomic Science, 24* (2), 94–6.

Miller, G. A. (1972). Lexical memory. *Proceedings of the American Philosophical Society, 16* (2), 140–4.

Miller, G. A. (1972). English verbs of motion: A case study in semantics and lexical memory. In A. W. Melton & E. Martin (Eds.), *Coding Processes in Human Memory*. Washington, D.C.: Winston, pp. 335–72.

Miller, G. A. (1972). Linguistic communication as a biological process. In J. W. S. Pringle (Ed.), *Biology and the Human Sciences*. Oxford: Oxford University Press, pp. 70–94.

Miller, G. A., & Buckhout, R. (1973). *Psychology: The Science of Mental Life*, 2nd ed. New York: Harper & Row.

Miller, G. A. (ed.). (1973). *Communication, Language, and Meaning*. New York: Basic Books.

Miller, G. A. (1974). Needed: A better theory of cognitive organization. *IEEE Transactions on Systems, Man, and Cybernetics, SMC-4*, 95–7.

Miller, G. A. (ed.). (1974). *Linguistic Communication: Perspectives for Research*. Report of the Study Group on Linguistic Communication to the National Institute of Education. Newark, Del.: International Reading Association.

Miller, G. A. (1974). Psychology, language, and levels of communication. In A. Silverstein (Ed.), *Human Communication: Theoretical Explorations*. Hillsdale, N.J.: Erlbaum, pp. 1–17.

Miller, G. A. (1974). Listen and hear. In H. R. Moskowitz, B. Scharf, & J. C. Stevens (Eds.), *Sensation and Measurement: Papers in Honor of S. S. Stevens*. Holland: D. Reidel, pp. 129–35.

Miller, G. A. (1974). Stanley Smith Stevens: 1906–1973. *American Journal of Psychology, 87*, 279–88.

Miller, G. A. (1974). Toward a third metaphor for psycholinguistics. In W. B. Weimer & D. S. Palermo (Eds.), *Cognition and the Symbolic Processes*. Hillsdale, N.J.: Erlbaum, pp. 397–413.

Miller, G. A. (1974). Human communication. In E. H. Kone & H. J. Jorday (Eds.), *The Greatest Adventure: Basic Research That Shapes Our Lives*. New York: Rockefeller University Press, pp. 254–65.

Miller, G. A. (1975). Some comments on competence and performance. *Annals of the New York Academy of Sciences, 263*, 201–4.

Miller, G. A. (1975). Stanley Smith Stevens: 1906–1973. *National Academy of Sciences Biographical Memoirs, 47*, 425–60.

Miller, G. A. (1975). Language development and education. In W. Kessen (Ed.), *Childhood in China*. New Haven, Conn.: Yale University Press, 175–84.

Miller, G. A., & Johnson-Laird, P. N. (1976). *Language and Perception*. Cambridge, Mass.: Harvard University Press.

Miller, G. A. (1977). Problems of communication. *Daedalus, 106* (4), 113–25.

Miller, G. A. (1977). *Spontaneous Apprentices: Children and Language*. New York: Seabury Press.

Halle, M., Bresnan, J., & Miller, G. A. (eds.). (1978). *Linguistic Theory and Psychological Reality*. Cambridge, Mass.: MIT Press.

Miller, G. A. (1978). Semantic relations among words. In M. Halle, J. Bresnan, & G. A. Miller (Eds.), *Linguistic Theory and Psychological Reality*. Cambridge, Mass.: MIT Press, pp. 60–118.

Miller, G. A. (1978). Practical and lexical knowledge. In E. Rosch & B. B. Lloyd (Eds.), *Cognition and Categorization*. Hillsdale, N.J.: Erlbaum, pp. 305–19.

Miller, G. A. (1978). On knowing the right word. *The National Elementary Principal, 57* (4), 36–40.

Miller, G. A. (1978). Reconsideration: Whorf's "Language, Thought and Reality." *Human Nature, 1* (6), 92–6.

Miller, G. A. (1978). Lexical meaning. In J. F. Kavanagh & W. Strange (Eds.), *Speech and Language in the Laboratory, School, and Clinic*. Cambridge, Mass.: MIT Press, pp. 394–436.

Miller, G. A. (1978). Some psychological implications of the verbs of motion. *Psychologica Belgica, 18* (1), 75–86.

Miller, G. A. (1978). The acquisition of word meaning. *Child Development, 49*, 999–1004.

Miller, G. A., & Lenneberg, E. (Eds.). (1978). *Psychology and Biology of Language and Thought: Essay in Honor of Eric Lenneberg*. New York: Academic Press.

Miller, G. A. (1978). Introduction. In G. A. Miller & E. Lenneberg (Eds.), *Psychology and Biology of Language and Thought: Essays in Honor of Eric Lenneberg*. New York: Academic Press, pp. 1–12.

Miller, G. A. (1978). Pastness. In G. A. Miller & E. Lenneberg (Eds.), *Psychology and Biology of Language and Thought: Essays in Honor of Eric Lenneberg*. New York: Academic Press, pp. 167–85.

Miller, G. A. (1978). Construction and selection in the mental representation of text. In J. Costermans (Ed.), *Structures cognitives et organisation du langage*. Cahirs de l'institut de linguistique de Louvain (CILL), *5* (1–2), 185–97.

Miller, G. A. (1978). Automated dictionaries. In J. M. Mays, A. S. Melmed, & S. Scribner (Eds.), *Testing, Teaching, and Learning: Report of a Conference on Research in Testing*. Washington, D.C.: National Institute of Education, U.S. Department of Health, Education, and Welfare, pp. 146–50.

Miller, G. A. (1979). Images and models, similes and metaphors. In A. Ortony (Ed.), *Metaphor and Thought*. New York: Cambridge University Press.

Miller, G. A., & Miller, K. J. (1979). Critical notice: John Lyons on semantics. *Quarterly Journal of Experimental Psychology, 31*, 711–35.

Miller, G. A. (1979). *Automated Dictionaries, Reading and Writing*, Chairman's report of a conference on educational uses of word processors with dictionaries, June 14–15, 1979. Washington, D.C.: National Institute of Education, December 1979.

Miller, G. A. (1980). Computerword: A non-Orwellian view. *The National Elementary Principal, 59* (2), 50–3.

Miller, G. A. (1980). Foreword to *Social Foundations of Cognition and Language: Essays in Honor of Jerome S. Bruner*. New York: Norton.

Miller, G. A. (1981). *Language and Speech*. New York: Freeman.

Miller, G. A., & Kwilosz, D. M. (1981). Interaction of modality and negation in English. In A. K. Joshi, B. L. Webber, & I. A. Sag (Eds.), *Elements of Discourse Understanding*. New York: Cambridge University Press, pp. 201–16.

Miller, G. A. (1981). Trends and debates in cognitive psychology. *Cognition, 10*, 215–25.

Miller, G. A. (1982). Some problems in the theory of demonstrative reference. In R. J. Jarvella & W. Klein (Eds.), *Speech, Place, and Action*. New York: Wiley, pp. 61–72.

Miller, G. A., & Cantor, N. (1982). Critical review of Nisbett and Ross, *Human Inference: Strategies and Shortcomings of Social Judgment*. *Social Cognition, 1*, 83–93.

Miller, G. A. (1983). Is scientific thinking different? *Bulletin of the American Academy of Arts and Sciences, 36* (5), 26–37.

Miller, G. A. (1983). The background of modern psychology. In J. Miller (Ed.), *States of Mind: Conversations with Psychological Investigators.* New York: Pantheon, pp. 12–29.

Miller, G. A. (1983). Introduction to *William James, The Principles of Psychology.* Cambridge, Mass.: Harvard University Press.

Miller, G. A. (1983). Informavores. In F. Machlup & U. Mansfield (Eds.), *The Study of Information: Interdisciplinary Messages.* New York: Wiley, pp. 111–13.

Miller, G. A. (1983). Thought, language, and communication. In F. Machlup & U. Mansfield (Eds.), *The Study of Information: Interdisciplinary Messages.* New York: Wiley, pp. 319–20.

Miller, G. A. (1983). Information theory in psychology. In F. Machlup & U. Mansfield (Eds.), *The Study of Information: Interdisciplinary Messages.* New York: Wiley, pp. 493–6.

Jorgensen, J., Miller, G. A., & Sperber, D. (1984). A test of the mention theory of irony. *Journal of Experimental Psychology: General, 113,* 112–20.

Miller, G. A., & Gazzaniga, M. S. (1984). The cognitive sciences. In M. Gazzaniga (Ed.), *Handbook of Cognitive Neuroscience.* New York: Plenum, pp. 3–11.

Miller, G. A. (1984). The test. *Science 84, 5* (9), 55–7.

Miller, G. A. (1984). Normal, pathological, and other states of mind. Review of A. W. Ellis, *Normality and Pathology in Cognitive Functions. Cognitive Neuropsychology, 1,* 267–77.

Miller, G. A. (1984). Some comments on the subjective lexicon. In D. Schiffrin (Ed.), *Meaning, Form, and Use in Context: Linguistic Applications.* Proceedings of the 35th Annual Georgetown University Round Table on Languages and Linguistics, 1984. Washington, D.C.: Georgetown University Press, pp. 303–12.

Miller, G. A. (1985). Dictionaries of the mind. *Proceedings, 23rd Annual Meeting of the Association for Computational Linguistics,* July 8–12, 1985. Chicago: University of Chicago Press, pp. 305–14.

Miller, G. A. (1985). The constitutive problem of psychology. In S. Koch & D. E. Leary (Eds.), *A Century of Psychology as Science.* New York: McGraw-Hill, pp. 40–5.

Miller, G. A., & Gildea, P. M. (1985). How to misread a dictionary. *AILA Bulletin, 2,* 13–26.

Miller, G. A. (1986). Dismembering cognition. In S. H. Hulse & B. F. Green, Jr. (Eds.), *One Hundred Years of Psychological Research in America: G. Stanley Hall and the Johns Hopkins Tradition.* Baltimore: Johns Hopkins University Press, pp. 277–98.

Name index

Alexander, C., 94
Allen, W., 90
Allport, G., 95
Almond, G., 95
Arabie, P., 48, 66
Argyle, M., 37
Attneave, F., 29

Baddeley, A., 250
Bartlett, F., 85, 248
Bateman, H., 17
Bauer, R., 95
Beebe-Center, J., 37
Berkeley, G., 224
Berlyne, D., 95
Bever, T., 101, 157
Birkhoff, G., 10
Black, F., 97
Bloomfield, L., 114–5
Blumenthal, A., 148–9
Boring, E., 5, 90, 93, 103
Boulding, K., 38
Bregman, A., 94, 103–4
Brooks, L., 84
Brown, R., 47, 94–5, 98, 102
Bruner, J., 11, 28, 47, 72, 85, 89, 90, 95, 100–2, 104, 108, 197
Buehler, K., 102
Bundy, M., 91–2
Burke, C., 11
Bush, R. R., 10
Bush, R., 10–11, 16, 39, 47
Butters, N., 250–2

Cantor, N., 264
Carey, S., 94
Carroll, J., 48, 94
Carson, D., 27
Cermak, L., 250–2
Chang, J., 48, 65

Chase, S., 77
Chomsky, N., 47, 82, 85–6, 91, 94–7, 100–4, 120–1, 143–7, 150, 198, 259–62
Churchland, P., 243
Clark, E., 199–201
Cohen, N., 252–3
Conklin, H., 97
Craik, F., 102, 251
Cummings, E., 95
Cunningham, J., 48

D'Arcais, I., 98
de Groot, A., 106
Deknatel, F., 95
Diene, Z., 94–5

Egan, J., 7
Estes, W., 11

Faverge, J., 23–4
Fechner, G., 3
Feller, W., 10
Festinger, L., 38
Fitts, P., 30
Flottorp, G., 7
Fodor, J., 101, 158–60, 242–3
Frake, C., 97
Frege, G., 210, 214
French, D., 94–5
Freud, S., 85
Frick, F., 7, 21–4, 32, 82, 95
Friedman, E., 27

Galambos, R., 7
Galanter, E., 1, 85
Gardner, H., 92
Gardner, J., 91
Garner, W., 1, 7, 10, 22, 24, 27, 29–30
Gazzaniga, M., 242, 254–5
Gerstenhaber, M., 37
Gibbon, E., 17

279

Gibson, J., 33, 86
Goodman, N., 37, 91, 94
Graham, C., 74
Grassman, G., 3
Green, B., 47
Green, D., 47
Greenfield, P., 94
Guillaume, P., 102

Hake, H., 22
Harris, K., 11
Harris, Z., 116, 120
Hartley, D., 37
Hartley, R., 21
Heinemann, E., 77–8
Held, R., 95
Helmholtz, H., 3, 75
Henry, J., 95
Hick, W., 25
Hirsh, I., 7
Hochberg, J., 29
Hovland, C., 48
Hughes, H., 94–5
Hull, C., 115
Hyman, R., 25

Ingres, J., 97
Inhelder, B., 94

Jaffe, J., 94
Jakobson, R., 94–5
James, W., 4, 76, 107–8
Jenkins, H., 83
Jenkins, J., 37–8
Johnson, S., 48
Johnson-Laird, P., 198–9, 259

Kahnemann, D., 98, 263–4
Kandel, E., 246
Katz, J., 101
Kennedy, R., 94
Koffka, K., 82
Kohler, W., 82–3
Kolers, P., 94, 103
Kruskal, J., 48, 66
Kuhn, T., 40–1

Lacan, J., 97
Lashley, K., 41–3, 243
Lawrence, D., 38
Leeper, R., 74
Lenneberg, E., 95–7, 154, 157, 243
Leonard, J., 25
Lettvin, J., 106
Levelt, P., 98
Levelt, W., 89, 100–2, 109
Licklider, J., 7, 16, 83

Lieberman, D., 236
Lockhart, R., 251
Luce, D., 47
Luria, A., 102
Lynch, K., 95

Mackay, D., 237
Mackworth, N., 94
Maclane, S., 10
Mandelbrot, B., 94
Mandler, G., 72
Markman, E., 199–202
Marr, D., 190, 240, 247
Maslow, A., 86
Maturnana, H., 106
Mayr, E., 95
McAlister, E., 29
McCarthy, J., 106, 170–4
McClelland, J., 247–8
McCullough, W., 106, 247
McGill, W., 1, 39
McNeill, D., 94, 98, 104
Mehler, J., 94, 101–3
Michotte, A., 102, 191
Miller, J., 95
Milner, B., 248–51
Minsky, M., 47, 106
Mischel, W., 95
Morgan, C., 7
Morgenstern, D., 9
Mosteller, F., 8–11, 47, 94
Myhill, J., 37

Neisser, U., 2, 32, 47, 72, 95, 107, 242–3
Newell, A., 47, 106
Newman, E., 5, 72, 103
Newton, I., 3
Nicely, P., 48–64
Nisbett, R., 263–4
Norman, D., 89, 94, 98, 100–4, 107
Nyquist, H., 21

Oppenheimer, J., 91
Osgood, C., 37, 74

Page, D., 95
Peak, H., 37
Piaget, J., 85, 96, 102
Pitts, W., 106
Pollack, R., 26, 29
Posner, M., 232
Postman, L., 28
Potter, M., 98
Preyer, W., 102
Pribram, K., 1, 37–8, 85
Putnam, H., 217–19, 242–3
Pylyshyn, Z., 236, 238–40

Quine, W., 8, 94, 205–6

Ratcliff, F., 7
Richards, I., 95
Rosch, E., 84
Rosenblith, W., 7, 95
Ross, L., 263–4
Rumelhart, D., 109, 247–8

Salton, G., 95
Savin, H., 94
Schlosberg, H., 74
Schwartz, R., 94
Selfridge, O., 27, 47, 83–5, 118
Selz, O., 106
Shannon, C., 8, 21, 26–7, 32, 76, 91
Shaw, J., 106
Shepard, R., 2, 72–3, 84
Shickman, J., 73
Simon, H., 47, 106, 242
Skinner, B., 5, 37, 72–3, 101, 103, 108
Slobin, D., 94
Soja, N., 203–7
Solomon, R., 72
Sperling, G., 2, 47–8, 84–5
Sperry, R., 237
Squire, L., 252–3
Sternberg, S., 47–8, 73, 84
Stevens, S., 4, 7–8, 22, 72–4, 83, 103, 107,
    197

Suppes, P., 16
Swets, J., 47

Teitelbaum, P., 72
Thurstone, L., 3
Tinbergen, N., 84
Toda, M., 94, 98
Torgerson, W., 47
Tversky, A., 98, 263–4

Van der Rohe, M., 97
Von Bekesy, G., 7, 103, 107
Von Neumann, J., 9, 91
Vygotsky, L., 102

Warrington, E., 250–2
Wason, P., 94
Waugh, N., 103
Weiner, N., 40, 91
Weir, R., 94
Weiskrantz, L., 250–2
Wertheimer, M., 82
Winston, P., 240
Wish, M., 61, 63
Woodbury, M., 16–17
Woodworth, R., 74–5
Wundt, W., 75–6, 104–5, 112–15, 210, 214

Zeaman, D., 11
Zeigarnik, B., 41
Zwislocki, J., 7

Subject index

absolute judgments, 22, 28–9, 31, 71–4, 77–8, 212, 227–8
acoustic confusability, 77, 120
additive distemy, 59–68
ambisyllabic consonants, 158–9
amnesia, 246, 248–54
anaphora, 219–21
arabic, broken plurals of, 171
articulatory features, 178–82
artificial intelligence, 190, 240, 258
assimilation, phonetic, 174–5, 179
assumption of mutual exclusivity, 199, 201–2, 206–7
auditory psychophysics, 8

basic grammatical relations, 147
behaviorism, 38, 82, 85, 91, 102, 108, 114–23, 153, 234
Bell Telephone Laboratories, 45–8, 50, 54

Carnegie Corporation, 91, 93
cellular models of behavior, 244–8
Center for Advanced Studies in Behavioral Science, 36
Center for Cognitive Studies, 85, 89–109, 153–4, 164–5, 197, 259
channel capacity, 20, 22–4, 28–32
channels, 49, 86
chunks, 72, 75, 77
coding, 20, 32
cognitive development, 198–208, 239
cognitive neuroscience, 230, 232, 235–43, 255
cognitive penetrability, 236, 238–9
cognitive psychology, 32–3, 73–9, 86–7, 100–7, 112, 235, 242–6, 250, 254–5, 258–9
cognitive science, 45, 68, 87, 210, 232–5, 241, 258–9, 264–7
communication, channels of, 20
communication, efficiency of, 20

competence–performance distinction, 121, 130, 145
computer models, 41–4, 77–9, 85, 97–8, 106, 267
computers, 104, 109, 233, 242
concepts, 187–94, 214
conceptual reference, 190, 217–18, 220–1, 224–5
conceptual representation, 187, 214
connectionism, 134, 245–7
consciousness, 233–4, 237
count noun/mass noun distinction, 203–9
cybernetics, 40–2

deep structure, 121–8, 130–1, 147–51
derivational theory of complexity, 112, 123–4, 149–50
difference equation, 12–17

ecological validity, 84, 86–7
epistemic systems, 235–8
e.s.p., 266–7
ethnoscience, 97

features, distinctive, 170–4
features, terminal, 175–9, 182

game theory, 9
generalized poisson distribution, 17
generative semantics, 131
gestalt psychology, 41, 82–3, 86, 117

Harvard University, 4, 48, 72–3, 81–5, 107, 112, 153, 197
higher mental processes, 93

illiterates, 155–7
immediate memory span, 123, 129, 211, 227

information, amount of, 19, 30–1
information, bits of, 20, 71–2
information, transmission of, 28, 71–2, 74
information theory, 3, 8, 19–33, 71–9, 100–1, 106
information theory, symposia on, 22, 83–4
initial state, 161
Institute for Advanced Study, 68
intentions, 40–3, 192–3
interdisciplinary studies, 91, 94–8, 265

Klamath, nasal assimilation in, 176–8

language, knowledge of, 97, 112
language, "secret," 173–4
language redundancy, 27–8
left cerebral dominance, 155–8
levels of analysis, 203, 233, 240–1, 247–8
levels of processing, 251–2
lexical concepts, architecture of, 128, 189, 192
lexical development, 197–209
lexical meaning, 189, 192–3, 211
lexical stress, 159
lexicon, 192, 197–8, 202
lexicon, structure of, 192, 198–9
Lincoln Lab at M.I.T., 240
linguistic concepts, psychological reality of, 105, 119, 129, 145–51
linguistic rules, 97, 120, 122, 134–5, 143–4
linguistics, 97, 104–5, 112–15, 143, 260–2
logic, 214, 221–2, 233–5, 261–3
logical form, 219–22, 261

magical number 7, 47, 211–12, 224–8
Markov chains, 1, 10–11, 82
mathematical models, 38–9
mathematical psychology, 3–18, 38–9, 83–4, 101
Memorial Hall, 4–7, 16, 48, 72–3, 93
memory, 226, 244–54
mental dichotomy, 187, 195
motion verbs, 187–9
motor skills, 30–1
multidimensional scaling, 46, 48, 50–3, 59–63
mutual exclusivity, 199–202

neural quantum, 8

object/substance distinction, 203–9
operant conditioning, 5–6

paradigms, 123, 267
parallel processing, 77–9

pattern perception, 83
phonemes, immanent structure of, 167, 174–82
phonetics, 167
phonological representation, 173–8
plans, 39–43, 85, 186–94
priming, 252–3
primitive concepts, conceptual decomposition to, 115, 187, 190–5, 198
principle of contrast, 199–202, 207
processing strategies, 157
proper noun/common noun distinction, 206
propositions, 129
psychoacoustic laboratory, 5–7, 36–7, 81
psycholinguistics, 3, 49–68, 100–1, 104–6, 118, 143–54, 213, 223
psychological space, 46–7
psychophysical scaling, 6

reaction time, 25–6, 31–2
reasoning, errors in, 263–4
recognition, 190–1, 253–4
reductionism, 112, 239, 244–5
redundancy, 20–1, 24, 27–31
Rockefeller University, 112, 230, 242

sequential dependencies, 24
short-term memory, 249
Sloan Foundation, viii
semantic components, 112, 192–3
semantic development, 197–209
semantic fields, 193
speech perception, 118–29, 157–8, 160–4, 167
speech perception, acoustic interference in, 26–31, 49–64, 118
speech production, 167–8
statistical learning theory, 10
Stat-Rat, 10–11
stimulus elements, 29
stochastic latency mechanisms, 17
stochastic process, 37
surface structure, 112, 121–3, 126, 133, 147–8
Swarthmore College, 83
syllabic structure, 158–9, 170–4
syllabification, 159, 171
syntactic processing models, 120, 130

talks at the Center, 164–5
taxonomic assumption, 203–4
Thursday afternoon colloquia, 94–6, 100, 109
top-down processing, 119, 213
TOTE, 1, 40–3

transformational grammar, 117, 120–3, 128,
  144–51, 213–15
transformational psycholinguistics, 144–51

units, 112, 115–17, 129, 170

word meaning, components of, 188, 199
word meaning, constraints on, 199–209

Yale University, 45–8

Zipf's law, 8